Biochemistry

Other books in the Biomedical Sciences Explained Series

0 7506 28790	Biological Foundations *N. Lawes*
0 7506 32542	Biology of Disease *W. Gilmore*
0 7506 31112	Cellular Pathology *D.J. Cook*
0 7506 28782	Clinical Biochemistry *R. Luxton*
0 7506 24574	Haematology *C.J. Pallister*
0 7506 32550	Human Genetics *A. Gardner, R.T. Howell and T. Davies*
0 7506 34138	Immunology *B.M. Hannigan*
0 7506 34677	Medical Physics *I. Trowbridge*
0 7506 32534	Molecular Genetics *J. Hancock*
0 7506 34154	Transfusion Science *J. Overfield, M. Dawson and D. Hamer*

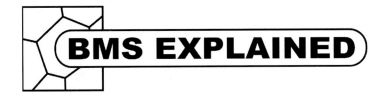

Biochemistry

James C. Blackstock BSc PhD CBiol MIBiol FIBMS
Senior Lecturer, School of Biological and Biomedical Sciences, Glasgow Caledonian University, Glasgow, Scotland

Series Editor:
C. J. Pallister PhD MSc FIBMS CBiol MIBiol CHSM
Principal Lecturer in Haematology, Department of Biological and Biomedical Sciences, University of the West of England, Bristol, UK

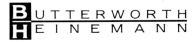

OXFORD BOSTON JOHANNESBURG MELBOURNE NEW DELHI SINGAPORE

Butterworth-Heinemann
Linacre House, Jordan Hill, Oxford OX2 8DP
225 Wildwood Avenue, Woburn, MA 01801-2041
A division of Reed Educational and Professional Publishing Ltd

 A member of the Reed Elsevier plc group

First published 1998

British Library Cataloguing in Publication Data
A catalogue record for this book is available from the British Library

Library of Congress Cataloguing in Publication Data
A catalogue record for this book is available from the Library of Congress

ISBN 0 7506 3256 9

Data manipulation by David Gregson Associates, Beccles, Suffolk
Printed and bound in Great Britain by The Bath Press plc, Avon

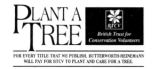

Contents

To Marja

Preface

Biochemistry is considered as an essential subject for students of the biomedical sciences. This concise textbook has been developed from my successful *Guide to Biochemistry* to meet the needs of the various biomedical disciplines. The format of the *Biomedical Sciences Explained* series offered opportunities to incorporate a significant amount of additional material and to demonstrate the relevance of some aspects of biochemistry to daily life.

The book is designed to be self-contained and is directed towards students of biomedical disciplines, which demand knowledge of molecular interactions and concepts. The text is viewed as providing a substantial molecular underpinning for the other textbooks in this series. The content has been carefully selected to provide a sound core of basic human and mammalian biochemical knowledge without impinging excessively on other members of the series. For example, molecular biology is restricted since a dedicated text on molecular genetics is programmed within the series. However, it is not desirable to exclude this topic entirely. Contrarily, some examples have been chosen from biomedical disciplines to demonstrate the application of biochemistry to these subject areas.

The focus is on an understanding of basic principles rather than extensive details which are not essential for healthcare specialists. The chapters are sequenced to provide a systematic, logical advancement into the subject matter. The later chapters assume an understanding of the earlier ones. It is hoped that the reader will feel capable of development within his/her chosen specialist subject from a position of molecular strength and thereby be comfortable in the reading of contemporary texts. Some readers will wish to explore further the issues raised within each chapter and so some reading suggestions from the associated literature have been included. Self-assessment questions and answers have been provided for the benefit of those readers who wish to test themselves progressively.

I am extremely grateful to Drs Joe Conner, Ruth Fulton and Peter F. Rebello of Caledonian University for their helpful advice. I am also very grateful to Myriam Brearley, Jane Campbell, Melanie Tait and Tim Brown of Butterworth-Heinemann for driving the project forward and Dr Chris Pallister of the University of the West of England for his fine editorship. Finally, I acknowledge the patience and support of my wife, Marja, during frequent bouts of frustration.

J. Blackstock

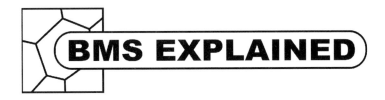

Series preface

The many disciplines that constitute the field of Biomedical Sciences have long provided excitement and challenge both for practitioners and for those who lead their education. This has never been truer than now as we ready ourselves to face the challenges of a new millennium. The exponential growth in biomedical enquiry and knowledge seen in recent years has been mirrored in the education and training of biomedical scientists. The burgeoning of modular BSc (Hons) Biomedical Sciences degrees and the adoption of graduate-only entry by the Institute of Biomedical Sciences and the Council for Professions Supplementary to Medicine have been important drivers of change.

The broad range of subject matter encompassed by the Biomedical Sciences has led to the design of modular BSc (Hons) Biomedical Sciences degrees that facilitate wider undergraduate choice and permit some degree of specialization. There is a much greater emphasis on self-directed learning and understanding of learning outcomes than hitherto.

Against this background, the large, expensive standard texts designed for single subject specialization over the duration of the degree and beyond, are much less useful for the modern student of biomedical sciences. Instead, there is a clear need for a series of short, affordable, introductory texts, which assume little prior knowledge and which are written in an accessible style. The *Biomedical Sciences Explained* series is specifically designed to meet this need.

Each book in the series is designed to meet the needs of a level 1 or 2 student and will have the following distinctive features:

- written by experienced academics in the biomedical sciences in a student-friendly and accessible style, with the trend towards student-centred and life-long learning firmly in mind;
- each chapter opens with a set of defined learning objectives and closes with self-assessment questions which check that the learning objectives have been met;
- aids to understanding such as potted histories of important scientists, descriptions of seminal experiments and background information appear as sideboxes;
- extensively illustrated with line diagrams, charts and tables wherever appropriate;
- use of unnecessary jargon is avoided. New terms are explained, either in the text or as sideboxes;
- written in an explanatory rather than a didactic style, emphasizing conceptual understanding rather than rote learning.

I sincerely hope that you find these books as helpful in your studies as they have been designed to be. Good luck and have fun!

C.J. Pallister

Acknowledgement of sources for figures and tables

Figure 2.4 adapted from Voet, D. and Voet, J.G. (1995). *Biochemistry*, 2nd ed. New York: Wiley, p. 864; Figure 2.8, adapted from Rawn, J.D. (1989). *Biochemistry*. Burlington: Patterson, p. 680; Figure 2.14, from Lake, J.A. (1985). *Ann. Rev. Biochem.* **54**, 509, by kind permission of author and Annual Reviews Inc.; Figure 2.15, adapted from Brimacombe, R. (1984). *TIBS* **9**, 274; Table 2.3, adapted from Szekely, M. (1980). *From DNA to Protein: The Transfer of Genetic Information*. London: MacMillan, p. 13; Table 2.5, adapted from Mathews, C.K. and van Holde, K.E. (1996). *Biochemistry*, 2nd ed. Menlo Park: Benjamin/Cummings, p. 101; Table 2.6, adapted from Kozak, M. (1983). *Microbiol. Rev.* **47**, 1–45; Figure 3.7, adapted from Prockop, D.J. and Kivirikko, K.I. (1984). *New Eng. J. Med.* **311**, 377; Figure 3.8, adapted from Branden, C. and Tooze, J. (1991). *Introduction to Protein Structure*. New York: Garland, pp. 20–55; Figure 3.9, from Dickerson, R.E. (1964). *The Proteins*, Vol. 2, 2nd ed. (Ed. H. Neurath). New York: Academic Press, p. 634, by kind permission of author and publisher; Figure 3.11, from Gordon-Smith, E.C. (1983). Biochemical aspects of haematology, in *Biochemical Aspects of Human Disease* (Eds R.S. Elkeles and A.S. Tavill). Oxford: Blackwell, p. 409, by kind permission of author and publisher; Figure 4.8, adapted from Mathews, C.K. and van Holde, K.E. (1996). *Biochemistry*, 2nd ed. Menlo Park: Benjamin/Cummings, p. 381; Figure 7.2, adapted from Zubay, G.L., Parson, W.W. and Vance, D.E. (1995). *Principles of Biochemistry*. Dubuque: Brown, p. 645; Figure 7.5, adapted from Hooper, N.M., Karran, E.H. and Turner, A.J. (1997). *Biochem. J.* **321**, 266; Figure 7.7, adapted from Alberts, B., Bray, D., Lewis, J., Raff, M., Roberts, K. and Watson, J.D. (1994). *Molecular Biology of the Cell*, 3rd ed. New York: Garland, pp. 966–996; Figure 7.8, adapted from Wolfe, S. (1993). *Molecular and Cellular Biology*. Belmont: Wadsworth, p. 287; Figure 7.9, adapted from Wolfe, S. (1993). *Molecular and Cellular Biology*. Belmont: Wadsworth, p. 283; Figure 8.7, adapted from Zhang, G., Liu, Y., Ruoho, A.E. and Hurley, J.H. (1997). *Nature* **386**, 250, and Fields, T.A. and Casey, P.J. (1997). *Biochem. J.* **321**, 564; Figure 8.10, adapted from Weigel, N.L. (1996). *Biochem. J.* **319**, 658; Figure 11.3, adapted from Garrett, R.H. and Grisham, C.M. (1995). *Biochemistry*. Fort Worth: Saunders, p. 640; Figure 11.5, adapted from Stryer, L. (1995). *Biochemistry*, 4th ed. New York: Freeman, p. 547; Figure 11.6, adapted from Stryer, L. (1995). *Biochemistry*, 4th ed. New York: Freeman, p. 548; Figure 12.7, adapted from Garrett, R.H. and Grisham, C.M. (1995). *Biochemistry*. Fort Worth: Saunders, pp. 785–791; Figure 13.4, adapted from Voet, D. and Voet, J.G. (1995). *Biochemistry*, 2nd ed. New York: Wiley, p. 994; Figure 13.5, adapted from Nierhus, K.H. (1996). *Nature* **379**, 491.

Chapter 1
Biological molecules

Learning objectives

After studying this chapter you should confidently be able to:

Differentiate between prokaryotic and eukaryotic cells.

Relate the biological importance of water to its physical and chemical properties.

Discuss the movement of water and ions through semipermeable membranes.

Explain the term pH, the concept of buffering and their biological significance.

Discuss the biologically important properties of carbon.

Discuss the stereochemistry of biological molecules.

Describe macromolecules as polymers of smaller molecules.

Describe hybrid molecules as conjugates of different classes of biological molecules.

Biochemistry is the investigation of the **chemical processes** which are responsible for the **state of living**. These studies are applications of the general scientific method of observe, measure, formulate and test hypotheses, reject failed propositions and investigate further those ideas of potential until substantial supportive evidence is acquired. All the knowledge presented in this textbook has been acquired through this process of detailed experimental investigation and rigorous scrutiny of the resultant data.

Living organisms continually effect functional activities which permit the organism to survive, grow and reproduce. Life depends on the ability to harness and use energy (Chapter 8). Without energy, the organism fails to maintain vitality and dies. Living organisms are composed of lifeless molecules. In biochemistry, the **structure**, the **organization** and the **potential activities** of these molecules are examined in an attempt to elucidate the features which make indispensible contributions to the complex life-giving assemblage.

The word **cell** was introduced to biology in 1665 by **Robert Hooke** in his collection of microscopic drawings, called *Micrographia*, which included a drawing of a thin slice of cork. He recorded the honeycomb structure of cork and referred to the compartments as cells by analogy to the cell of a prisoner or monk. The term, however, has been retained not to describe the voids remaining after the disintegration of cell cytoplasm (observed by Hooke) but the living contents normally resident between these plant cell walls. Today, the cell may be defined as the simplest integrated unit in living systems capable of independent survival.

By the early nineteenth century, recognition was given to cells as life forms and their organization into more complex multicellular organisms. In 1839, **Theodor Schwann**, a zoologist, published *Mikroskopische Untersuchungen*, which also contained figures supplied by **Mathias Schleiden**, a botanist, to record that plants and animals are composed of similar cells. Twenty years later, **Rudolf Virchow** announced 'omnis cellula e cellula', i.e. all cells arise from pre-existing cells.

Water is a vital substance. A 70 kg man contains approximately 40 litres of water and his death will ensue when about 20% of the body water is lost. Body water is generally not in large pools but is highly partitioned by aggregates of water-hating (**hydrophobic**) molecules which coalesce to form **membranes** (Chapter 6). Membranes package complex arrays of molecules which constitute **cells**. Collections of appropriate types of cells constitute **tissues**.

Despite the wide variety of cell types, most cells can be classified according to their **size and complexity** into one of two categories:

- **prokaryotes** in which the genetic material is not enclosed by an intracellular membrane;
- **eukaryotes** in which the genetic material is contained within a well-formed discrete nucleus.

These terms are derived from Greek (*karyon* = kernel, as in a nut; *pro-* = before; *eu-* = well).

A definitive feature of **prokaryotic cells** is their **lack of membrane-bound structures** although layers of internal membranes may arise from the outer membrane called the **plasma membrane**. In contrast, **eukaryotic cells** contain numerous **membrane-bound organelles**, e.g. mitochondria and lysosomes. The term organelle refers to an organized or specialized structure within a cell. Another discriminating feature of prokaryotic cells is that they lack the intracellular framework called the **cytoskeleton**, their structure being maintained by the cell wall. Although the size of cells of both categories are variable, in general, prokaryotic cells range from 0.1 to 3 µm whereas the dimensions of most eukaryotic cells are 10–20 µm. **Prokaryotic organisms** may be subdivided into three morphologically distinct groups:

- **bacteria** which are micro-organisms encompassed by a rigid cell wall;
- **mycoplasmas**, minute micro-organisms which lack rigid cell walls and give rise to small colonies on media enriched with body fluids;
- **cyanobacteria** which have the capacity to utilize the electromagnetic energy of sunlight by the possession of a membranous photosynthetic apparatus.

Eukaryotic cells may be:

- **unicellular organisms**, e.g. yeast, protozoa;
- **aggregated** to constitute the tissues, e.g. kidney and liver, of multicellular organisms.

This chapter considers the properties and roles of the two major constituents of biological systems, water and carbon-containing molecules.

Water

Water has been selected by nature as the biological solvent because of its physical properties, which are markedly different from the solvents commonly used by chemists. Water has a higher:

- **melting point,** $0°C$ compared with $-117°C$ for ethanol;
- **boiling point,** $100°C$ compared with $78°C$ for ethanol;
- **heat of vaporization,** i.e. the amount of heat energy required to change 1 g of solvent from its liquid state into the gaseous state. The value for water is $2260 \, \mathrm{J\,g^{-1}}$ compared with $854 \, \mathrm{J\,g^{-1}}$ for ethanol. The heat of vaporization is a direct measure of the energy required to overcome the forces of attraction between molecules in the liquid phase;
- **dielectric constant,** i.e. the capacity to store electrical potential energy in an electric field. The value for water is 78.5 compared with 24.3 for ethanol.

These higher values are due to the structure of water.

Structure of water

In water, one oxygen atom bonds with two hydrogen atoms (Figure 1.1). Each O–H bond is formed by a **sharing of electrons** and is therefore a **covalent bond.** However, the more **electropositive** oxygen nucleus attracts the electrons more strongly than the hydrogen atom which results in a slight negative charge (δ^-) in the region of the oxygen atom and a slight positive charge (δ^+) in the region of the hydrogen atom. This means that the water molecule, although it has no net charge, has two regions of **partial positivity** and one region of **partial negativity** which results in the molecule being an **electric dipole,** i.e. **polar.**

When two molecules of water are in close proximity, **electrostatic attraction** occurs between the partial negative charge on the oxygen atom of one water molecule and a partial positive charge on a hydrogen atom of its neighbour. This is accompanied by a redistribution of the electronic charges in both water molecules which enhances the attraction. This form of electrostatic attraction, called a **hydrogen bond,** is not unique to water and has an important role in determining the structures of macromolecules. The arrangement of the electrons around the oxygen atom potentially allows the binding of four adjacent water molecules to any water molecule.

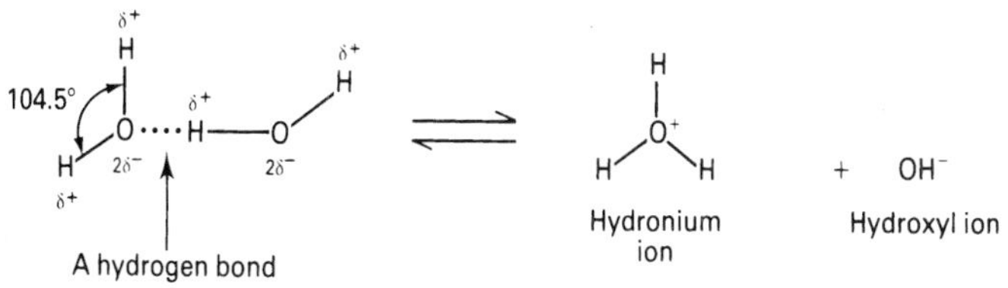

Figure 1.1 *The structure and ionization of water*

As a result of its polarity, **water** is a powerful solvent for ionic substances, e.g. salts, and for polar, non-ionic substances, e.g. sugars and amines. An **ion** is an atom or group of atoms which has lost or gained one or more orbital electrons. When an ionic solute dissolves in a solvent, the bonds between the molecules or ions of the solute are abolished, the bonds between the molecules of the solvent are destroyed and new bondings between the molecules of the solvent and the ions of the solute form. To remain in solution, these replacement bonds must balance both the attractions between solvent molecules and between solute molecules. Therefore, when a solute dissolves in water, electrostatic attractions within the solute are separated by the specific alignment of water dipoles, i.e. δ^- oxygen atoms of water molecules are attracted to the positive charges of the solute and δ^+ hydrogen atoms of the water molecules are similarly attracted to the negative charges of the solute. These orientations result in the solute becoming surrounded by specifically aligned water molecules, the encompassing arrangement being called a **hydration shell**.

With polar (but non-ionic) substances, solubility is determined by water molecules readily forming hydrogen bonds with the polar groups on these substances.

The structure of water is dynamic. The hydrogen bonding in water is transient; about every 10 picoseconds (1×10^{-12} s) each randomly located water molecule changes position, straining its hydrogen bonds and causing a collapse of the hydrogen bonding arrangement. This is immediately followed by the formation of a hydrogen bond with another neighbouring water molecule. This creates an internal motion in which water molecules constantly regenerate their hydrogen bonding, thus producing **fluidity**. The interlinking of the water molecules by hydrogen bonds is responsible for the **internal cohesion of water** resulting in its physical properties.

Osmosis and osmotic pressure

Osmosis is a biologically important example of a property of a solution which is dependent upon the number of solute molecules present, i.e. its concentration, rather than upon the chemical reactivity of the solute. All biological membranes are termed **semipermeable** because they can select which molecules or ions they will allow to pass through.

When a semipermeable membrane (either a natural or artificial one, e.g. cellophane) separates two aqueous solutions of different concentrations of solute molecules, the membrane may retain the solute but permit water molecules to freely pass through it. Osmosis is the net movement of water through a semipermeable membrane from the solution of lower concentration into the solution of higher concentration and with time may equalize the concentrations across the membrane.

The **plasma membranes of cells** perform as semipermeable membranes in that they retain solutions of protein (and other) molecules within the cell but are readily permeable to water. The result is that water freely passes into and out of the cell according to the concentration gradient for water molecules across the membrane, the gradient being determined by both extracellular and intracellular conditions. The direction of flow is to dilute the more concentrated solution.

Osmotic pressure is defined as the pressure developed when solutions of different concentration of the same solute are separated by a membrane permeable to only the solvent. Alternatively, osmotic pressure can be considered as the pressure required to be applied on one side of the membrane to prevent osmosis. Within the human body (and other multicellular animals), proteins and other molecules/ions occur in significant concentrations in the extracellular fluids as well as within the cell, so the concentration of water across the plasma membrane is carefully balanced. Because of the impact of numbers of molecules, cells minimize the osmotic pressure generated by their cytosolic (Chapter 7) contents by **polymerization** of small molecules into longer chains, e.g. glucose is stored as glycogen.

Cell volume

The **volume** of a **eukaryotic cell** is not fixed but is subject to dynamic changes, under the influence of nutrients, hormones and osmotic variation. These fluctuations influence **cell function**. The effects of cell volume have been most extensively studied in the liver cell (hepatocyte) where volume changes lead to alterations in the intracellular chemical processes, called **cellular metabolism** (Chapter 8):

- **cell swelling** inhibits the breakdown of glycogen, glucose and proteins but stimulates the synthesis of glycogen (Chapter 9) and protein (Chapter 13);
- **cell shrinkage** stimulates glycogen, glucose and protein degradation but glycogen and protein synthesis are inhibited.

There is evidence that these changes are triggered by **chemical messengers**, called **hormones**, acting between cells in different locations in the body. Hormones effect volume changes by influencing the activity of **plasma membrane ion-transport systems** (Chapter 7). In hepatocytes, the hormone **insulin** stimulates the cellular accumulation of potassium, sodium and chloride ions and consequently the cell volume increases. Another hormone, **glucagon**, a single 29-amino acid residue polypeptide chain also activates ion-transport systems but results in a loss of intracellular K^+, Na^+ and Cl^- from hepatocytes and the cell shrinks. Under the influence of different hormones, hepatocyte volume may vary by as much as 20%. Cell volume changes also affect cellular metabolism in the longer term by modifying the biosynthesis of enzymes (Chapter 13), e.g. phospho*enol*pyruvate carboxykinase in gluconeogenesis (Chapter 9), but vice versa, alterations in gene expression may influence cellular volume.

pH and buffering

In water, the electron of the hydrogen atom is attracted to the nucleus of the oxygen atom and so there is a tendency for the **hydrogen nucleus (a proton)** to dissociate from the water molecule. This proton will be attracted to the oxygen of another water molecule to which it is hydrogen bonded, forming a **hydronium ion** (H_3O^+) and a hydroxyl ion (Figure 1.1). The hydronium ion is usually considered to be a hydrated proton or hydrogen ion and is therefore designated by H^+. The concentration of H^+ ions in pure water at 25°C is $1 \times 10^{-7}\,\text{mol}\,l^{-1}$.

Hydrogen ion concentration values are cumbersome figures to use since they contain negative powers of 10. In 1909, Sörenson introduced the term, **pH**. This expresses the $[H^+]$ of an aqueous solution as a logarithmic function. The pH of a solution equals the negative of the logarithm to the base 10 of its hydrogen ion concentration, i.e. $\textbf{pH} = -\textbf{log}_{10}\textbf{[H}^+\textbf{]}$. pH offers a convenient mech-

About **two-thirds of the total body water** is found inside the cells. This is termed the **intracellular fluid compartment (ICF)** whilst the remainder lies outside cells and is called the **extracellular fluid compartment (ECF)**. Blood plasma together with interstitial fluid constitute the ECF. These compartments are in contact and water can pass freely between them. Any water loss from the plasma causes an increase in the osmotic pressure of the ECF and consequently movement of water from the ICF into the ECF to equalize the osmotic pressure between the two compartments. The replacement of lost water by drinking pure water causes the osmotic pressure of plasma to fall. Water now passes from the ECF into the ICF in an attempt to balance the osmotic pressure and if the uptake of water is sufficently large, the cell will swell and may burst.

Intracellular fluid loss may cause **cellular dysfunction** which may manifest itself at the whole organism level as lethargy and confusion. Loss of ECF may result in circulatory collapse and kidney failure. Movements of these fluids also alters the concentrations of ions in these compartments. Of particular importance for the well-being of the individual are intracellular K^+ and extracellular Na^+ levels.

Table 1.1 *The pH scale*

$[H^+]$ (mol l^{-1})	pH	$[OH^-]$ (mol l^{-1})	pOH	Acidity or basicity
1.0 (10^0)	0	10^{-14}	14	↑
0.1 (10^{-1})	1	10^{-13}	13	
10^{-4}	4	10^{-10}	10	Increasing | acidity
10^{-7}	7	10^{-7}	7	Neutral
10^{-10}	10	10^{-4}	4	Increasing |basicity
10^{-13}	13	10^{-1}	1	
10^{-14}	14	10^0	0	↓

anism of expressing a wide range of $[H^+]$ in small positive numbers. The letter p is used to denote the negative logarithm to the base 10 of the concentration.

The **pH scale** from 0 to 14 covers all the hydrogen ion concentrations (Table 1.1) found in dilute aqueous solutions and biological systems. Pure water has a pH of 7 which is considered to be **neutrality**. When pH is less than 7, the solution is **acidic** and when pH is more than 7, the solution is **basic** or **alkaline**. Because of the logarithmic function, a change of one pH unit represents a 10-fold difference in hydrogen ion concentration. Measurements of pH can be easily performed using a **pH meter**.

Most **macromolecules** exist within the cell in a charged state, i.e. they are **ionized**. The ionic state is determined by the concentration of hydrogen ions in the aqueous medium. Any alteration in the $[H^+]$ of this environment may affect the state of ionization of these molecules and thus result in a change in their structural shape which may lead to a modification in their biological activity, e.g. the effect of $[H^+]$ on enzymes (Chapter 4). Cells and body fluids of living organisms employ buffer systems to regulate the free $[H^+]$ within the limits which allow normal function of their constituent biomolecules.

In the laboratory, buffer systems are employed to enable:

- **the preparation of biological materials** which retain their biological activity *in vitro* for further investigation;

- **the investigation of biochemical reactions** which often involve proton transfer;

- **the control of pH** in microbiological, cell and tissue culture media;

Buffer systems are based on the **interactions** of:

- **monoprotic acids and bases,** where usually one component is strong and the other is weak;

- **polyprotic weak acids and strong bases.**

Acids and bases can be identified as monoprotic or polyprotic

---

Calculate the pH of a solution in which the hydrogen ion concentration is 4.2×10^{-4} mol l^{-1}.
$[H^+] = 4.2 \times 10^{-4}$ mol l^{-1} and pH $= -\log_{10}[H^+]$;
pH $= -\log(4.2 \times 10^{-4})$.
Take log by calculator:
pH $= -(-3.38)$;
pH $= 3.38$ (pH is normally quoted to two decimal places).

Calculate the hydrogen ion concentration in a solution of pH 8.32.
pH $= 8.32$ and pH $= -\log_{10}[H^+]$;
$8.32 = -\log_{10}[H^+]$;
$\log_{10}[H^+] = -8.32$.
Take antilog:
$[H^+] = 4.79 \times 10^{-9}$ mol l^{-1};
i.e. the $[H^+]$ in a solution of pH 8.32 $= 4.79 \times 10^{-9}$ mol l^{-1}.

depending upon the numbers of dissociable protons the acid contains or the number of protons with which the base can combine.

According to the Brönsted and Lowry theory of acids and bases, their interaction involves the transfer **of a proton** from an acid to a base:

$$\underset{\text{monoprotic acid}}{HA^+} + \underset{\text{base}}{B} \rightleftharpoons \underset{\substack{\text{monoprotic} \\ \text{conjugate acid}}}{BH^+} + \underset{\text{conjugate base}}{A^-}$$

The events occurring during this interaction can be followed on a plot of change in pH during the dropwise addition of one component to a fixed volume of the other component. The plot is called a **titration curve**. The events which occur during the interaction depend upon the nature of the components, i.e. whether both the acid and base are strong or one component is strong and the other weak, or both weak.

During the titration of a **weak acid**, HA, **with a strong base** (OH⁻), the interaction can be represented as:

$$\underset{\text{weak acid}}{HA} + \underset{\text{strong base}}{OH^-} \rightleftharpoons H_2O + \underset{\text{conjugate base}}{A^-}$$

However, in this case, the product of the interaction is the relatively stronger conjugate base of the weak acid which can accept protons from the water and thereby effect the reverse reaction. During the initial stages of this titration, weak acid is being removed to produce its conjugate base which is actively reconstituting the weak acid and thereby repressing the dissociation of the weak acid. The effect of this process on the pH of any mixture of solutions of weak acid and its conjugate base can be calculated using the **Henderson–Hasselbalch equation**:

$$pH = pK_a + \log_{10} \frac{[\text{base}]}{[\text{acid}]}$$

This allows the pH to be calculated for any mixture in which both weak acid and its conjugate base are present using pK_a values.

The interaction of a **weak base** (B) **and a strong acid** (HCl) can be represented as:

$$\underset{\text{weak base}}{B} + HCl \rightleftharpoons \underset{\text{conjugate acid}}{BH^+} + Cl^-$$

The relatively stronger conjugate acid formed can release H⁺ and thereby reverse the reaction. So during the initial stages of this titration, the process of removing the weak base is being hampered by the dissociation of the BH⁺. The effect of this process on the pH of any mixture of weak base and its conjugate acid can be calculated from the Henderson–Hasselbalch equation.

The **strength of an acid or base** refers to the efficiency with which an acid donates protons or a base accepts protons. With respect to strength, there are two general classes of acids and bases: **strong** and **weak**. Strong acids and bases are ones which are almost completely dissociated in dilute aqueous media. Weak acids and bases are ones which are only partially dissociated in these media. The strength of an acid or a base is most frequently determined by a **dissociation constant, K**.

For an acid, HA:

$$HA + H_2O \rightleftharpoons H^+ + A^-$$

the equilibrium constant, K_{eq} is the mathematical product of the concentrations of the substances formed by a chemical reaction divided by the product of the concentrations of the reactants in that reaction.

$$\therefore K_{eq} = \frac{[H^+][A^-]}{[HA][H_2O]}$$

$$\therefore K_{eq}[H_2O] = \frac{[H^+][A^-]}{[HA]}$$

$K_{eq}[H_2O]$ equals a new constant called K_a, **the acid dissociation constant**.

$$\therefore K_a = \frac{[H^+][A^-]}{[HA]}$$

For weak acids and bases, there is a **gradation of strength**, i.e. some are weaker than others as shown by K_a (or pK_a) or K_b (or pK_b); e.g. formic acid with $K_a = 1.77 \times 10^{-4}$ ($pK_a = 3.75$) is more acidic than acetic acid ($K_a = 1.76 \times 10^{-5}$ and $pK_a = 4.75$).

Figure 1.2   *Interaction of aqueous*
solutions of monoprotic acids and
bases: (a) titration of a weak acid with a
strong base; (b) titration of a weak base
with a strong acid

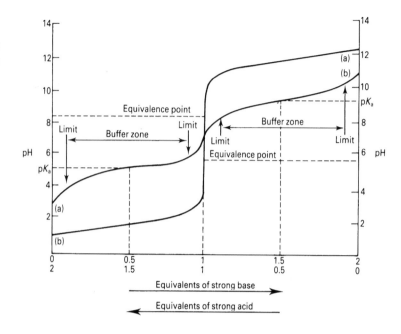

Examples of the titration curve obtained when a **weak acid is titrated with strong base** and a **weak base is titrated with strong acid** are shown in Figure 1.2. Because of the **gradation of strength** found in weak acids and weak bases, Figure 1.2a represents the actual plot of only one weak acid (0.1 mol l^{-1} acetic acid with 0.1 mol l^{-1} NaOH) although the shape is characteristic of weak acid–strong base titrations in general. Similarly, Figure 1.2b represents the plot of one weak base (NH_3) with equimolar HCl. The points to note from these titrations are:

- The **equivalence points differ from pH 7** due to the basicity of the conjugate base ion (or the acidity of the conjugate acid ion).
- The **initial parts** of these titration curves are **sigmoidal** in shape.
- The **point of inflection** per titration curve centres on a region in which the addition of strong base (or strong acid) results in a small change in pH. A solution which resists a change in pH on the addition of strong acid or base is called a **buffer solution**.

When half an equivalent quantity of titrant (strong base or acid) has been added, there is a point of inflection. Here, one half of the weak acid (or weak base) will have interacted with the strong base (or strong acid) whilst the other half has not. From the Henderson–Hasselbalch equation:

$$pH = pK_a + \log_{10} \frac{[base]}{[acid]}$$

at the half-equivalence point, [acid] = [conjugate base] = x {or [base] = [conjugate acid] = x}.

$$\therefore \mathbf{pH} = pK_a + \log\frac{x}{x} = pK_a + \log 1 = pK_a + 0 = \mathbf{pK_a}$$

The pK_a value of the weak acid or conjugate acid of the weak base can therefore be obtained from the appropriate titration curve.

If acid or base is added in drops of uniform volume, the further from the half-equivalence point in the titration curve, the greater the effect of the addition, i.e. less buffering (Figure 1.2). The limits of the buffer zone correspond to weak acid–conjugate base or weak base–conjugate acid mixtures in which the [acid] is 10 times that of the [base], i.e. [acid]/[base] = 10 : 1 or in which [base]/[acid] = 10 : 1. Applying these values to the Henderson–Hasselbalch equation:

$$pH = pK_a + \log_{10}\frac{[base]}{[acid]} = pK_a + \log\frac{1}{10} = pK_a - 1$$

$$pH = pK_a + \log_{10}\frac{[base]}{[acid]} = pK_a + \log\frac{10}{1} = pK_a + 1$$

The buffer zone is defined by the region within $\mathbf{pK_a - 1}$ to $\mathbf{pK_a + 1}$.

Biological media contain many **polyprotic components**. At physiological pH, many substances exist as ionic species, e.g. amino acids, nucleotides, triacylglycerols and phosphoacylglycerols. In their titration, a number of progressive steps are observed, the number being equal to the number of dissociable protons. The dissociation of one acidic species is completed before any appreciable dissociation of its product, called an **amphiprotic conjugate base** since it may act as a base or an acid. Each step terminates at an equivalence point. The pH at half-equivalence represents a pK_a value but since there is a half-equivalence point per step, each pK_a is identified by a subscript, e.g. pK_{a1}, pK_{a2} etc. pK_{a1} represents the most acidic pK_a value with others being in order of decreasing acidity.

Buffering mixtures are usually selected on the basis of their effectiveness at the pH of interest and their non-interference with the substances under study.

Carbon-containing molecules

There are 92 naturally occurring chemical elements of which living cells contain only approximately 27. The actual number depends on the type of cell and species of the organism. Over 99% of the mass of most cells is composed of only six elements which are called the **major elements**. The other constituent elements are the

Table 1.2 *The elements found in living cells*

Major elements	
Element	*Symbol*
Carbon	C
Hydrogen	H
Nitrogen	N
Oxygen	O
Phosphorus	P
Sulphur	S

Minor elements	
Element	*Symbol*
Arsenic	As
Boron	B
Calcium	Ca
Chlorine	Cl
Chromium	Cr
Cobalt	Co
Copper	Cu
Fluorine	F
Iodine	I
Iron	Fe
Magnesium	Mg
Manganese	Mn
Molybdenum	Mo
Nickel	Ni
Potassium	K
Selenium	Se
Silicon	Si
Sodium	Na
Tin	Sn
Vanadium	V
Zinc	Zn

minor elements (Table 1.2). Apart from water, the vast majority of cellular molecules contain **carbon**.

Carbon

Carbon (atomic number 6, atomic weight 12) is a small atom which has four electrons in its outer electronic orbital enabling it to participate in electron-sharing with up to four other atoms. The outer electrons of carbon are arranged around the carbon nucleus as in a **tetrahedron**, a pyramid with triangular faces (Figure 1.3). A bond formed by the sharing of electrons is a **covalent bond**.

A carbon atom can share each electron with a hydrogen atom to form **single bonds** or it may share multiple electrons, e.g. two electrons shared with oxygen to form a **double bond**. It is possible for carbon to share three electrons with certain atoms, e.g. nitrogen, but this is rare in biological systems. One of the most important properties of carbon is its ability to form covalent bonds with other carbon atoms to form **chains** or **rings** which are the basis of large and complex molecules. The formation of bonds requires energy, e.g. C–H bonding needs 414 kJ mol^{-1}, C–C bonding 343 kJ mol^{-1}, C–O bonding 351 kJ mol^{-1}, C=C bonding 615 kJ mol^{-1} and C=O bonding 686 kJ mol^{-1}.

Carbon atoms when bonded to each other by single bonds have the ability to rotate unless they are restricted by the attachment of large or charged groups. Rotation enables an organic molecule to assume different shapes called conformations. Carbon–carbon double bonds:

- **are shorter than single bonds;**
- **limit rotation;**
- **increase rigidity**, important in large molecules;
- **change the angle between any two electrons**, affecting the conformation of the molecule. This has a major impact on the biological activity of the molecule since its activity often involves a shape-dependent interaction with another molecule.

The chains and rings may have bonding arrangements in which single and double bonds alternate giving rise to a **conjugated bond system**. In this system, the bonding electrons move within the molecule increasing the stability of the structure. This phenomenon is called **resonance stabilization** and the structure is constantly shifting between the two representations shown in Figure 1.4.

Functional biological molecules are derived from the ability of carbon to bond covalently to nitrogen, hydrogen, oxygen and sulphur. For convenience, biological molecules have been considered initially as derivatives of long, branched or unbranched chains or rings of carbon atoms. **Hydrogen atoms** which are bonded to these carbon atoms may be replaced by N, O and S atoms to constitute functional groups, e.g. amine, aldehyde, carbonyl and sulphydryl (thiol). This results in the great chemical variation found in biological molecules. Functional groups can alter the electron distribution and bond angles, and contribute considerably to chemical reactivity. Biological molecules often contain more than one functional group, frequently of different kinds. Such molecules are said to be **polyfunctional** with each type of group displaying its own chemical characteristics and contributing to the overall chemical properties of the molecule. For example, amino acids contain at least one amino group and one carboxyl group which determine a number of the chemical properties of the amino acid.

Stereochemistry

The bonding of four different groups to a carbon atom results in two possible tetrahedral structures (Figure 1.5a). Since the illustrated molecules have identical composition but different structures, they are called **isomers**. Isomers which differ in the spatial arrangement of the atoms in the molecules are called **stereoisomers**. Neither of the structures has a plane or centre of symmetry and the term asymmetric was applied. This term has been superseded by **chirality**, indicating that the stereoisomers can be considered as right- or left-handed. Consider your hands. One hand cannot be exactly superimposed on the other or on its mirror image because your thumbs will be on opposite sides. A molecule that cannot be superimposed on its mirror image is called a **chiral molecule** (Figure 1.5b). When a carbon atom has up to three different groups attached to it, the spatial arrangement permits the molecular structure to be superimposed on its mirror image and the molecule is said to be **achiral** (Figure 1.5c).

With chiral molecules, when one of them is viewed in a mirror, its reflection would show the other stereoisomer. These stereoisomers are called mirror images or **enantiomers**. Enantiomers are optically active. One rotates the plane of polarized light to the right (clockwise) and is called the **dextrorotatory** stereoisomer. The other

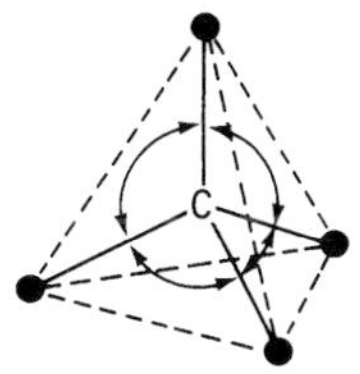

Iron is essential for almost all eukaryotes mainly because it is a component of the iron-dependent **ribonucleoside-diphosphate reductase**, an enzyme which converts ribonucleotides into deoxyribonucleotides. It also has numerous significant roles including being involved in oxygen transport, electron transfer reactions and detoxification.

In man, **iron** is absorbed mainly through the action of mucosal cells located in the duodenum of the gastrointestinal tract. Only about 5–10% of dietary iron (1–2 mg per day) is absorbed, with haem and ferrous iron being preferred to non-haem and ferric iron.

Figure 1.3 *The tetrahedral arrangement of electrons in carbon:* ●, *outer electron;* – – –, *outline of tetrahedron;* ———, *distance from nucleus to electron, 0.154 nm;* ↶, *angle between two electrons, 109.5°*

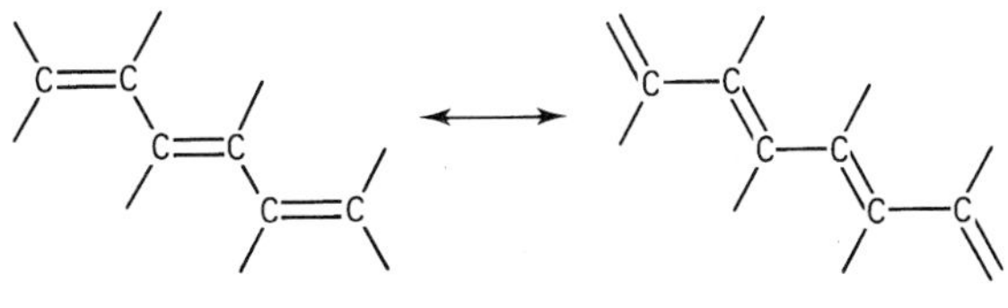

Figure 1.4 *Resonance stabilization of conjugated bond systems*

Figure 1.5 *Stereochemistry; (a) the tetrahedral structures formed by the bonding of four different groups to carbon; (b) a chiral molecule; (c) an achiral molecule*

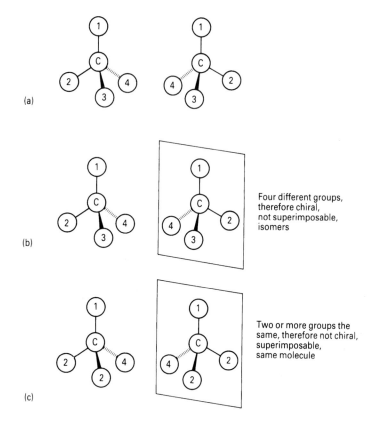

Four different groups, therefore chiral, not superimposable, isomers

Two or more groups the same, therefore not chiral, superimposable, same molecule

rotates the plane of polarized light to the left (anticlockwise) to the same extent and is called the **laevorotatory** stereoisomer. A mixture of each enantiomer in equal proportions is optically inactive (racemic).

The positions of atoms and groups around a chiral carbon atom are not however related to the direction of the plane of polarized light in a simple manner. The direction can change by varying the wavelength of light. Until the 1940s when specialized techniques based on **X-ray diffraction studies** were introduced, there was no means of accurately relating structure to optical activity. Nevertheless, a German chemist, Emil Fischer, in 1891, arbitrarily and correctly assigned a molecular structure to the dextrorotatory form of glyceraldehyde and called it D-glyceraldehyde. The laevo-rotatory isomer was called L-glyceraldehyde (Figure 1.6). Today, glyceraldehyde remains the basis of the stereochemical configuration of biological molecules. Stereoisomers of all chiral molecules have structural configurations related to one form of glyceraldehyde and are designated D and L irrespective of their optical activity. Optical activity is denoted by (+) for dextrorotatory and (−) for laevorotatory.

Chirality is of biological importance since many biomolecules contain chiral centres. Nature appears selective in that virtually all

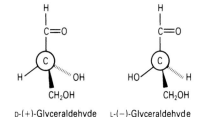

D-(+)-Glyceraldehyde   L-(−)-Glyceraldehyde

Figure 1.6 *The stereochemistry of glyceraldehyde*

proteins and polysaccharides of higher organisms are composed of L-amino acids and D-monosaccharides respectively. This selectivity is due to the additional stability these configurations confer on polymeric molecules.

Macromolecules

Macromolecules (Greek *makros* = long) are constructed by the chemical linkage of small molecules to form **polymerized chains**. The small building-block molecules are called **monomers** and individually have certain biological activities/functions. The linkage, unique to each type of macromolecule, is formed by a **condensation reaction**, an energy-requiring process (Figure 1.7).

The sizes of molecules are compared by consideration of their **molecular mass**. The unit of mass employed is the **dalton** (Da) or kilodalton (1000 Da or 1 kDa) where 1 Da equals the weight of one hydrogen atom, i.e. 1.66×10^{-24} g.

There are **four major classes** of biological molecules:

- **nucleic acids,** which are the largest macromolecules with molecular masses extending to the billion dalton range;
- **proteins,** the molecular masses of which range from thousands to millions of daltons;
- **carbohydrates,** the molecular masses of which are usually within the range quoted for proteins;
- **lipids** are relatively small (about 300–1500 Da) but large numbers of certain lipid molecules frequently associate to form very large structures such as the basic structure of cellular membranes.

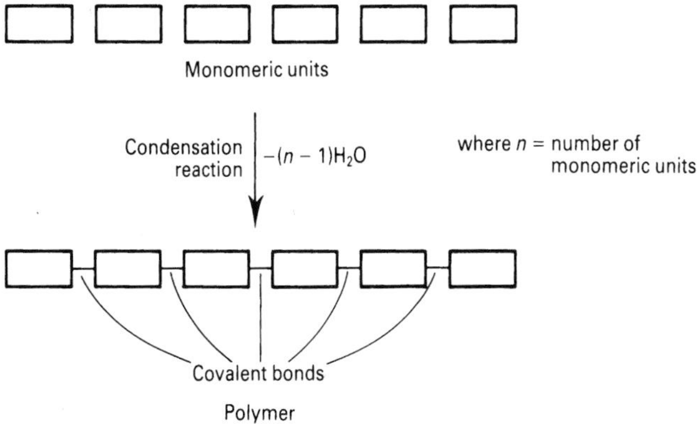

The RS system of stereochemical configuration was developed in 1956 to overcome the major problem associated with the DL nomenclature, namely that it may be ambiguous for compounds with multiple chiral centres. The RS system compares the substituent atoms or groups on an asymmetric tetrahedral carbon atom. Each type of functional group is assigned a **priority rating** according to defined rules. The priority listing includes $-OR > -OH > NH_2 > COOH > CHO > CH_2OH > CH_3 > H$. A molecular model of the chiral carbon atom is viewed with the group of the lowest priority orientated to be the furthest from the observer, e.g. H in glyceraldehyde. The priority ratings of the other three substituents are then considered. If the priorities decrease in a clockwise direction, the configuration is termed R (Latin, *rectus* = right). If the priorities descend in an anticlockwise direction, the configuration is S (Latin, *sinistrus* = left). Therefore, R-glyceraldehyde is synonymous with D-glyceraldehyde. The RS system enables the stereochemical configuration of compounds containing numerous chiral centres to be accurately described, e.g. (2S,3R)-threonine.

Figure 1.7 *Construction of macromolecules from building-block molecules*

Table 1.3 *Functions of macromolecules*

Carbohydrates	Proteins	Nucleic acids	Lipids
Energy-yielding fuel	Enzymes	Genetic material	Structural components
Structural	Structural	Transmission of genetic	of membranes
Protection	Transport	information	Energy-yielding fuel
Components of proteoglycans,	Hormones	Protein synthesis	Steroid hormones
glycoproteins and glycolipids	Gene regulation	Components of cell organelles	Insulation
Adherence	Protection		Protection
Turnover of glycoproteins	Toxins		Vitamins

Table 1.4 *Comparison of classes of macromolecules*

Feature	Carbohydrate	Protein	Nucleic acids
Monomeric units	Monosaccharides	Amino acids	Nucleotides
Covalent bond formed by condensation reaction	Glycosidic	Peptide	Phosphodiester
Number of major monomeric units	6	20	8
Nomenclature of multiple units			
2–10 units	Oligosaccharide	Oligopeptide	Oligonucleotide
>10 units	Polysaccharide	Polypeptide	Polynucleotide
Occurrence of hydrogen bonds	Intra- and intermolecular	Intra- and intermolecular	Intra- and intermolecular
Hydrolytic enzyme	Glycosidases	Peptidases	Nucleases

The **functions** of macromolecules are listed briefly in Table 1.3. Further details follow in subsequent chapters.

Table 1.4 highlights the key features of macromolecule construction. As an example, polymeric carbohydrates are composed of monosaccharides linked by **glycosidic bonds** to form multiple units which, if relatively small, are called **oligosaccharides**, and, if larger, are called **polysaccharides**. An oligosaccharide may be described as a disaccharide, trisaccharide or tetrasaccharide, etc. according to the number of monomeric units. Similar nomenclature is employed for proteins and nucleic acids. Most macromolecules contain only a small number of different **monomeric units**, e.g. glycogen contains only one monomeric unit, namely D-glucose, and deoxyribonucleic acid (DNA) contains only four different nucleotides.

The **precise shape** of the polymeric structure is conferred by the nature of the covalent bond and additional bonds such as hydrogen bonds. Additional bonding may occur between certain atoms or functional groups of the same polymeric chain called **intra-molecular bonds** or between adjacent chains called **inter-molecular bonds**. The polymeric structure can be degraded back to its monomeric units by **hydrolysis**, the addition of the elements of water to the groups which are involved in the covalent linkages. In biological systems, this is achieved by the action of enzymes.

The classes of biological macromolecules are not mutually exclusive and may interact to produce **hybrid** or **conjugate molecules**. By way of an example, protein and carbohydrate may form **proteoglycans** or **glycoproteins**. Proteoglycans are primarily carbohydrate in nature but contain protein associated with carbohydrate chains through both covalent and non-covalent bonding (Chapter 5). Glycoproteins contain a much lower percentage of carbohydrate which is branched and linked to the polypeptide chain by covalent bonds only. Proteins which function either on the surface of the cell membrane or extracellularly tend to be **glycosylated** whereas intracellular proteins tend to be devoid of carbohydrate. Other hybrid molecules are glycolipids, lipoproteins and nucleoproteins.

Finally, it should be noted that biological activity is not confined to monomeric units, large polymeric chains or hybrid molecules. There are many examples of biologically active oligomers, e.g. glutathione, a tripeptide, functions in the maintenance of membrane integrity.

Suggested further reading

Häussinger, D. (1996). The role of cellular hydration in the regulation of cell function. *Biochemical Journal* 313, 697–710.

Hegstrom, R.A. and Kondepudi, D.K. (1990). The handedness of the universe. *Scientific American* 262, 108–115.

Sarma, J.A.R.P., Nangia, A., Desiraju, G.R., Zass, E. and Dunitz, J.D. (1997). Even odder carbons. *Nature* 387, 464–465.

Welch, G.R. (1995). T.H. Huxley and the 'Protoplasmic Theory of Life': 100 years later. *Trends in Biochemical Sciences* 20, 481–485.

Welch, G.R. (1995). Schrödinger's 'What is Life?' A 50-year reflection. *Trends in Biochemical Sciences* 20, 45–48.

Montgomery, R. and Swenson, C.A. (1976). *Qualitative Problems in the Biochemical Sciences*. San Francisco: Freeman.

Self-assessment questions

1. Write the structures of the following carbon-containing compounds: (a) methylamine; (b) acetaldehyde; (c) acetone; (d) phenylamine; (e) dimethyl ether.
2. (a) What is a semipermeable membrane?
   (b) If a $0.1 \, mol \, l^{-1}$ solution of the protein, albumin, is placed on the left side of a biological membrane and $0.01 \, mol \, l^{-1}$ solution of the same protein is placed on the right side, in which direction does water move?

During the period from 1957 to 1961, about 10,000 people worldwide including about 480 people in Britain were born with missing or deformed limbs after their mothers ingested the drug **thalidomide** to treat morning sickness and nausea during pregnancy. In 1979, a report suggested that the stereochemistry of the drug was crucial. Thalidomide may exist as two enantiomers. Animals treated with R(+)-thalidomide produced normal neonates whereas those which had received the S(−)-enantiomer gave birth to deformed offspring. The prescribed preparation had contained both enantiomers.

However, the report was based on rodent experiments. Rodents are generally insensitive to the **teratogenic** effects of thalidomide. Earlier work with New Zealand white rabbits, a sensitive species, had not demonstrated any difference in the teratogenicity of R(+)- and S(−)-thalidomide. In 1995, it was reported that in man there is rapid interconversion between the two enantiomers. An equilibrium in the blood was established in which both forms were present at similar concentrations irrespective of which enantiomer is initially employed. This suggests that the use of pure R(+)-thalidomide would not have altered the outcome of its original therapeutic use.

3. Calculate the pH of solutions with the following hydrogen ion concentrations:
   (a) $8 \times 10^{-4} \, mol \, l^{-1}$; (b) $4 \times 10^{-8} \, mol \, l^{-1}$; (c) $6 \times 10^{-10} \, mol \, l^{-1}$.

4. Calculate the hydrogen ion concentration in solutions of the following pH:
   (a) $pH = 3.45$; (b) $pH = 6.82$; (c) $pH = 9.31$.

5. Determine the relative concentrations of sodium acetate and acetic acid required to produce a buffer solution of pH 5.5 (pK_a of acetic acid $= 4.75$).

6. In your laboratory, you have available a $0.1 \, mol \, l^{-1}$ solution of NaOH and $0.1 \, mol \, l^{-1}$ solutions of HCl, N-[2-hydroxyethyl] piperazine-N'-[2-ethanesulphonic acid] (HEPES, $pK_a = 7.5$), 2-[N-morpholino] ethanesulphonic acid (MES, $pK_a = 6.1$) and triethanolamine (TEA, $pK_a = 7.8$). Assuming that the above solutions are used without dilution by the addition of water, how would you prepare 100 ml of a buffer solution to hold the pH essentially constant at pH 6.50 in an acid-producing enzymic reaction?

7. Distinguish between 'intra-molecular' and 'inter-molecular' bonds.

8. Draw the structures of the stereoisomers of glyceraldehyde.

9. How does water dissolve non-ionic, polar molecules?

10. What effects do the hormones, insulin and glucagon have on the volume of liver cells?

Key Concepts and Facts

Cells
- Prokaryotic cells do not have their genetic material enclosed by a nuclear membrane and lack discrete membrane-bound structures.
- Eukaryotic cells may be aggregated into tissues.

Water
- Water has characteristic physical properties when compared with other solvents.
- The water molecule is an electric dipole.
- Water molecules interact with each other through hydrogen bonding.
- Osmotic pressure is dependent upon the concentration differences between solutions separated by a semi-permeable membrane.
- Cell volume influences cellular metabolism.
- The pH of a solution influences the biological behaviour of ionic molecules.
- Buffer systems are composed of mixtures of acids and bases in which one component is weak.

Carbon
- The carbon atom is the basis of biological molecules.
- Carbon atoms can form chains or rings.
- Many biological molecules may exist in different stereo-chemical configurations.
- Macromolecules are formed by the condensation of small building-block molecules.
- There are four classes of biological molecules.
- The classes of biological macromolecules are not exclusive.

Answers to questions (Chapter 1)

1. (a) CH_3-NH_2; (b) $CH_3-\underset{\underset{H}{|}}{C}=O$; (c) $CH_3-\underset{\underset{CH_3}{|}}{C}=O$; (d) $CH=CH$;

(e) CH_3-O-CH_3.

2. One capable of selecting the molecules/ions which can pass through it.
(b) To the left side.

3. (a) pH = 3.10; (b) pH = 7.40; (c) pH = 9.22.

4. (a) 3.55×10^{-4} mol l^{-1}; (b) 1.51×10^{-7} mol l^{-1};
(c) 4.90×10^{-10} mol l^{-1}.

5. From the Henderson–Hasselbalch equation:

$$pH = pK_a + \log\frac{[acetate]}{[acetic\ acid]}$$

$$\therefore 5.55 = 4.75 + \log\frac{[acetate]}{[acetic\ acid]} \qquad \therefore 0.8 = \log\frac{[acetate]}{[acetic\ acid]}$$

$$\therefore \frac{[acetate]}{[acetic\ acid]} = antilog\ 0.80 \qquad \therefore \frac{[acetate]}{[acetic\ acid]} = \frac{6.31}{1}$$

∴ Relative concentration of acetate to acetic acid is 6.31 to 1.

6. Use NaOH (strong base) with one other solution; exclude HCl as strong acid–strong base mixtures do not act as buffers; select from weak acids using buffer zone = $pK_a - 1$ to $pK_a + 1$; MES/NaOH and HEPES/NaOH can function at the required pH but only MES can protect against acid production since pH 6.50 is at the $pK_a - 1$ end of the buffer zone for HEPES. (Consider the titration curve):
Final volume = 100 ml; note solutions are equimolar; let the initial volume of MES = x ml, and of NaOH = y ml; on mixing, final volume of MES = $x - y$ ml.

From the Henderson–Hasselbalch equation:

$$pH = pK_a + \log\frac{[conj.\ base]}{[acid]}$$

$$\therefore 6.50 = 6.10 + \log\frac{y}{(x-y)} \qquad \therefore 0.40 = \log\frac{y}{(x-y)}$$

$$\therefore \frac{y}{(x-y)} = antilog\ 0.40 = 2.51 \qquad \therefore y = 2.51(x-y)$$

But $x + y = 100$ ml

$$\therefore x = 100 - y \qquad \therefore y = 2.51[(100-y)-y]$$

$$\therefore y = (2.51 \times 100) - 2.51y - 2.51y \qquad \therefore y = 251 - 5.02y$$

$$\therefore 6.02y = 251; y = 41.7$$

But $x = 100 - y = 58.3$.

You require 58.3 ml of MES solution and 41.7 ml of NaOH solution to make your buffer.

7. Intra-molecular bonds are formed between functional groups on the same polymeric chain whereas inter-molecular bonds link different polymeric chains.
8. See Figure 1.6.
9. By forming hydrogen bonds with the polar groups on these molecules.
10. Insulin causes the cells to swell and glucagon causes shrinkage.

Chapter 2
Nucleic acids

Learning objectives

After studying this chapter you should confidently be able to:

Describe the central dogma of molecular biology.

Describe the structure of nucleotides and polynucleotide chains.

Describe the major structural features of double-stranded DNA.

Appreciate that DNA can assume different conformations.

Discuss the development of a method for sequencing of polynucleotide chains.

Discuss the importance of denaturation and renaturation of nucleic acids.

Describe the distinctive structural features of the major forms of RNA.

Relate protein structure to the structure of mRNA through the genetic code.

Describe ribosome subunits as nucleoproteins.

The important **cellular functions of nucleic acids** may be summarized by reference to the **central dogma of molecular biology** (Figure 2.1). Nucleic acids exist as two different types:

- **deoxyribonucleic acid (DNA),** the reservoir of genetic information in all living forms;
- **ribonucleic acid (RNA),** of which there are three main forms: mRNA, tRNA and rRNA.

DNA contains the instructions for all chemical processes within the organism. The information is held in the sequence of deoxynucleotides contained within its structure analogous to the way the sequence of the letters in a written word imparts certain information to the reader. DNA is the only biological molecule capable of **direct self-replication** so that, during the process of cell division,

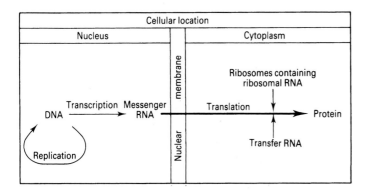

Figure 2.1 *The central dogma of molecular biology in eukaryotic cells*

each daughter cell will receive deoxyribonucleotide sequences containing identical information.

The manifestation of this information is the **proteins** manufactured by the cell. In prokaryotic and eukaryotic cells, the information for **protein synthesis** must be transported from the DNA to the **ribosomes**. This is the function of **messenger RNA** (mRNA) which also conveys the instructions through the nuclear envelope of eukaryotic cells. The synthesis of mRNA occurs by **transcription**. The ribonucleotide sequence of the mRNA is complementary to the deoxyribonucleotide sequence of the DNA and is **translated** into the amino acid sequence of the protein, a process involving the ribosomes of the cell. Translation involves numerous molecules of **transfer RNA** (tRNA) which deliver and insert amino acids, according to the instructions, into growing polypeptide chains. **Ribosomal RNAs** also play an important role in protein synthesis (Chapter 13). The flow of genetic information in cells is therefore DNA → RNA → protein.

A **stretch of DNA** which is transcribed and then employed as a template in protein synthesis was termed a **gene**. The entire genetic information of a cell is termed its **genome** irrespective of its location (Chapter 7). Only approximately 30% of the nuclear genome may serve as genes, the other 70% being termed **extragenic** DNA. Recent advances in molecular biology have resulted in the broadening of the definition of a gene. Today, a gene is defined as a sequence of genomic DNA which performs a specific function. The gene need not be translated or transcribed to function. Genes have been classified into three classes:

- **protein-coding genes** are transcribed into RNA which is translated into protein;
- **RNA-specifying genes** are transcribed into RNA;
- **regulatory genes** are neither transcribed nor translated but function in the control of transcription. Note that protein-coding gene products may also function in regulation.

The entire **protein-coding gene** will not be expressed in the final

An **exception to the central dogma of molecular biology** is the storage of genetic information in RNA molecules in certain viruses e.g. human immunodeficiency virus (HIV). When such viruses enter susceptible cells, the RNA genome is copied into a DNA replica by an enzyme called **reverse transcriptase**. The DNA product remains dormant within the host cell until transcription is initiated. The genetic material of viral origin is then expressed according to the rules of the central dogma. The RNA viruses, called **retroviruses**, represent a variation , not a violation, of the rules of the central dogma.

The **human genome** contains within its 23 pairs of chromosomes, an estimated 80,000 genes and 3 billion base-pairs. Inheritance of defective genes leads to loss, or alteration in the structure, of the resultant proteins. It is estimated that about **4000 human diseases** result from such defects with about 2–5% of the world's population being afflicted by these debilitating or fatal inherited conditions. Following the identification of the defective gene, pre-natal diagnostic tests have been developed for some conditions, e.g. **cystic fibrosis** (gene identified in 1989) and **Duchenne muscular dystrophy** (1986). Further study of defective genes has elucidate some of the mechanisms by which a defective copy of a gene results in disease.

In **cystic fibrosis**, a dysfunction in all exocrine glands causes abnormal mucus production. This results from a specific deletion of the codon for the amino acid phenylalanine at position 508 in the primary structure of a transmembrane protein which regulates the passage of chloride ions through the plasma membranes of cells. **Duchenne muscular dystrophy**, characterized by proximal limb weakness, is the result of the absence from muscle cells of a cytoskeletal protein called **dystrophin**, encoded within the X-chromosome.

protein product. **In eukaryotic cells** (but not prokaryotic cells), the product of transcription, called the **primary RNA transcript** or **heterogeneous nuclear RNA** (hnRNA) or **pre-messenger RNA** (pre-mRNA), contains additional sequences which are excised in the processing of the RNA transcript to form mRNA. The sequences are called **intervening sequences** or **introns**. All nucleotide sequences which remain in the mRNA following splicing are referred to as **exons**. Exons (or parts of exons) are translated from the mRNA template in the ribosome during protein synthesis. The terms intron and exon are used to describe nucleotide sequences at the levels of both DNA and RNA.

This chapter considers the structure of nucleotides, their polymerization into polynucleotide chains, the structure of DNA and RNAs, some properties of nucleic acids, DNA-sequencing techniques and the genetic code.

Nucleotides

Ribonucleotides and **deoxyribonucleotides** are the building blocks of RNA and DNA respectively.

The structure of nucleotides

Nucleotides (Figure 2.2) have **three component parts**:

- a **heterocyclic ring**, which is a derivative of either **pyrimidine or purine**. A purine can be considered as a pyrimidine ring to which a five-membered imidazole ring has been fused. It is these nitrogenous bases which are responsible for the important biological properties of nucleic acids;
- a **pentose sugar**, either D-ribose or **2-deoxy-D-ribose**;
- a **phosphate group**.

Each of the components contributes to the chemistry of the monomer.

By convention, **numbering** of the atoms in a pyrimidine is clockwise whereas in purines the six-membered ring is numbered anticlockwise. The interaction of either pentose with a nitrogenous base gives rise to a **nucleoside**, either a ribonucleoside or deoxyribonucleoside. The bond is named according to carbohydrate nomenclature. The **β-glycosidic bond** involves the C-1 atom of the sugar and either the N-1 atom of a pyrimidine or the N-9 atom of a purine and so is either a C-$1'$ → N-1 or C-$1'$ → N-9 glycosidic linkage, the prime superscipt denoting the carbon atoms of the sugar.

The suffix **-idine** indicates that the nucleoside contains a pyrimidine base whereas **-osine** denotes the presence of a purine base.

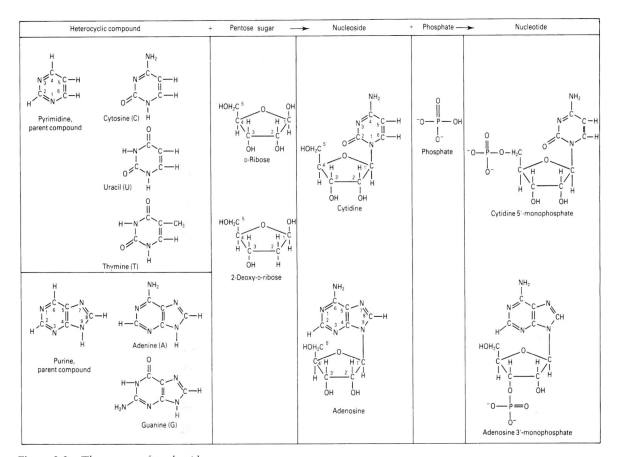

Figure 2.2   *The nature of nucleotides*

Nucleoside nomenclature is clarified in Table 2.1 which shows the one-letter code for each nitrogenous base. Because thymine is a major base of DNA but rarely occurs in RNA, the ribonucleoside is called ribosylthymine whilst thymidine refers to the deoxyribonucleoside.

The addition of one, two or three **phosphate groups** to the sugar of a nucleoside by **ester linkage** (alcoholic-OH + acid → ester) derives a **nucleotide**. The nomenclature of the nucleotide is based upon the name of the nucleoside plus the position and number of

Table 2.1   *Nomenclature of nucleosides*

Base	One-letter code	Ribonucleoside	Deoxyribonucleoside
Cytosine	C	Cytidine	Deoxycytidine
Uracil	U	Uridine	Deoxyuridine
Thymine	T	Ribosylthymine	Thymidine
Adenine	A	Adenosine	Deoxyadenosine
Guanine	G	Guanosine	Deoxyguanosine

The **Human Genome Project** is an international collaborative project which aims **to map and determine the sequence of all the genes** present in the nucleus of a human cell. Such a plan should facilitate the identification of genes which may play a role in the development of cancer, age-related diseases or malfunction of the immune system. The strategy is that once a problem gene is identified, it may be possible to excise it (or part of it) from the genome or block its effects.

Progeria is a number of syndromes afflicting the young, which are characterized by an accelerated rate of aging. In progeria patients, it has been demonstrated that there is an enhanced production of aberrant proteins reaching levels found in the elderly. Following the identification of a **regulatory gene**, there is the expectation that it may be possible to achieve a reduced rate of synthesis of these abnormal proteins not only in progeria but also in the normally ageing individual.

the phosphate groups, e.g. adenosine $3'$-monophosphate, cytidine-$5'$-triphosphate. Phosphorylation may occur at the $2'$, $3'$ or $5'$ positions of a ribonucleoside and at the $3'$ or $5'$ positions of a deoxyribonucleoside. However, it is the $5'$-nucleotides which are of major biological importance. The nucleoside $5'$-monophosphates are sometimes referred to as adenylate, uridylate, thymidylate etc. because of the presence of the phosphate group. $5'$-Ribonucleotides are denoted as NMP, NDP and NTP whereas $5'$-deoxyribonucleotides are denoted as dNMP etc., e.g. adenosine-$5'$-triphosphate (ATP), deoxyadenosine-$5'$-triphosphate (d-ATP).

Polynucleotide chains

Identification of the component pentose sugar confirms whether the polynucleotide chain is RNA or DNA. RNA and DNA contain the following **major heterocyclic bases:**

- **the same two purine bases,** adenine (A) and guanine (G);
- **the pyrimidine base,** cytosine;
- **a second pyrimidine base,** uracil (present in RNA), or its 5-methyl derivative called thymine (present in DNA).

In addition to the major bases, DNA and RNA also contain altered or less common bases called **minor bases.** In DNA, the minor bases are usually methylated derivatives of the major bases, e.g. 7-methylguanine, which play a specific role in the functioning of the polynucleotide. In RNA, minor bases are predominantly found in tRNAs and are mainly modified versions of major bases, e.g. 5,6-dihydrouracil.

Individual monomeric nucleotides are **polymerized** by the formation of **phosphodiester linkages** (Chapter 1) so that RNA may be described as a linear polyribonucleotide having a ribose–phosphate backbone with $3',5'$-**phosphodiester internucleotide links** (Figure 2.3a). Strands of DNA may similarly be described as a polydeoxyribonucleotide having a deoxyribose–phosphate backbone with $3',5'$-phosphodiester internucleotide links (Figure 2.3b).

Linear nucleic acids have two ends, termed the **$5'$-end** and **$3'$-end**. Because the biosynthesis of nucleic acids utilizes nucleoside $5'$-triphosphates, the $5'$-end exhibits a terminal phosphate group whereas a terminal hydroxyl group is located at the $3'$-end. The terms, **upstream** and **downstream** may be applied to nucleotide sequences towards the $5'$-end and $3'$-end respectively. The size of nucleic acids means their structures are usually written in the convenient form of a **one-letter code** with the $5'$-end on the left and the $3'$-end on the right. The tetraribonucleotide in Figure 2.3 may be denoted as AGCU and its deoxyribonucleotide counterpart as AGCT.

Single **phosphorus–oxygen bonds** permit rotation of the nucleoside moieties. Rotation about the glycosidic bond within the

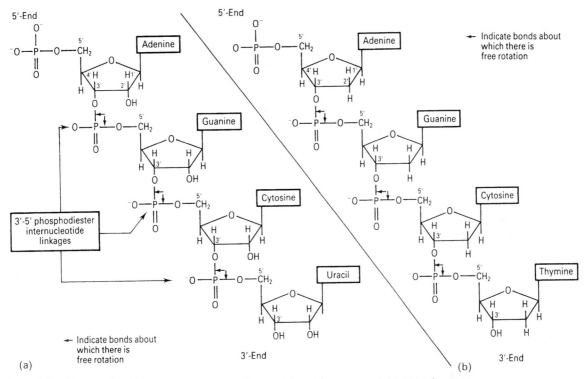

Figure 2.3 *Tetranucleotide sequences representing nucleic acid structure: (a) RNA; (b) DNA*

nucleoside is limited by potential steric hindrances so that in most double helical structures (Z-DNA is an exception), only one steric conformation called the *anti* conformation is found (Figure 2.4).

Some properties of nucleotides

At physiological pH, the phosphate groups, but not the heterocyclic bases, are ionized. All heterocyclic bases found in nucleic acids may exist in two forms, depending on the pH of their environment. Changing between forms, called **tautomerism**, involves proton exchange between atoms in the molecule. Keto–enol tautomerism, also called lactam–lactim tautomerism (Figure 2.5), results from the electron-withdrawing effect of the oxygen atom creating slight electropositivity in the imino-hydrogen atom which migrates to the electronegative oxygen to produce an enol group. At physiological pH, the bases of nucleic acids are in the keto form which promotes hydrogen-bonded base-pairing. Local intracellular pH variations therefore may effect deviations from normal base-pairing arrangements.

All **nucleic acids** demonstrate an **absorption maxima** at approximately 260 nm. The precise value for a given nucleic acid depends upon its base composition since the absorption of ultraviolet light is

> **Nucleotides perform other important functions** in addition to their important roles as the building blocks of nucleic acids. Certain **coenzymes**, e.g. NAD^+, FAD and coenzyme A (Chapter 4), contain nucleotide structures. The chemical form in which **energy** is carried and from which it is released in the cell is ATP, a nucleotide. Some nucleotides are involved in carbohydrate biosynthesis as **glycosyl carriers**, e.g. UDP-glucose in glycogen biosynthesis (Chapter 10). **Cyclic nucleotides**, e.g. cAMP, have an intracellular role in signal transduction.

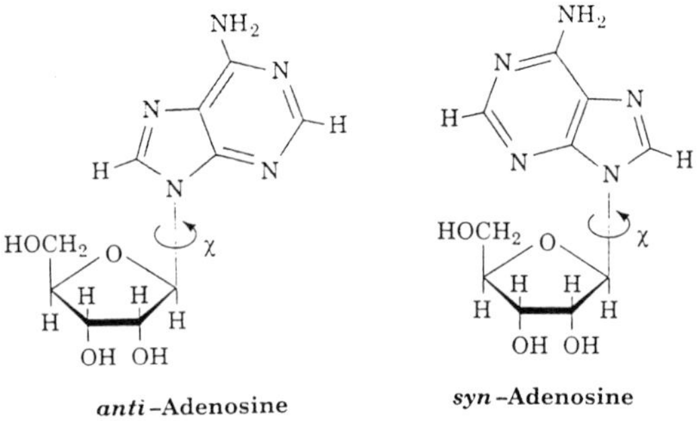

Figure 2.4 *The permissible steric conformations of adenosine*

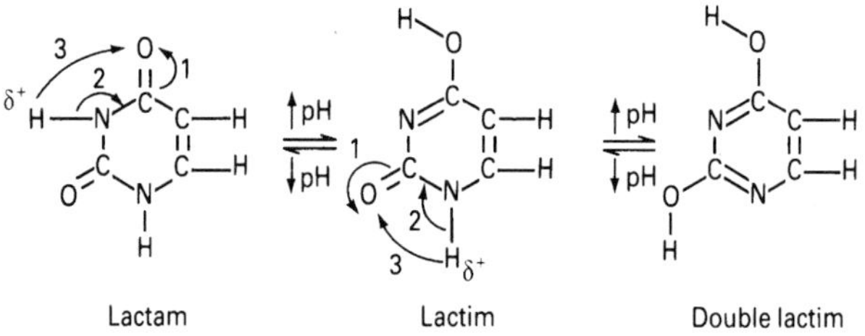

anti-Adenosine   *syn*-Adenosine

Lactam   Lactim   Double lactim

Figure 2.5 *Tautomerism of uracil*

a property conferred by the conjugated bond systems of the heterocyclic bases, each of which absorbs at different wavelengths (Table 2.2).

DNA

DNA is the storage molecule for genetic information. The sequence of nucleotides is responsible ultimately for every cellular activity.

The structure of DNA

Table 2.2 *The absorption maxima of heterocyclic bases of nucleic acids at pH 7.0*

Heterocyclic base	Absorption maximum/ maxima (nm)
Adenine	260
Guanine	246, 276
Cytosine	268
Uracil	258
Thymine	266

The **size** of DNA, recorded either as molecular mass or in terms of numbers of base pairs, varies according to its source (Table 2.3). In the late 1940s, **chemical analysis** of the base composition of DNA from various sources by Edwin Chargaff revealed that the relative amounts of the heterocyclic bases varied between species (Table 2.4) but were constant within a species irrespective of age and tissue of origin. The ratios A/T, G/C and purine/pyrimidine approximate to one and thus:

• A = T, i.e. the number of adenine residues equals thymine residues;

Table 2.3 *The size of DNA in different organisms*

Organism	Molecular mass (Da)	Base-pairs
SV40 virus	3×10^6	5×10^3
Adenovirus	1.4×10^7	2.1×10^4
Escherichia coli	2.2×10^9	4.6×10^6
Mouse cells	1.5×10^{12}	2.3×10^9
Human cells	1.8×19^{12}	2.8×10^9

Table 2.4 *Base equivalence in DNA from various sources*

Organism	Base composition (mol.%)				Base ratios			
	A	G	C*	T	$\frac{A}{T}$	$\frac{G}{C}$	$\frac{A+G}{T+C}$	$\frac{G+C}{A+T}$
Human	30.4	19.6	20.6	30.1	1.01	0.95	0.99	0.66
Ox	29.0	21.2	22.5	28.7	1.01	0.94	0.98	0.76
Rat	28.6	21.4	21.5	28.4	1.01	0.99	1.00	0.75
Salmon	28.9	22.4	21.6	27.1	1.07	1.04	1.05	0.79
Carrot	26.7	23.1	23.2	26.9	0.99	1.00	0.99	0.86
Wheatgerm	27.3	22.7	22.8	27.1	1.01	1.00	1.00	0.84
Yeast	31.7	18.3	17.4	32.6	0.97	1.05	1.00	0.56
E. coli	24.7	26.0	25.7	23.6	1.05	1.10	1.03	1.07
Staphylococcus aureus	30.8	21.0	19.0	29.2	1.05	1.11	1.07	0.67

* Including 5-methylcytosine if present.

- **G = C**, i.e. the number of guanine residues equals cytosine residues;
- **A + G = T + C**, i.e. the number of purine residues equals pyrimidine residues.

These parameters have become known as **Chargaff's rules**. The ratio $G + C/A + T$ indicates the characteristic chemical composition of DNA from a given organism.

With the exception of single-stranded DNA viruses, DNA occurs as a **double-helical (duplex)** molecule. In 1953, Watson and Crick constructed **a model of DNA** compatible with the available data from low resolution X-ray diffraction studies, chemical data on base composition, knowledge of the three-dimensional structure of nucleotides and knowledge of the stereochemistry of base-pairing. Base-pairing is the result of the ability of the bases to interact by the formation of **hydrogen bonds** (Chapter 1). Thymine may form two hydrogen bonds with adenine while cytosine may form three hydrogen bonds with guanine (Figure 2.6).

The **key features of the Watson–Crick model** of DNA (Figure 2.7) are as follows:

Figure 2.6 *Dimensions of hydrogen bonding of nucleotide pairs: (a) thymine to adenine; (b) cytosine to guanine*

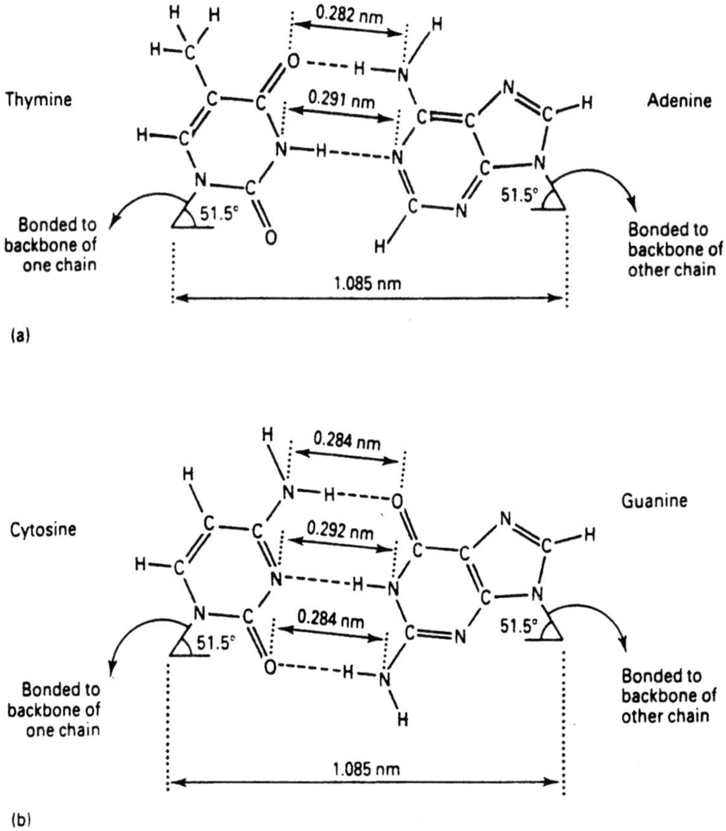

(a)

(b)

- Two polynucleotide chains are arranged with the sugar–phosphate backbone on the outside and the bases on the inside located perpendicular to the axis of the duplex.

- The two chains of the DNA duplex are antiparallel, i.e the 3′,5′-phosphodiester internucleotide linkages in each chain lie in opposing directions.

- The two polynucleotide strands are complementary in that the thymine always pairs with adenine and cytosine always pairs with guanine. This arrangement explains why the DNA duplex contains equimolar amounts of purines and pyrimidines as indicated by chemical analysis. Any other combination of bases (non-Watson–Crick base-pairing) would distort significantly the double helix since their insertion would create a ruffling of the sugar–phosphate backbone.

- The DNA duplex is a right-handed helix. This means that when the molecule is viewed from one end, the top surface of the helix spirals towards the right. Each turn of the helix contains 10 base-pairs, measures 3.4 nm in length and corresponds to the major periodicity attained by X-ray diffraction. The distance of 0.34 nm

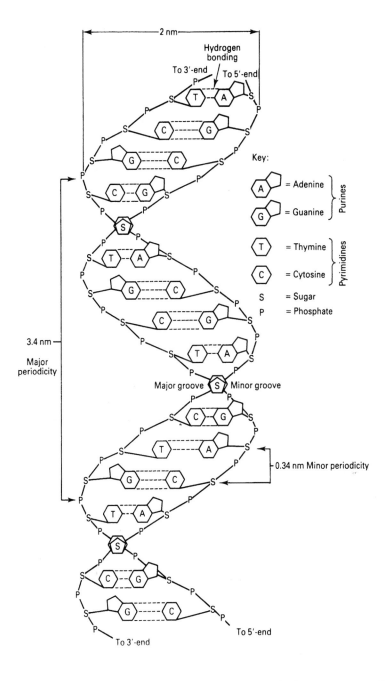

occupied by one nucleotide is consistent with the experimental minor periodicity.

- **The two helical strands are held together by the hydrogen bonds** between complementary base-pairs.
- **Additional stability** may result from vertical hydrophobic interactions between adjacent non-polar heterocyclic bases which create stacking throughout the duplex structure.

- **The crossing of the antiparallel chains creates external helical grooves** of different dimensions called **major** and **minor grooves.** The major grooves are the major sites of contact with DNA-binding proteins through hydrogen bonding between the protein and exposed base functional groups. In the minor grooves, protein–DNA contacts are not excluded but are less frequent because the positions of potential hydrogen-bonding groups make them less recognizable to the hydrogen-bond donor and acceptor groups of the protein.

The **Watson–Crick model** also suggested a possible mechanism for DNA replication. Replication may proceed through:

- **the separation of the two chains;**
- **the use of each of the separated chains as a template** to arrange nucleotides in order according to the rules of base-pairing;
- **the synthesis of new chains complementary to each of the existent strands** by joining the nucleotides arranged in sequence.

This hypothesis was experimentally confirmed by Meselson and Stahl in 1957.

DNA can assume different **conformations**, called A-DNA, B-DNA, C-DNA and Z-DNA (zigzag), depending upon the chemical microenvironment, e.g. humidity and salt concentrations, the cations of which interact varyingly with the phosphates. These forms exhibit differences in, for example, major and minor periodicities, dimensions of major and minor grooves, and numbers of base-pairs per helical turn (Table 2.5).

The Watson–Crick model represents the most stable form, **B-DNA,** which is the predominant intracellular form and the major conformation of DNA in aqueous solution. Certain regions of B-DNA containing alternate purine and pyrimidine residues may adopt the only left-handed helical form, Z-DNA. This transformation involves the *N*-glycosyl bonds of purines rotating 180° from the *anti* to the *syn* conformation (Figure 2.4). This 'flipping' of the ring causes the pyrimidines to flip to maintain

Table 2.5 *Comparison of some structural features of B-DNA and Z-DNA*

Feature	B-DNA	Z-DNA
Helix	Right-handed	Left-handed
Base-pairs per helical turn	10	12
Major periodicity	3.4 nm	4.5 nm
Minor periodicity	0.34 nm	0.37 nm
Major groove	Wide	Flat
Minor groove	Narrow	Narrow
Glycosidic bond conformation	*Anti*	*Anti* for pyrimidines, *syn* for purines

normal base-pairing. This process may be important in the regulation of gene expression by the switching on and off of genes, co-ordinated events which govern all cellular activities.

The DNA molecules of prokaryotes and numerous viruses are **circular** in that each chain is continuous. To enhance packaging *in vivo*, the axis of the duplex may be twisted into a **supercoil or superhelix** (Figure 2.8) which may be either right-handed or left-handed. Only a helix which is circular or fixed at both ends can form a stable supercoil. The number of crossover points varies with the source of DNA.

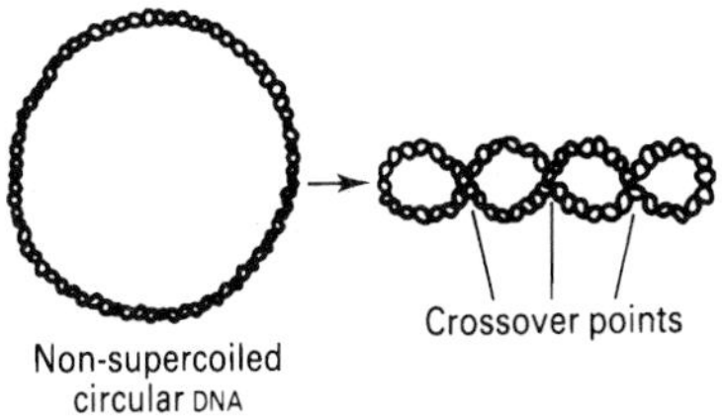

Figure 2.8 *An example of supercoiling of DNA*

The sequencing of DNA

The **sequence of nucleotides** along a polynucleotide chain is termed the **primary structure**. DNA molecules of natural origin tend to be immense (Table 2.3) and impossible to sequence as a complete structure.Three developments in the late 1970s made the elucidation of the primary structure of DNA feasible:

- **availability of sufficient quantities of identical DNA molecules** through gene cloning techniques;
- **development of sequencing techniques** capable of processing relatively large polynucleotides. Until 1977, sequencing could be performed on oligonucleotides up to 10 nucleotides long but was difficult and time-consuming;
- **development of a method for the precise cleavage of DNA.** Such cleavage can be obtained through the use of site-specific **restriction endonucleases**. The cleavage products, called **restriction fragments**, are then sequenced.

Rapid DNA sequencing may be performed by:

- the **dideoxy sequencing method** of Sanger and Coulson, which is now the favoured method because of its simplicity and its adaption into an automated system;
- the **chemical cleavage method** of Maxam and Gilbert (not described herein).

The **dideoxy sequencing method** exploits the ability of a key enzyme in the replication of DNA, **DNA polymerase,** which positions nucleotides into a growing nucleotide chain according to a pre-existing template. The dideoxy sequencing method utilizes *in vitro* the polymerase activity of *Escherichia coli* **DNA polymerase I.** Since DNA polymerase I also contains an exonuclease activity (it removes one nucleotide at a time from the 5'-end) at a separate catalytic site, the enzyme has been subjected to proteolytic cleavage into two fragments. The polymerase activity is contained within the **Klenow fragment** of the enzyme and this fragment is employed to synthesize a collection of radioactively labelled fragments through

Restriction endonucleases are enzymes which *in vivo* protect certain micro-organisms from **viral** infection by the destruction of the foreign DNA molecules. Since this phenomenon is called **host-controlled restriction**, the enzymes are referred to as restriction endonucleases. Hundreds of restriction endonucleases have been purified from a wide variety of micro-organisms. Since the destruction of bacterial DNA would be lethal, the corresponding sequences in the microbial DNA are protected by the methylation of adenine or cytosine residues.

Restriction endonucleases have been classified into Types I, II and III according to differences in their modes of action. Type I enzymes recognize a specific nucleotide sequence but cleave less specifically at a distance of over 1000 base-pairs from the recognition site. Type II enzymes have cleavage sites which are specific and within or close to their recognition sites. Type III enzyme cleavage sites lie 24–26 base-pairs downstream of their recognition sites. Also, Types I and III endonucleases catalyse the methylation of DNA whereas Type II enzymes demonstrate only endonucleolytic cleavage.

Type II enzymes are valuable since they cleave their substrates in a very precise manner. They recognize specific **short palindromic sequences** (four to six base-pairs long) in DNA and cut at least one strand. A palindrome is a word or sentence which reads alike backward and forward as exemplified in the British place-names Glenelg and Notton. The cleavage sites are symmetrical and produce either linear (blunt-end) or staggered (cohesive-end) incisions. Cohesive ends are valuable in the insertion of a foreign gene into a bacterial or eukaryotic genome for gene cloning.

the controlled inhibition of the replication process by the addition of **dideoxyribonucleotides** (containing 2,3-dideoxyribose) to the growing strand. Since a 3′-OH group is not available, the elongation process is halted (Figure 2.9). The **template** is a single-strand copy of the DNA to be sequenced to which a single-strand primer complementary to the preceding template bases is hybridized through hydrogen-bonding arrangements.

For each determination (Figure 2.10), four reaction mixtures are employed, each containing all four dNTPs, one of which is labelled, e.g. dGTP, dCTP, dTTP and $[\alpha\text{-}^{32}\text{P}]$-dATP plus one different dideoxyribonucleotide (ddNTP). Each reaction mixture generates oligonucleotide chains of varying length which all terminate with the same base. The duplex chains may be separated by **denaturation** (disruption of the hydrogen bonds). The newly synthesized sequences are then separated according to size by **polyacrylamide** (for up to several hundred nucleotides in length) **or agarose** (for longer polynucleotide strands) **gel electrophoresis.** Since a radioactively labelled dNTP was present in the four reaction mixtures, all new oligonucleotide chains may be detected by **autoradiography.**

Visualization by autoradiography requires an **X-ray film** to be laid on the gel. The disintegrations from the radiolabelled ^{32}P will blacken the emulsion of the film to produce a pattern. Since all four reaction mixtures are electrophoresed adjacently in the same gel, the DNA sequence can be read directly from the autoradiogram (X-ray film) starting at the fastest (smallest) fragment located at the bottom of the film. A DNA segment containing 500 nucleotides may be sequenced in one experiment by this method.

The technique has been continually refined and currently may involve the use of:

- **fluorescent tags;**

- **bacteriophage T7 DNA polymerase** which is less sensitive to the presence of ddNTPs than the Klenow fragment and improves the banding (more even intensities which aids automated reading systems);

- **taq polymerase** (DNA polymerase from the thermophilic bacteria, *Thermus aquaticus*) which is stable at 90°C and may be employed successfully at temperatures which prevent hydrogen bonding between strands. The formation of duplex structures would interfere with elongation of the chain.

A **fluorescent dye** may be attached to the primer at its 5′-end and the primers are used in four separate reactions. The reaction products are electrophoresed in adjacent lanes and the order of fluorescent fragments in the gel is recorded by a **laser-activated fluorescence detection system.** In an alternative method, each dideoxynucleotide may be tagged with a dye which fluoresces at a different wavelength. A single reaction is conducted in the presence of the tagged dideoxynucleotides and the resultant fragment

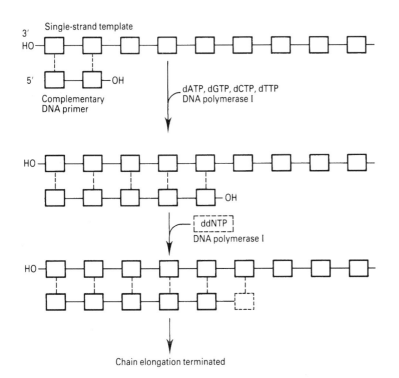

Figure 2.9 *Dideoxyribonucleotide-induced termination of DNA synthesis*

Single-strand template

3′
HO—

Complementary DNA primer

5′

dATP, dGTP, dCTP, dTTP
DNA polymerase I

ddNTP
DNA polymerase I

Chain elongation terminated

mixture is electrophoresed in a **single** gel lane. The terminal base is identified by its **fluorescence emission**. These modifications to the method are the basis of **automated systems** which can identify about 10,000 bases per day.

Some properties of DNA

The properties of DNA discussed in this section are:

- **denaturation** which is the **unfolding** of duplex strands into single chains;
- **renaturation** which is the **reforming** of duplex strands from partially or completely separated strands.

Denaturation occurs when a solution of double-stranded DNA is subjected to extremes of pH or heat. A decrease in viscosity and an increase in ultraviolet (UV) light absorption are recorded. The heterocyclic bases contain the conjugated ring systems which absorb the light energy. Because in double-stranded DNA the bases are highly ordered due to hydrogen bonding and stacking hydrophobic interactions, the UV absorption at 260 nm of the duplex structure is lower than for the random conformation of single-stranded DNA.

The **heat denaturation of DNA** may be referred to as **melting** because, since hydrogen bonds mutually re-inforce, the denaturation occurs over a small temperature range. The temperature at

Gene cloning involves the production *in vitro* of new DNA molecules which contain novel combinations of genes or oligonucleotides and the propagation of such **recombinant DNA molecules** by the exploitation *in vivo* of the replicative mechanisms of bacteria and some eukaryotic organisms. The technique has permitted the alteration of the genome of organisms so that they produce substances of little intrinsic value but of great medical or economic value to mankind, e.g the α- and β-interferons (antiviral agents), insulin, somatostatin, somatotropin (hormones), Factor VIII (a coagulation factor), actinorhodin (an antibiotic), tomatoes resistant to bruise-damage (used for tomato purée), maize resistant to infection, pesticide-resistant soya beans etc.

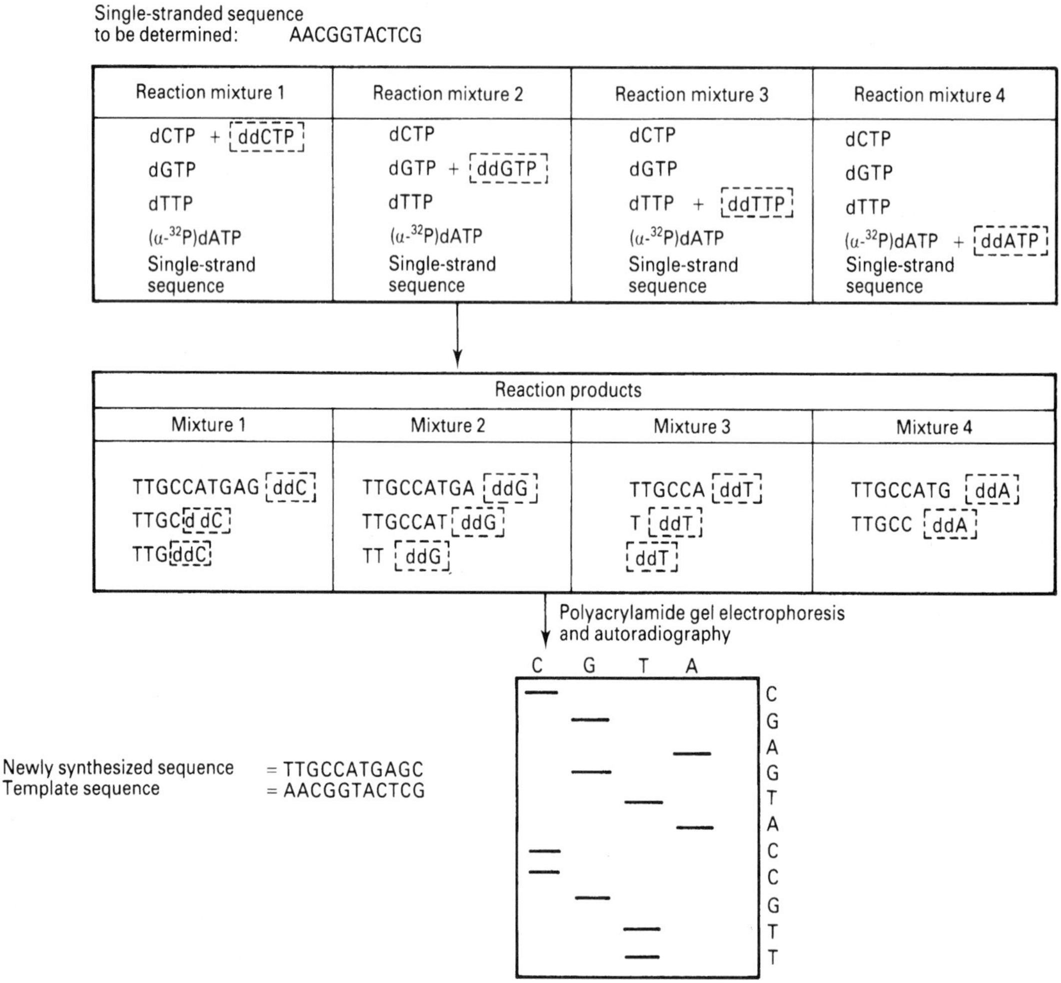

Single-stranded sequence
to be determined: AACGGTACTCG

Reaction mixture 1	Reaction mixture 2	Reaction mixture 3	Reaction mixture 4
dCTP + [ddCTP]	dCTP	dCTP	dCTP
dGTP	dGTP + [ddGTP]	dGTP	dGTP
dTTP	dTTP	dTTP + [ddTTP]	dTTP
(α-^{32}P)dATP	(α-^{32}P)dATP	(α-^{32}P)dATP	(α-^{32}P)dATP + [ddATP]
Single-strand sequence	Single-strand sequence	Single-strand sequence	Single-strand sequence

Reaction products

Mixture 1	Mixture 2	Mixture 3	Mixture 4
TTGCCATGAG [ddC]	TTGCCATGA [ddG]	TTGCCA [ddT]	TTGCCATG [ddA]
TTGC[ddC]	TTGCCAT [ddG]	T [ddT]	TTGCC [ddA]
TTG[ddC]	TT [ddG]	[ddT]	

Polyacrylamide gel electrophoresis
and autoradiography

Newly synthesized sequence   = TTGCCATGAGC
Template sequence   = AACGGTACTCG

Figure 2.10   *The Sanger dideoxy method of DNA sequencing*

which 50% of the DNA is denatured is termed the **transition or melting temperature**, T_m (Figure 2.11a). The T_m value of DNA depends upon its $G + C/A + T$ **ratio** (Table 2.4), the higher this ratio the higher the T_m value (Figure 2.11b). The importance of the $G + C$ content reflects the triple hydrogen bonding in this base-pair (Figure 2.6) which requires a higher temperature for its disruption.

Denatured DNA molecules from different species may interact with each other to create **hybrid duplexes** in which regions of a DNA strand from one species have base-paired with a disparate DNA strand. Such **hybridizations** permit the identification of like genes within different species and the determination of evolutionary relationships between species. Hybridization may also occur between a single DNA strand and an RNA molecule; the process is called DNA–RNA hybridization. Such techniques have proved valuable in the isolation and purification of genes and their corresponding RNAs.

If the denaturation of the DNA is incomplete with about 12 intact consecutive base-pairs, a return to favourable conditions (neutral pH, room temperature) permits the partially separated strands to re-form the duplex structure spontaneously, a process called **renaturation**. If the denaturation is complete, renaturation may occur but at a markedly lower rate since complementary sequences must align through collisions before the re-formation of the duplex. Renaturation tends to occur at 20–25°C below the T_m value.

On the basis of DNA renaturation data, additional genomic sequences have been identified in eukaryotes. The DNA renatures at different times:

- **Almost immediately,** about 10% of mouse DNA containing a thousand to several million copies per cell of almost identical sequences of less than 10 base-pairs renatures. This class is called **highly repetitive DNA**. It is believed that highly repetitive DNA has a role in the alignment of homologous chromosomes during meiosis (the formation of germ cells) or their post-meiotic recombination. The number of such repeats varies from individual to individual.

- **Next to reassociate** is ~20% of the mouse DNA composed of sequences up to several hundred base-pairs which are repeated up to over 1000 times. This class is called **moderately repetitive DNA.**

- **Last to reassociate** are sequences present as a **single copy** per cell and classified as **unique DNA**. Unique DNA sequences may however be repeated a few times and account for ~70% of cellular DNA.

Moderately repetitive DNA sequences are interspersed with massive sections of unique DNA.

After isopycnic gradient centrifugation, highly repetitive DNA is found as a minor band (a satellite) next to the main band of

Electrophoresis is the migration of ions in an electric field. The technique is widely employed for the analytical (and sometimes the preparative) separation of proteins and nucleic acids. Modern electrophoretic techniques utilize a system in which the ions migrate through an **immobilized support**, e.g. cellulose acetate strips, polyacrylamide gel or agarose gel. The support is selected on the basis of its **matrix** through which the ions must pass. Large charged molecules may be entirely retarded by using a support with too small pores.

The sample mixture is applied to the support, the ends of which are in contact with an appropriate buffer solution contained within separate reservoirs. The pH of the buffer is selected to ensure that the components of the sample will be differentially charged. The electrical circuit is completed by placing an electrode into each reservoir. A stable direct electric current is provided by a power-pack located between the electrodes.

When the current is applied, the positive ions of the sample will move towards the negative electrode (cathode) and negative ions will migrate towards the anode. Depending upon the degree of charge per ion at the selected pH, the ions migrate at different rates to form discrete bands. Upon completion of the separation, the bands are usually visualized, e.g. by staining or autoradiography. A variety of electrophoretic and band-locating techniques is available.

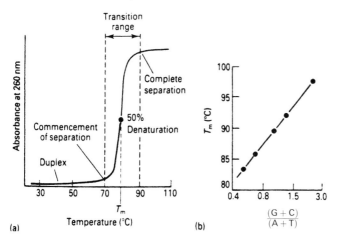

Figure 2.11 *Denaturation of DNA: (a) a melting curve profile of DNA; (b) the relationship between* T_m *and (G + C) content*

In **isopycnic (equilibrium density) gradient centrifugation**, isolated DNA is mixed with a concentrated solution ($>6\,mol\,l^{-1}$) of caesium chloride (CsCl) in a centrifuge tube and subjected to centrifugation at 140,000g for 20 h. During the centrifugation, the gravitational force draws the caesium ions towards the bottom of the tube until an equilibrium is achieved due to the sedimentation of the ions being opposed by their diffusion. The gradient so formed is continuous between the highest CsCl concentration at the bottom of the tube and the lowest concentration at the top of the tube. During gradient formation, individual DNA molecules migrate downwards or upwards in the salt solution until their sedimentation/ buoyancy is counterbalanced by the density of the gradient. Like molecules experience like forces to form a narrow band of molecules across the tube. Heavier DNA will migrate to an equilibrium position lower in the CsCl gradient than lighter DNA.

chromosomal DNA and therefore it is also termed **satellite DNA**. Derived from this term, **minisatellite DNA** is generally used to refer to extragenic adjoining (tandem) repeat units of 9–100 base pairs (b.p.). Short tandem repeat (STR) describes tandem repeats units of 3–5 b.p. The human genome contains over 300,000 STRs, e.g. $(GTG)_5$, $(GATA)_4$. **Microsatellite DNA** has tandem repeats units of 2 b.p. Microsatellites are employed as synthetic genomic probes.

RNA

The function of RNA resides within the entire process of protein synthesis, i.e. from DNA to protein. There are **three major classes of RNA**:

- **Messenger RNA** (mRNA) molecules are produced directly (in prokaryotic cells) or indirectly (in eukaryotic cells) from the nucleotide sequences of the DNA. A mRNA molecule serves as the 'messenger' that directs the sequence of the amino acids during the assembly of a protein molecule on the ribosome.
- **Transfer RNA** (tRNA) molecules carry 'activated' amino acids through the cell cytoplasm to the ribosomes and position the amino acids into the growing polypeptide chain according to the message of the mRNA.
- **Ribosomal RNA** (rRNA) molecules are an integral part of the structure of the ribosome.

RNA is synthesized during transcription by enzymes called **DNA-dependent RNA polymerases** (often abbreviated to RNA polymerases). These enzymes use ribonucleoside triphosphates as substrates and DNA as a template. Transcription involves both protein-coding genes and RNA-specifying genes. The enzyme responsible for transcription in bacteria is one type of DNA-dependent RNA polymerase. However, in eukaryotes, there are three DNA-dependent enzymes:

- **RNA polymerase I** (Pol I) transcribes genes specifying rRNAs;
- **RNA polymerase II** (Pol II) transcribes protein-coding genes and some snRNAs, e.g. U2;
- **RNA polymerase III** (Pol III) transcribes genes specifying tRNAs and some snRNAs, e.g. U6.

In duplex DNA, the strand to which the RNA polymerase binds, and is used as a template, is termed the **antisense strand**. The other strand, which is not copied, is termed the **sense strand** since its nucleotide sequence is the same as the RNA transcript except for their thymine/uracil content. In reading the antisense strand, the RNA polymerase moves along it in a $3' \rightarrow 5'$ direction.

Some **physical characteristics of RNA** isolated from a prokaryote are listed in Table 2.6. Traditionally RNAs are differentiated by

Table 2.6   *RNA molecules in* E. coli

Type	Approximate relative amount (%)	Sedimentation coefficient (S)	Molecular mass (kDa)	Number of nucleotides
Messenger RNA (mRNA)	2	Heterogeneous		
Transfer RNA (tRNA)	16	4	24–31	73–94
Ribosomal RNA (rRNA)	82	23	1200	2904
		16	560	1541
		5	36	120

their **rate of sedimentation** in a centrifugal field (expressed in Svedberg units, denoted as S). Except in certain viruses, RNAs are single-stranded molecules and, in contrast to DNA, exhibit significant variations in the proportions of bases. However, RNA molecules do contain regions of base-pairing induced by hydrogen bonding. As much as 70% of the bases may participate in base-pairing. Denaturation and renaturation of RNA molecules, similar to that of DNA, occur due to their regions of hydrogen bonding. Bases which happen to lie side-by-side but which are not complementary may be looped out to facilitate the pairing of other bases.

Other forms of RNA include:

- **Heterogeneous nuclear RNA** (hnRNA) molecules, commonly called the primary RNA transcripts or pre-mRNA. In eukaryotic cells, mRNA is not produced directly from the DNA. The products of transcription in these cells are hnRNAs which contain transcribed introns and exons. Pre-mRNAs undergo capping, tailing and splicing to generate mature mRNA molecules.

- **Small nuclear RNA** (snRNA) molecules, which are about 60–300 nucleotides in length and contain numerous copies of several highly conserved sequences. They are found only in eukaryotic cells and are involved in the editing of RNA transcripts into mRNA.

- **Guide RNA** (gRNA) molecules, which consist of 60–80 ribonucleotides and have 3'-oligo(U) tails (cf. mRNA below). gRNA molecules were isolated from the mitochondria of trypanosomes (a protozoan) where they function in the editing of mitochondrial RNA transcripts.

Messenger RNA

Although **mRNA** is present only in small amounts, mRNA accounts for the largest number of individual RNA molecules in the cytoplasm of a cell. The process of the transcription of DNA involves base-pairing in which uracil pairs with adenine of the

DNA template. The primary structure of a mRNA molecule is thereby complementary to that of a region of one strand of the DNA molecule. When a particular protein is no longer required by the cell, synthesis of the mRNA is inhibited to conserve materials and the mRNA template is degraded by ribonucleases. Therefore, mRNAs have short intracellular life-spans generally measured in minutes for prokaryotic mRNAs or hours for eukaryotic mRNAs. This accounts for the relatively low amount present in the cell at any given time.

Prokaryotic mRNA may contain the information for the synthesis of several proteins. These mRNAs are called **polycistronic**. The term **cistron** originated in viral genetics and refers to a functional genetic unit of a length of DNA which contains a genetic message for protein synthesis. Polycistronic mRNAs have only been found in prokaryotic cells.

In prokaryotes, alignment of amino acids seldom commences at the 5′-end of the mRNA but at a nucleotide sequence located within the molecule. The frontal untranslated RNA bases constitute the **leader** section (Figure 2.12a). Additional untranslated sequences may be found at the 5′- and 3′-ends. Within polycistronic mRNA, such sequences of 1–400 bases may also be located internally and are termed **spacers or intercistronic regions**.

Eukaryotic mRNA exhibits three distinctive structural features (Figure 2.12b):

- **All are monocistronic.**
- **All have a 5′-cap** consisting of a single residue of **7-methyl-guanosine** linked uniquely through a **5′–5′ triphosphate bridge** to the first nucleotide which is methylated at the 2′-OH position. The cap promotes translation by increasing mRNA binding to the 40S ribosomal subunit and by binding the initiation factors involved in protein synthesis.

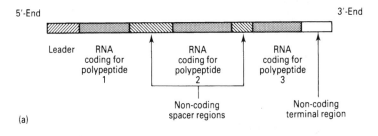

(a)

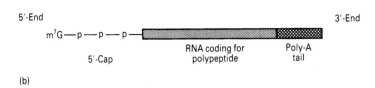

Figure 2.12 *Comparative structures of messenger RNA: (a) polycistronic prokaryotic RNA transcript; (b) monocistronic eukaryotic mRNA*

(b)

- **Most RNAs have a poly (A) tail** of 100–200 consecutive adenine residues at the 3′-end. It is believed that the poly (A) tail is important in transporting mRNA from the nucleus to the cytoplasm. Poly (A) tails are not essential for translation since they are absent in several translatable mRNAs, e.g. histone mRNA.

The 5′-cap and the poly (A) tail are added by specific enzymes as **post-transcriptional modifications** to pre-mRNA molecules but not to rRNA or tRNA.

Transfer RNA

Transfer RNAs are the smallest RNA molecules. Their biological roles are the delivery and positioning of amino acids in the correct order in the growing polypeptide chain according to the mRNA template. Each amino acid has at least one specific tRNA molecule: leucine, arginine and serine have the maximum of six different tRNAs. In 1965, the first primary sequence of a tRNA, that of yeast alanine tRNA, was attained. Since certain regions of the sequence would be complementary if the chain was folded in a particular manner, the structure was presented as the two-dimensional cloverleaf diagram (Figure 2.13a). In actuality, the three-dimensional structure determined by X-ray crystallography resembles an inverted letter L (Figure 2.13b).

All tRNA molecules demonstrate similar structural features:

- **tRNAs contain a number of minor bases,** e.g. inosine, pseudo-uridine, in addition to the major bases. Pseudo-uridine is the most abundant modified nucleoside in RNA. In addition to its occurrence in tRNA where it was first discovered, it is also found in rRNA and in several snRNAs;
- **at the 5′-end,** a guanosine or cytidine residue is located;
- **at the 3′-end,** tRNAs contain the trinucleotide sequence CCA. Attachment of the amino acid for which the tRNA is specific occurs through esterification involving the 3′-OH group;
- **tRNAs exhibit regions of base-pairing.** Non-hydrogen-bonded areas create four loops, i.e. loop I (containing 5,6-dihydrouridine), loop II (the anticodon loop), loop III (the variable loop) and loop IV (containing ribosylthymine).

Variability in tRNA size (Table 2.6) results from differences in the numbers of nucleotides contained within loop I and/or loop III. Amino acids are correctly positoned by base-pairing between nucleotide triplets on the mRNA, called **codons**, and a defined nucleotide triplet on the tRNA, called an **anticodon**, contained within loop II.

In numerous cases, the first two bases seem to determine the amino acid to be included. Using scale models of various

Affinity chromatography may be employed in the **preparation of mRNA**. This method exploits the poly (A) sequence at the 3′-end of most eukaryotic mRNAs to isolate mRNA from other cytoplasmic components. The poly (A) tail will hybridize with a poly (U) sequence through hydrogen bonding.

A **chromatographic column** is packed with **agarose beads** (or cellulose) to which a poly (U) nucleotide sequence is covalently attached. The poly (A) tails of mRNAs in a cytoplasmic preparation specifically bind to the complementary poly (U) sequences in conditions of high salt concentration and low temperature and the mRNAs are retained on the column. Non-interactive mixture components do not bind to the beads and pass directly through the column. By reducing the salt concentration and raising the temperature, the hydrogen bonding between the heterocyclic bases is weakened and mRNAs will be released from the agarose bead attachment.

Affinity chromatography may be adapted to isolate a particular mRNA by the attachment of a DNA strand which is complementary to the desired mRNA base sequence. Other cytoplasmic mRNAs will pass through the column leaving the mRNA of interest attached to the bead for subsequent release from the DNA–RNA hybrid.

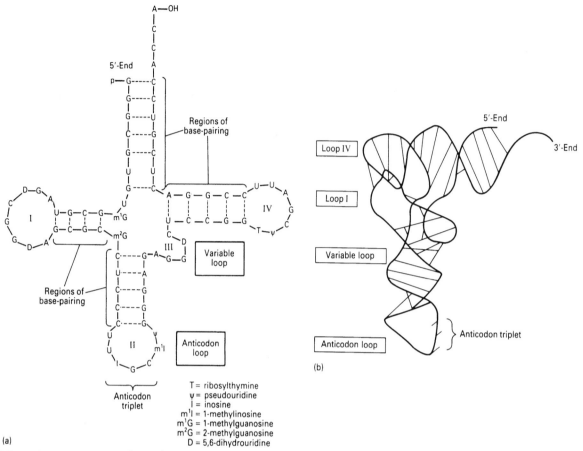

Figure 2.13 *Structure of transfer RNA: (a) the cloverleaf diagram of yeast alanine tRNA; (b) the three-dimensional conformation of yeast phenylalanine tRNA*

base-pairing arrangements, it was demonstrated that **non-Watson–Crick base-pairing** is permissible in the 3′-position of the codon since steric constraints inherent within the DNA duplex do not apply. The phenomenon is called **wobble**. The base inosine (I) frequently found in the 5′-position of the anticodon may pair with A or C or U. Also, G may pair with U. Because of its hydrogen-bonding permutations, inosine maximizes the number of codons with which the particular tRNA can bind. Wobble therefore reduces the number of specific tRNA molecules needed by the cell.

The genetic code

The information contained in the base sequence of the mRNA template is interpreted in sequences of three bases; **each codon represents one amino acid.** Therefore, the unit of information is the codon. Since there are four major bases in mRNA, 64 (i.e. 4^3) different codons are possible. The 64 triplets constitute **the genetic code** (Table 2.7).

Table 2.7 *The genetic code in prokaryotic cells*

Amino acid	mRNA codon*
Alanine	GCU, GCC, GCA, GCG
Arginine	CGU, CGC, CGA, CGG, AGA, AGG
Asparagine	AAU, AAC
Aspartic acid	GAU, GAC
Cysteine	UGU, UGC
Glutamic acid	GAA, GAG
Glutamine	CAA, CAG
Glycine	GGU, GGC, GGA, GGG
Histidine	CAU, CAC
Isoleucine	AUU, AUC, AUA
Leucine	CUU, CUC, CUA, CUG, UUA, UUG
Lysine	AAA, AAG
Methionine	AUG
Phenylalanine	UUU, UUC
Proline	CCU, CCC, CCA, CCG
Serine	UCU, UCC, UCA, UCG, AGU, AGC
Threonine	ACU, ACC, ACA, ACG
Tryptophan	UGG
Tyrosine	UAU, UAC
Valine	GUU, GUC, GUA, GUG
Start	AUG, GUG†
Stop	UAA, UAG, UGA

* The mRNA is read from the 5′-end which is indicated by the first letter. The third letter is the 3′-end of the codon.
† The use of GUG in initiation is very rare.

All codons have been assigned to **amino acids or punctuation signals**. Three triplets, i.e. UAA, UAG and UGA, are not complemented by anticodons on tRNAs and serve as **stop signals**, i.e. to signal that the polypeptide chain has been completed. Of the other 61 triplets which have complementary tRNAs, AUG and GUG, the codons for methionine and valine respectively, have additional roles as **start signals** in the initiation of protein synthesis. Since there are only 20 amino acids which occur in proteins, most amino acids are specified by more than one codon, i.e. the code is degenerate. The genetic code applies to prokaryotes and eukaryotic nuclear mRNAs but not to mitochondrial mRNAs. Therefore, the genetic code is quasi-universal!

Ribosomal RNA

Ribosomal RNA is the most abundant of the RNAs in the cell (Table 2.6). In prokaryotic cells, there are three species of rRNA each of which is present within each 25 nm long 70S ribosome. Ribosomes consist of two subunits, designated **large** and **small** (Figure 2.14).

Huntington's disease is a dominantly heritable disorder of the central nervous system and is characterized by progressive irregular involuntary movements of the extremities and the face, disturbed speech and dementia. In common with a number of hereditary neurodegenerative diseases which also involve progressive and fatal loss of specific neurones, the gene which renders the patient susceptible to the condition, on transcription produces a mRNA containing repetitions of the codon CAG. This results in an encoded protein with abnormally long stretches of residues of the amino acid, glutamine.

The polyglutamine expansion in the protein does not render the protein non-functional but harmful. The normal protein is called **huntingtin**. The more glutamine repeats the more strongly the protein binds to **huntingtin-associated protein-1** (HAP-1). Apart from the above, the role of HAP-1 in Huntington's disease remains unclear.

In *Escherichia coli*, the **large subunit** (50S, 1.6×10^6 Da) consists of 34 proteins (designated L1–L34) ranging in molecular mass from 5.4 kDa to 29.4 kDa and one molecule each of 23S and 5S rRNA. The proteins occur singly except for four molecules of L7 and L12. Ten methylated bases and three **pseudo-uridine** residues are found in 23S rRNA but 5S rRNA, located on the central protuberance, lacks minor bases. The **small subunit** (30S, 9×10^5 Da) consists of 21 proteins (designated S1–S21) ranging in molecular mass from 8.3 kDa to 61.2 kDa and a single molecule of 16S rRNA which contains nine methylated bases. The secondary structures of 16S and 23S rRNA have been elucidated (Figure 2.15). The flexibility of the polynucleotide chain creates the potential for a large amount of intrastrand sequence complementarity leading to areas of hydrogen bonding. Palindromic sequences may give rise to tight folding of the rRNA structure to create structures called **hairpins**. Almost half of the bases in 16S rRNA are base-paired with non-Watson–Crick base-pairings featuring, e.g. G–U, G–A, A–C pairs. In prokaryotic ribosomes, about two-thirds of their weight is due to their rRNA content.

In **eukaryotic cells**, the ribosomal architecture is similar but a fourth rRNA (5.8S) and a larger number of proteins have been identified. Eukaryotic ribosomes, e.g. from rat liver cytosol, are larger (80S):

- The **large subunit** (60S, 2.8×10^6 Da) consists of 49 proteins and three rRNA molecules, i.e. 5S (120 nucleotides), 5.8S (160 nucleotides) and 28S (4718 nucleotides) rRNA.
- The **small subunit** (40S, 1.3×10^6 Da) consists of 33 proteins and 18S rRNA (1874 nucleotides).

In eukaryotic ribosomes, about 60% of their weight is due to rRNA.

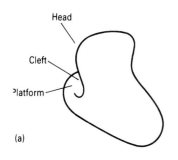
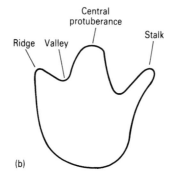
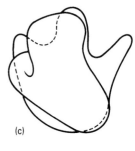

Figure 2.14   *The 70S ribosome of* Escherichia coli: *(a) the small (30S) subunit; (b) the large (50S) subunit; (c) the intact ribosome. (Reproduced with permission from the* Annual Review of Biochemistry, *Vol. 54, © 1985 by Annual Reviews Inc.)*

RNA sequencing

RNA may be rapidly sequenced by essentially the same methods employed in DNA sequencing. Firstly, the RNA chain is converted into a complementary strand of DNA (cDNA) by the enzyme **reverse transcriptase**. The resultant cDNA may then be sequenced by the **dideoxy sequencing method** (or the chemical cleavage method).

Suggested further reading

Dickerson, R.E. (1992). DNA structures from A to Z. *Methods in Enzymology* **211**, 67–111.

Jordan, E. and Collins, F.S. (1996): A march of genetic maps. *Nature* **380**, 111–112.

Wahl, M.C. and Sundaralingam, M. (1997). C–H···O hydrogen bonding in biology. *Trends in Biochemical Sciences* **22**, 97–102.

Watson, J.D. and Crick, F. (1953). Molecular structure of nucleic acids. *Nature* **171**, 737–738.

Watson, J.D. and Crick, F. (1953). Genetic implications of the structure of deoxyribonucleic acid. *Nature* **171**, 964–967.

Bishop, M.J. and Rawlings, C.J. (1996). *DNA and Protein Sequence Analysis: A Practical Approach*. Oxford: IRL Press.

Lewin, B. (1997). *Genes VI*. Oxford: Oxford University Press.

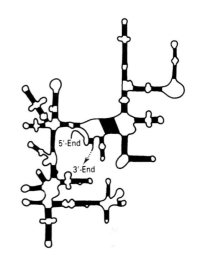

Figure 2.15 *A section of the secondary structure of 16S rRNA.* ▬▬, *Regions of hydrogen bonding (hairpins);* ▭, *regions of non-complementary bases*

Self-assessment questions

1. How does the conformation of the glycosidic bond of nucleotides affect the structure of DNA?
2. Which forms of RNA are found in eukaryotic cells but not in prokaryotic cells?
3. What forces stabilize the DNA duplex structure?
4. What will be the sequence of the resultant oligopeptide when a mRNA of sequence AUGGAAGAUAAAGCUUAC is translated?
5. You wish to make the newly synthesized DNA, but not the RNA, in actively dividing cells to fluoresce. Which nucleoside in the culture medium should you tag with a fluorescent label?
6. A double-stranded DNA molecule is 50% heat-denatured at 87°C. What is its base composition in mole per cent?
7. The oligodeoxynucleotide chain dGCATCAACG was subjected to sequencing by the chain termination method. Draw a diagram of the banding pattern you would expect to obtain from gel electrophoresis.
8. On base analysis, a viral DNA is found to have the following base composition in mole per cent: A = 40; G = 15; C = 20; T = 25. What do you conclude about the structure of this DNA?

9. When double-stranded DNA denatures, why is there an increase in the absorbance of UV light?
10. How would you prepare a sample of gRNA?

Key Concepts and Facts

Nucleotides
- Nucleotides are composed of a heterocyclic base, a pentose sugar and a phosphate group.
- Ribonucleotides and deoxyribonucleotides are the building blocks of RNA and DNA respectively.

Polynucleotide Chains
- Polynucleotide chains have a pentose–phosphate backbone with $3',5'$-phosphodiester internucleotide linkages.
- Single polynucleotide chains are flexible structures due to the rotation of phosphorus–oxygen bonds.
- Polynucleotide chains have a $5'$-end and a $3'$-end.

DNA
- DNA is the storage molecule for genetic material.
- In most organisms, DNA constitutes the genome.
- Deoxyribonucleic acid contains the pyrimidine base, thymine.
- DNA replicates through a semiconservative mechanism.
- DNA may be sequenced by the dideoxy method.
- The deoxynucleotide sequence of genes determines the amino acid sequence of proteins.

RNA
- RNA functions in the transfer of genetic information from the nucleus to the ribosome.
- Ribonucleic acid contains the pyrimidine base, uracil, and minor heterocyclic bases.
- There are three major forms of RNA: mRNA, tRNA and rRNA.
- RNA is produced by the transcription of DNA.
- Proteins are produced by ribosomal translation of mRNA.
- The anticodons of tRNAs are complementary to the codons of mRNAs.
- The genetic code is degenerate and quasi-universal.
- Ribosomes are composed of rRNA and protein molecules.

Answers to questions (Chapter 2)

1. The *anti*-conformation of the bond is found in B-DNA and most other DNAs whilst the *syn*-conformation occurs only in Z-DNA.
2. hnRNA, snRNA and gRNA.
3. Hydrogen bonding and hydrophobic interactions between stacked heterocyclic bases.
4. Glutamylaspartyllysylalanyltyrosine. AUG = start.
5. Thymidine (dT) will be incorporated only into DNA.
6. Refer to Figure 2.12. $(G+C)/(A+T) = 0.8$ ∴ $(G+C) = 0.8/1.8 = 0.44$. The base composition is approximately $G = C = 22\%$ and $A = T = 33\%$.
7. The Sanger dideoxy method is sometimes called the chain termination method as opposed to the Maxam–Gilbert chemical cleavage method. The pattern follows:

C   G   T   A

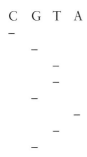

Note: Template is GCATCAACG. Pattern reads from the bottom: CGTAGTTGC.
8. It is single-stranded because the A/T and G/C ratios do not equal 1.
9. During denaturation, there is a loss of base stacking and therefore loss of interactions between the planar bases.
10. By affinity chromatography of the mitochondrial preparation employing agarose beads with covalently attached poly (A) sequences.

Chapter 3
Proteins

Learning objectives

After studying this chapter you should confidently be able to:

State various functions of proteins.

Describe the general properties and classification of the amino acids found in proteins.

Discuss the nature of the interactions which occur in proteins.

Describe the reasons for, and the strategies applied to, protein sequencing.

Discuss the salient features of the fundamental protein structures described as secondary structure.

Discuss the structure of fibrillar collagens.

Describe the motifs and conformations which constitute tertiary structure.

Discuss the key features of the oxygen-transporting proteins, myoglobin and haemoglobin.

Describe the major structural features of antibody molecules.

Proteins are the most abundant macromolecules found within cells. A protein may be considered as a unique polymer of amino acids (Chapter 1). The different constituent amino acids determine the overall chemical and structural properties of a protein. There are over 300 catalogued amino acids but only 20 (plus a few derivatives) occur in proteins. Some proteins may contain derivatives of common amino acids, e.g. collagen contains 5-hydroxylysine and hydroxyprolines. Such derivatives are produced in reactions located in the endoplasmic reticulum during or subsequent to ribosomal protein synthesis. These reactions are termed **co- or post-translational modifications** (Chapter 13).

Proteins perform a wide variety of functions. They serve as:

- **Biochemical catalysts** called **enzymes**, e.g. hexokinase catalyses the phosphorylation of (addition of a phosphate group to) glucose (Chapter 9).

- **Structural components**, e.g. **microtubules** of the cytoskeleton (Chapter 7) are cylinders composed of two forms of the protein **tubulin**. The protective coats of viruses are proteins. Structural proteins are insoluble in water.

- **Transport proteins** which bind and carry specific molecules or ions from one organ to another, e.g. **haemoglobin** carries oxygen from the lungs to the peripheral tissues where it is employed intracellularly in oxidative processes. Other transport proteins may function in the transport of substances across cell membranes.

- **Hormones.** Hormones are substances which act as **chemical messengers** between cells in different parts of the body with the result that the activity of the recipient cell is modified. Some hormones are proteins, e.g. **insulin** is composed of an A-chain of 21 amino acid residues linked by two disulphide bridges to a B-chain of 30 amino acid residues. Other proteins act as hormone receptor molecules.

- **Antibodies. Immunoglobulins** are a family of proteins which have the biological role of affording protection to higher animals against invading bacteria or extracellular viruses and foreign proteins.

- **Regulatory proteins. Repressor proteins** regulate the expression of genes contained within the chromosomes.

This chapter considers in detail the nature and properties of amino acids and their polymerization into polypeptide chains. The various conformations found at the different levels of structure exhibited by native proteins will be discussed with reference to named examples.

Amino acids

Amino acids are the **building blocks** of proteins. Some amino acids which do not occur in proteins may function in cellular metabolism, e.g. citrulline and ornithine (Chapter 13).

Amino acids in proteins

Proline, an imino acid, is usually included along with the amino acids because of its occurence in proteins. The **amino acids found in proteins** may be referred to by the use of one-letter or three-letter codes (Table 3.1) and exhibit the following general properties:

- All are **α-amino acids** of the L-series (Chapter 1). D-amino acids occur alongside L-amino acids in some peptide antibiotics, e.g.

The Dutch chemist, **Gerardus Mulder**, is accredited with the adoption of the word **protein**, in 1838. Mulder had been studying the properties of a substance from milk and eggs which coagulated upon heating. This substance was common to animal tissues and plant juices. Mulder considered the substance to be of primary importance to all living organisms. The name protein (Greek *proteios* = of first quality) was actually suggested to him by the Swedish chemist, Baron Jöns Jakob Berzelius, who had earlier discovered the elements selenium (1817), silicon (1824) and thorium (1828).

The **first amino acid** to be discovered was asparagine from asparagus tissue in 1806. The first amino acid to be identified from protein was leucine by Proust in 1819. Cystine (two cysteine molecules linked by a disulphide bond) was extracted from urinary calculi in 1810 but it was not obtained from protein until 1899. The last amino acid to be discovered in protein was threonine in 1936. However, the proline derivative, 3-hydroxy-proline, present in collagen was not identified until 1962.

The naming of amino acids has not been systematic. Glycine was thus named because it tastes sweet (Greek *glycos* = sweet). Tyrosine was first isolated from cheese (Greek *tyros* = cheese) and glutamic acid was found in wheat gluten.

Table 3.1 *The R groups of the amino acids found in proteins*

Aliphatic	Hydroxy	Acidic, neutral amides	Basic	Sulphur	Aromatic	Imino
Glycine (Gly, G) H–	Serine (Ser, S) HO–CH₂–	Aspartic acid (Asp, D) $HO-\underset{\parallel O}{C}-CH_2-$	Arginine (Arg, R) $H_2N-\underset{\parallel NH}{C}-NH-CH_2-CH_2-CH_2-$	Cysteine (CySH, C) HS–CH₂–	Phenylalanine (Phe, F) (benzene ring) –CH₂–	Proline (Pro, P) (pyrrolidine ring) CH–COOH
Alanine (Ala, A) CH₃–	Threonine (Thr, T) $CH_3-\underset{\mid OH}{CH}-$	Asparagine (Asn, N) $H_2N-\underset{\parallel O}{C}-CH_2-$	Histidine (His, H) (imidazole ring) $CH=C-CH_2-$	Methionine (Met, M) CH₃–S–CH₂–CH₂–	Tryptophan (Trp, W) (indole ring) $C-CH_2-$	
Valine (Val, V) $CH_3-\underset{\mid CH_3}{CH}-$	Tyrosine (Tyr, Y) HO–(benzene ring)–CH₂–	Glutamic acid (Glu, E) $HO-\underset{\parallel O}{C}-CH_2-CH_2-$	Lysine (Lys, K) H₂N–CH₂–CH₂–CH₂–CH₂–CH₂–			
Leucine (Leu, L) $CH_3-CH-CH_2-$ $\quad\;\; \mid$ $\quad\; CH_3$		Glutamine (Gln, Q) $H_2N-\underset{\parallel O}{C}-CH_2-CH_2-$				
Isoleucine (Ile, I) $CH_3-CH_2-\underset{\mid CH_3}{CH}-$						

valinomycin and actinomycin D, and in the peptidoglycan of the bacterial cell wall (Figure 5.9b).

- **All** (except proline) **conform to a general formula** (Figure 3.1) in which an amino group and a carboxylic acid group are attached to the α-carbon (C^α) atom.
- **The R group,** also called the side chain (Table 3.1), determines the properties of individual amino acids. Many proteins lack some amino acids.
- **All** (except glycine) **contain a chiral α-carbon atom** (Chapter 1). These amino acids exhibit optical activity, e.g. alanine is dextrorotatory, phenylalanine is laevorotatory.

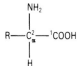

Figure 3.1 *General formula of L-α-amino acids (nature of R groups given in Table 3.1)*

Tyrosine, tryptophan and phenylalanine absorb light in the ultraviolet region because of the conjugated double-bond system of their aromatic rings. The absorption coefficient of tryptophan and tyrosine at a wavelength of 280 nm is large enough to allow the exploitation of this property in their estimation either in free form or as residues in polypeptide chains.

The **amino acids** may be **classified** into four main classes according to the tendency of their R groups to interact with water at pH 7.0 (Table 3.2):

- **Non-polar amino acids** do not interact with or bind water and are called **hydrophobic** (water-hating).
- **Neutral amino acids.** Their uncharged polar R groups may bind water through hydrogen-bond formation (Chapter 1) and are **hydrophilic** (water-loving) amino acids.
- **Acidic amino acids** are hydrophilic and have polar R groups which, at pH 7.0, carry a negative charge. Asparagine and glutamine are considered as amide derivatives of aspartic acid and glutamic acid respectively.

Table 3.2 *Classification of amino acids according to R group properties at pH 7.0*

R groups of amino acids			
Non-polar (hydrophobic)	*Polar (hydrophilic)*		
	Uncharged	*Acidic*	*Basic*
Alanine	Asparagine	Aspartic acid	Arginine
Cysteine	Glutamine	Glutamic acid	Histidine
Isoleucine	Glycine		Lysine
Leucine	Serine		
Methionine	Threonine		
Proline	Tyrosine		
Phenylalanine	Tryptophan		
Valine			

- **Basic amino acids** are hydrophilic amino acids, the R groups of which may accept protons to become positively charged.

Ionic properties of amino acids

The ionization characteristics of the amino acids in aqueous media are denoted by their pK_a values (Table 3.3). Observe the similarity in values for pK_{a1} of the α-carboxyl group and the pK_a of the α-amino group of different amino acids. Amino acids respond to changes in their aqueous environment in accordance with the **acid–base principles** (Chapter 1). In aqueous solutions at pH 1, the amino acid is fully protonated. Titration of this amino acid by the addition of one equivalent of equimolar base will release a proton from the carboxylic acid group. The addition of a second equivalent of equimolar base deprotonates the amino group. For example, alanine at low pH is fully protonated and carries a net charge of $+1$. Increasing the pH by the addition of one equivalent of base results in the complete ionization of the carboxyl group and the entire molecule exhibits no net charge. The addition of a second equivalent of base causes the removal of the proton from the NH_3^+

Table 3.3   *The pK values of groups occurring in the common amino acids*

Amino acid	pK_{a1} α-COOH	pK_{a2} R-COOH	α-NH$_2$	Other R	pK_{a3} α-NH$_2$	R-NH$_2$	Other R
Glycine	2.34	—	9.60	—	—	—	—
Alanine	2.34	—	9.69	—	—	—	—
Valine	2.32	—	9.62	—	—	—	—
Leucine	2.36	—	9.60	—	—	—	—
Isoleucine	2.36	—	9.60	—	—	—	—
Serine	2.21	—	9.15	—	—	—	—
Threonine	2.09	—	9.10	—	—	—	—
Tyrosine	2.20	—	9.11	—	—	—	10.07
Aspartic acid	1.88	3.65	—	—	9.60	—	—
Asparagine	2.02	—	8.80	—	—	—	—
Glutamic acid	2.19	4.25	—	—	9.67	—	—
Glutamine	2.17	—	9.13	—	—	—	—
Arginine	2.17	—	9.04	—	—	12.48	—
Histidine	1.82	—	—	6.00	9.17	—	—
Lysine	2.18	—	8.95	—	—	10.53	—
Cysteine	1.96	—	—	8.18	10.28	—	—
Methionine	2.28	—	9.21	—	—	—	—
Phenylalanine	1.83	—	9.13	—	—	—	—
Tryptophan	2.83	—	9.39	—	—	—	—
Proline	1.99	—	10.60	—	—	—	—

group of alanine which now has a net charge of -1. Thus the amino acids display amphoteric behaviour, i.e. they are capable of acting as an acid or base. The parameters pK_{a1} and pK_{a2} can be determined at the appropriate half-equivalence point.

With **neutral and monoamino-dicarboxylic acids** at the first equivalence point, the positive charge balances the negative charge. The molecules are therefore in their dipolar ionic state and are called **zwitterions** (German for hybrid ion). Since their net charge is 0, the zwitterions cannot migrate in an electric field, e.g. during the technique of electrophoresis (Chapter 2). This pH at which a molecule exhibits no net charge is termed its **isoelectric point (pI)**.

The **titrations of amino acids with dissociable R groups** conform to the same principles but require three equivalents of bases. The pI of any amino acid can be calculated according to the following formulae:

- **amino acids** other than basic amino acids: $pI = 0.5(pK_{a1} + pK_{a2})$;
- **basic amino acids**: $pI = 0.5(pK_{a2} + pK_{a3})$.

Protein structure

Chemical bonding between two amino acids is responsible for:

- **the construction of a polypeptide chain** (Chapter 1);
- **the conformation adopted by the polypeptide chain.**

The linear sequence of amino acids linked by **peptide bonds** along a polypeptide chain is the **first level** of the structural organization of proteins and is referred to as the **primary structure**. Hydrogen bonds involving peptide bond atoms, although individually weak, are responsible for the fundamental ordered shapes of the **second level** of protein structure described as **secondary structure**. Hydrogen bonds between R-group atoms along with **van der Waals' forces, ionic bonds, hydrophobic interactions** and **disulphide bonds** within a polypeptide chain, i.e. intra-molecular bonds, contribute to the stability of the protein structure at the **third level** described as **tertiary structure**. The types of bonds which maintain the tertiary structures of proteins are also responsible for the spatial arrangement of protein subunits through inter-molecular bonding. This is the **fourth level** of protein structure, found only in oligomeric proteins, described as **quaternary structure**.

Bonding in proteins

The peptide bond is formed when two amino acids link together by a **condensation reaction** in which one amino acid donates its carbonyl group and the other contributes an amino group. One end of the **dipeptide** exhibits a free amino group and is called the

---

Ion exchange chromatography is commonly conducted using **chromatographic columns** or **cartridges** although thin-layer plate systems have been developed. Ion-exchange chromatography separates molecules on the basis of their **net charge**. Positively or negatively charged functional groups, e.g. diethylaminoethyl, sulphonate or carboxylate groups, are covalently bonded to a porous **solid matrix**, e.g. acrylic, agarose, silica or styrene divinylbenzene, to yield a **cation or anion exchanger**. When a solution containing charged molecules is applied to a column of an exchanger of the opposite charge, known as the **stationary phase**, the charged molecules bind through ionic interactions to the charged groups of the exchanger. Neutral or similarly charged molecules pass through the column unhindered in the solvent, known as the **mobile phase**. The binding of the charged molecules is reversible and bound molecules are usually eluted by a buffer composed of an increased salt concentration and/or different pH which progressively weakens the ionic bonding.

Different ion exchangers are available to suit different requirements. Selection of the appropriate ion exchanger depends upon the properties of the molecules of interest. With amphoteric molecules, the separation strategy is based upon the pl and molecular stability at various pH values. At pHs greater than its pl, the desired molecule will be negatively charged; at pHs below its pl, the molecule will be positively charged. So if the molecule is stable above its pl value, an anion exchanger is used or, conversely, if it is stable below its pl value, a cation exchanger is employed.

Ion-exchange chromatography is used in a variety of separations and purifications of biological molecules, e.g. proteins, peptides, amino acids, nucleotides and iso-enzymes. It is also used in the deionization of water or solutions of non-ionic substances, and for ultrapurification of buffers and ionic reagents etc.

N-terminus. The other end displays a free carboxyl group and is called the **C-terminus.**

The **geometry of the peptide bond** (Figure 3.2a) is important. The C–N bond length in the peptide bond is shorter than the 0.145 nm recorded for a single covalent C–N bond. This is a result of the propensity of the oxygen atom to withdraw electrons. The electrons associated with the C–N bond and the C=O group resonate between two structures (Figure 3.2b) to create a **partial double bond character** (about 40%) for the C–N single bond and an equal **partial single bond character** for the C=O double bond. As a result of resonance stabilization, the rotation of the C–N single bond is restricted so that six atoms are rigidly positioned in the same plane, i.e. they are **coplanar.** The bond usually has a *trans* configuration (Figure 3.2c). Because proteins are composed of only L-amino acids, the R groups on each of the C$^\alpha$ atoms are arranged on opposite

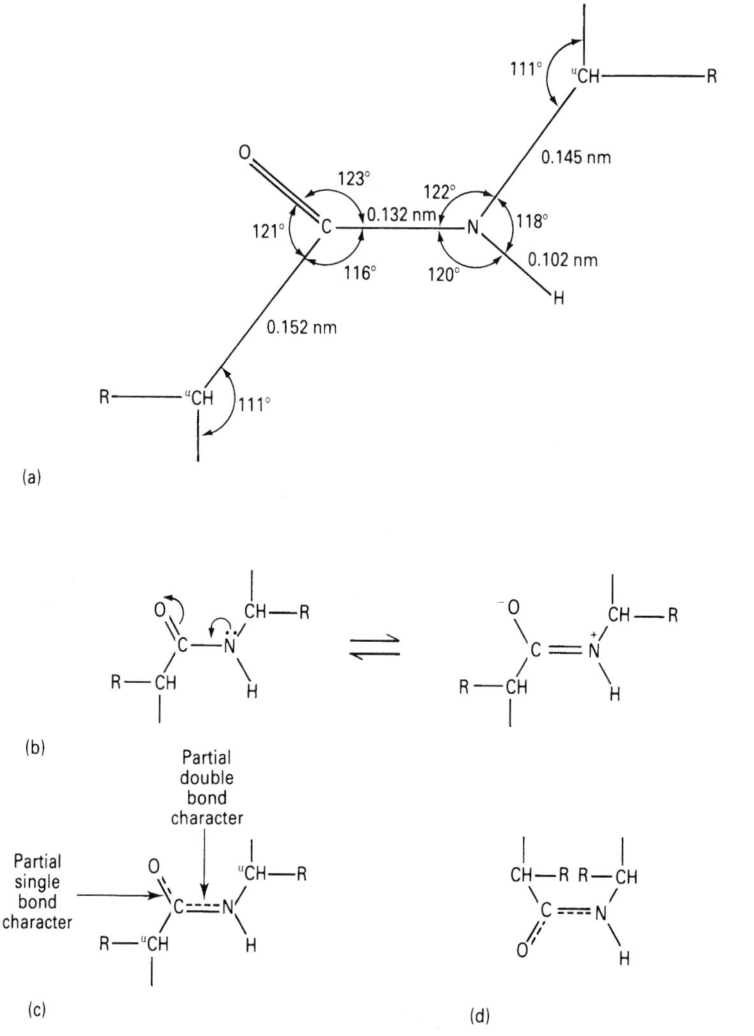

(a)

(b)

(c)

(d)

Figure 3.2 *Architecture of the peptide bond: (a) geometry; (b) resonance structures; (c)* trans *configuration; (d)* cis *configuration*

sides of the framework. This arrangement minimizes steric interaction of the bulky R groups in comparison with a *cis* configuration (Figure 3.2d). However, in peptide bonds involving the amide nitrogen of proline the *cis* configuration creates only slightly more steric hindrance than the *trans* configuration with the result that about 10% of prolyl residues in proteins appear to be in the *cis* configuration.

Since the imino group (N–H) of the peptide bond has no significant tendency to protonate at physiological pH, **the ionic properties of a protein** are the result of:

- R group ionizations;
- ionizations of the *N*-terminal amino group;
- ionizations of the *C*-terminal carboxyl groups.

Although the peptide bond cannot rotate freely, the C^α atom serves as a pivot on which the coplanar groups may rotate (Figure 3.3).

Hydrogen bonding in proteins may occur between groups associated with different peptide bonds (Figure 3.4a) or between appropriate R groups. The nitrogen atom tends to draw the electron away from its hydrogen atom so that the hydrogen atom has a slight positive charge (δ^+). The oxygen atom has a tendency to attract electrons from the carbon atom so that the oxygen atom is slightly electronegative (δ^-). Hydrogen bonding results from **electron sharing** between the oxygen and hydrogen atoms which produces a further redistribution of the electronic arrangement within the C=O and N–H groups thereby enhancing the attraction (Figure 3.4b). In addition, the electron-withdrawing properties of oxygen and nitrogen may render a hydrogen electropositive (δ^+) so that it may interact with an appositely positioned δ^- oxygen or nitrogen atom on another R group. Examples of participating groups include the hydroxyl groups of serine, threonine and tyrosine, the amino hydrogens and carbonyl oxygens of asparagine and glutamine and the heterocyclic nitrogens of histidine.

Van der Waals' forces are inter-molecular forces caused by the influence of neighbouring molecules upon each other. The **electron clouds** surrounding the atoms of a molecule are constantly redistributing their electronic charge densities. These fluctuations induce an electric dipole in the atoms of a neighbouring molecule so that when two uncharged atoms approach each other, the variations in the positions of electrons around one nucleus may create a transient, opposite dipole in the neighbouring atom. The two dipoles are weakly attracted to each other and consequently bring the nuclei closer. As they move closer, the electron clouds begin to overlap causing repulsion of each other and they ultimately take up an intermediate position where the attractive forces balance the repulsive forces. Such forces operate over very short distances.

Ionic bonds, also called salt bonds or salt bridges, result from the

Gel filtration chromatography, also called size-exclusion chromatography, separates molecules on the basis of their **size**. The stationary phase is a gel of porous spherical beads, e.g. agarose, dextran or polyacrylamide. The beads are manufactured to contain pores of a particular size range. Separation happens when molecules of different sizes contained within the mobile phase are passed through a column or cartridge containing such a gel. Small molecules diffuse into the gel pores and therefore are included, with the consequence that their passage through the column is retarded. Large molecules do not enter the pores (i.e. are excluded) and rapidly pass through the column in the mobile phase. Consequently, molecules of varying molecular weights can be separated within the gel matrix as they pass through the column and are eluted from the column in order of decreasing molecular size. The desired molecules should therefore fall within the fractionation range of the gel. Resolution depends upon particle size, pore size, flow rate, column length and diameter, and sample volume.

Applications of the technique include fractionation of proteins and polysaccharides, determination of the molecular weights of proteins, and purification of nucleic acids and plasmids.

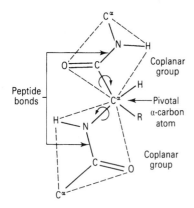

Figure 3.3 *Rotation around C^α–C and C^α–N bonds*

opposite charges on the R groups of certain amino acids. At physiological pH, the R groups of aspartate and glutamate carry a negative charge due to deprotonation but the R groups of arginine and lysine are protonated and bear a positive charge. Oppositely charged amino acids may attract each other to bring regions of the polypeptide chain(s) into adjacency with attendant stability (Figure 3.4c).

Hydrophobic interactions occur when the R groups of non-polar amino acid residues (Table 3.2), which do not permit hydrogen bonding with water, weakly associate by their mutual hydrophobic properties to provide a sanctuary from an aqueous environment (Figure 3.4d). Hydrophobic interactions mainly involve the aliphatic and aromatic amino acids. The hydrophobic effect is the major force driving the folding of proteins.

Disulphide bonds, or bridges, are covalent bonds and are the strongest of the fundamental bonds which contribute to the conformation of the protein. The R group of cysteine terminates in a free sulphydryl group. Pertinently positioned cysteinyl residues of proteins may dimerize on enzymic oxidation to form a disulphide bond (Figure 3.4e).

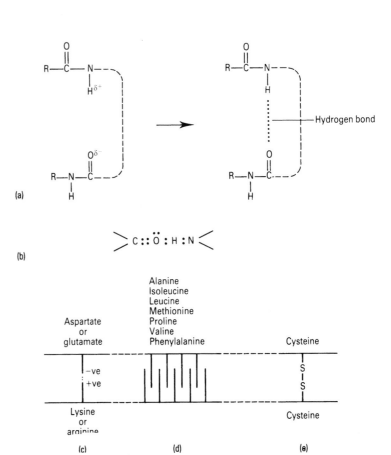

Figure 3.4 *Some bonds occurring in proteins: (a) hydrogen bonding in proteins involving peptide bonds; (b) electron distribution in hydrogen bonding; (c) ionic bonds; (d) hydrophobic interactions; (e) disulphide bonds*

Glycoproteins

Glycoproteins are proteins to which one or more monosaccharide or oligosaccharide groups are attached. Two classes of oligosaccharides are found in glycoproteins:

- **N-linked oligosaccharides** in which the attachment is through the amide group of asparagine.
- **O-linked oligosaccharides** in which the attachment is through the hydroxyl group of amino acids such as serine, threonine and hydroxylysine.

The potential for oligosaccharide diversity is large but the biosynthesis of N-linked oligosaccharides is relatively simple, involving a structured set of consecutive enzymic reactions which in effect minimize the range of oligosaccharides found in glycoproteins.

Denaturation and renaturation

Denaturation is the destruction of the molecular conformation of the native protein and results in the loss of its biological activity. A number of physical agents, e.g. heat and ultraviolet radiation, disrupt hydrogen bonds and ionic bonds because of increased molecular vibration. These bonds may also be affected by chemical agents, e.g. ionic reagents. The **slow removal** of some denaturing agents, e.g. removal of $8\,mol\,l^{-1}$ urea by dialysis, may enable the protein to recover its biological conformation and function. This process is termed **renaturation**.

Primary structure

The **determination of the amino acid sequence** of a protein is important for a number of reasons which include:

- **Understanding** of the way(s) in which a protein achieves its **biological function**.
- **Understanding of the effects of mutations.** Mutations, resulting in either single or multiple amino acid substitutions or deletions, may change the properties of the protein. Altered protein functioning may have serious consequences on the well-being of the afflicted individual.
- **Recognition of similar proteins in different organisms** may contribute to the subsequent deduction of evolutionary relationships between organisms.
- **Recognition of conserved sequences** within different proteins with similar functions. Such identifications assist the study of structure–function relationships.

Affinity chromatography involves unique stereospecific interactions between molecules. The technique is an important **one-step purification procedure**. A ligand is covalently bonded to a solid matrix, e.g. agarose beads, and packed into a chromatographic column to act as the stationary phase. A mixture of biomolecules including the desired component is applied to the column. Substances without affinity for the ligand pass through the column in the mobile phase. The component of interest has an affinity with the ligand, to which it binds non-covalently and specifically. Elution is accomplished by changing the pH and/or salt concentration or applying organic solvents or a competing molecule.

Affinity chromatography may be used in the preparation of various biological molecules. Some examples of protein purifications are as follows, shown with an appropriate ligand **in bold**: an enzyme – **the specific substrate, a competitive inhibitor, a coenzyme**; a protein – **a specific antibody**; hormone receptor – **the hormone**; an IgG antibody of subclass 1, 2 or 4 – **protein A** from the cell walls of some strains of *Staphylococcus aureus*; albumin and some serine proteases – **cibacron blue**, a dye; bacterial endotoxins – **polymyxin**, a polypeptide antibiotic; sulphydryl-containing proteins – **organomercurial substances**; polynucleotide polymerase – **heparin**; *cis*-diol containing glycoproteins – **boronate**.

- Identification of repetitive sequences within different proteins, which may allow the grouping of proteins into families.
- Verification of previously unknown proteins.

The direct method

The **original strategy** for the direct determination of the amino acid sequence of any protein was based on the pioneering work of Frederick Sanger who, in 1953, successfully elucidated the primary structure of the hormone insulin. The determination of the primary structure requires relatively large quantities of pure protein (>1 mg) so that different aliquots may be used for the various necessary chemical techniques. Initially, the number of polypeptide chains in the protein must be determined. Then the numbers of residues of each constituent amino acid in each separated chain must be established. Each polypeptide chain requires fragmentation by several carefully selected proteolytic enzymes, then the resultant oligopeptides are separated and the amino acid sequences of individual oligopeptides determined. The complete primary structure of the polypeptide chain may be deduced from the component oligopeptide sequences by the method of overlapping sequences. The method of overlapping sequences requires digestion by at least two enzymes since the sequence of the products of the action of one appropriate enzyme must overlap the sequences of peptides generated by another enzyme.

The indirect method

Since the advent of **gene cloning** and **DNA sequencing techniques** (Chapter 2), primary sequences of proteins are usually determined indirectly from DNA or complementary DNA (cDNA) sequences, the latter being generated by reverse transcriptase action on a purified RNA molecule. The DNA sequence established in the laboratory is converted into a **codon sequence**. The genetic code (Table 2.7) is applied to translate the codons into start, amino acid residue and stop sequences. The codon AUG, which is ATG on the sense strand of the DNA duplex, is the major start codon. The identity and order of the amino acid residues are read from Table 2.7 until a stop triplet of UAA, UAG or UGA (TAA, TAG and TGA on the sense strand) is reached.

The **advantages of employing DNA sequences** to establish primary protein sequences are that:

- the protein does not require isolation;
- very small quantities of nucleic acid are employed;
- the shorter duration of the entire sequencing process;
- the cost of sequencing is substantially reduced.

However, further experimental evidence is required to confirm that the sequence does relate to an expressed and functional protein.

Secondary structure

Protein conformation may be defined as the arrangement in space of its constituent atoms which determine the overall shape of the molecule. The conformation of the protein arises from the bonding arrangements within its structure. If the protein contained only peptide bonds, all proteins would be random in shape due to C^{α}–C and C^{α}–N bond rotations. Investigations on a large number of proteins have indicated that proteins are highly organized structures with defined shapes. The early studies of conformation were dominated by the technique of **X-ray diffraction** performed on crystals of protein (X-ray crystallography). This technique offered a view of the relative positions of the atoms within a structure. Proton nuclear magnetic resonance (^{1}H-NMR) has been a useful subsequent development.

The X-ray diffraction studies of the 1940s highlighted general features regarding the shape of the protein. The distances between major recurrent features is termed the **major periodicity** and between minor recurrent features is the **minor periodicity**. X-ray diffraction creates the impression that each atom in the protein molecule is firmly fixed in position. This view of a static structure has been replaced by an appreciation of the dynamic nature of the molecule in which the atoms of the protein are in a state of constant motion. Therefore, X-ray diffraction studies produce an average position around which each atom moves.

From the knowledge of the dimensions and characteristics of framework bonds, scale models were constructed in the 1940s to define the geometric relationship of neighbouring amino acid residues. In 1951, Pauling and Corey proposed the two fundamental structures of proteins:

- the α-helical chain;
- the β-conformation.

The α-helical chain

The **α-keratins** are long, thin, water-insoluble fibrous proteins found in hair, wool, feathers and the outer layer of skin. The α-keratins are an early example of proteins whose secondary structure is that of an α-helix. The characteristics of an α-helix in α-keratins are:

- **The framework** of the polypeptide chain is arranged in a helical coil of 3.6 amino acid residues per turn (Figure 3.5a).
- The **α-helix is right-handed** and composed of L-amino acids. Left-handed α-helices cannot be formed using L-amino acids

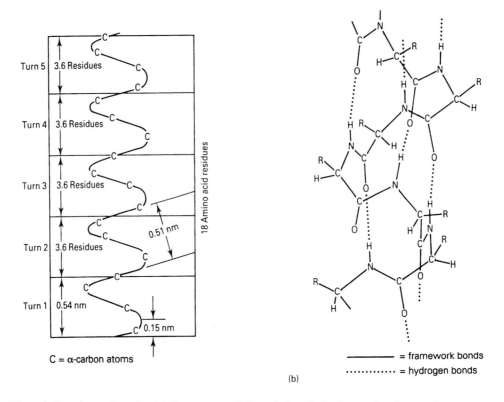

Figure 3.5 *The α-helix of an α-keratin: (a) dimensions of the α-helix; (b) hydrogen bonding and R group positions*

because of steric interactions involving the R groups, except when the α-helical stretch is very short, e.g. three to five residues in length.

- **The degree of rotation** for all C^α–C bonds is $-47°$ whilst that of all C^α–N bonds is $-57°$. This combination results in a very stable structure because the C=O group and the N–H group of the peptide bond are thereby in an orientation which promotes the formation of a network of intrachain hydrogen bonds.

- **Hydrogen bonds** occur between the carbonyl group of one peptide bond and the imino hydrogen atom of the third peptide bond along the chain (Figure 3.5b). The hydrogen bonds run parallel to the chain. Although individually weak, hydrogen bonds collectively reinforce each other, directing this folding pattern.

- **The R groups** of the amino acids extend outwards from the helix to minimize their molecular interactions which would increase the molecular energy level and destabilize the structure.

The accuracy of this model was later confirmed by X-ray diffraction studies on the protein from hair which demonstrated a **major periodicity of 0.50–0.55 nm** which closely corresponds to the

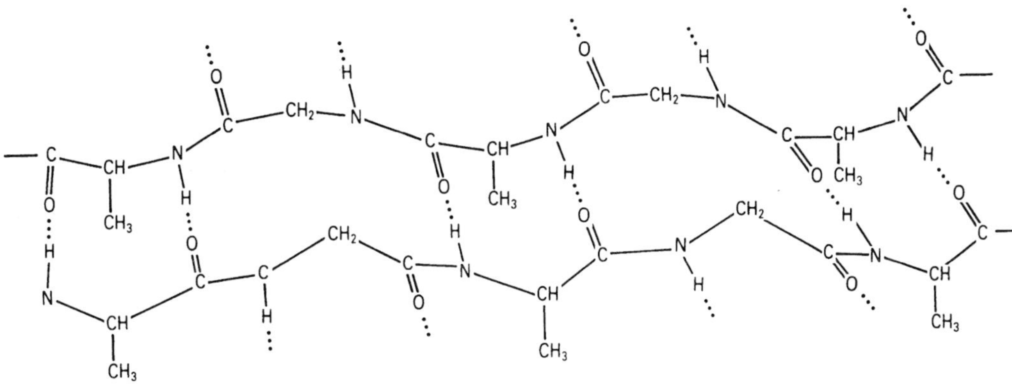

Figure 3.6 *The β-conformation or β-pleated sheet, showing the positions of groups and hydrogen bonds in an antiparallel β-conformation*

length of one turn of the helix (Figure 3.5a). The **minor periodicity of 0.15 nm** from the diffraction studies corresponds to the distance per residue. The dimensions observed in some other proteins vary from these although their structures are stable. An α-helix creates a long, thin, rod-like molecule.

The β-conformation

The **β-conformation** was based originally on an elongated α-helix. The α-keratin on treatment with steam at 100°C stretches, due to disruption of the hydrogen bonds, to almost twice its native length. This form is unstable due to R group steric interaction. The major periodicity was estimated as **0.7 nm**, the same value as that of **fibroin**, the major protein constituent of silk. Fibroin, however, is a stable structure because it contains very small R groups: alanine or serine alternating with glycine along the polypeptide chain (Figure 3.6). This extended structure is **sheet-like** and is stabilized by hydrogen bonds perpendicular to the chains. β-Sheets may be **parallel** or **antiparallel** and are formed by the folding of the polypeptide chain.

Prediction of secondary structure

The primary structures of proteins have been employed as a basis for attempts to predict the secondary structures of proteins. **Tables of the relative frequency** with which an amino acid residue lies in a particular conformation have been constructed. In decreasing orders of frequency for all quoted structures, methionyl, glutamyl, leucyl, alanyl, glutaminyl, lysyl, histidyl and cysteinyl residues promote the formation and stability of an α-helix, whilst phenyl-alanyl, tryptophanyl, isoleucyl, valyl, threonyl and tyrosyl residues reduce helix stability and favour the β-conformation. Aspartyl,

Bovine spongiform encephalopathy (BSE) was responsible for the death of over 150,000 cattle in Great Britain in the period of 1986–93. BSE, **scrapie** of sheep and the human diseases of **Creutzfeldt–Jakob disease (CJD)** and **kuru** are members of the family of **prion diseases**. The term **prion** was introduced to distinguish the causative pathogen from viruses and viroids and to stress its proteinaceous and infectious character. Substantial evidence indicates that prions are novel pathogens composed entirely of protein. Forms of prion protein (PrP) have been discovered and its gene has been mapped to the short arm of human chromosome 20. PrP is a normal cellular protein of 27–30 kDa, designated PrP^c. The infectious form, PrP^{Sc} (from scrapie), differs from PrP^c by its high β-sheet content, its insolubility in detergents and its tendency to aggregate, and its relative resistance to degradation. The transformation from PrP^c to PrP^{Sc} is a post-translational process in which some α-helices are converted into β-sheets.

Mutations in the human PrP genes are believed to be responsible for inherited prion diseases, e.g. familial CJD, Gerstmann–Sträussler–Scheinker disease (GSS) and fatal familial insomnia (FFI). More than 18 different mutations have so far been identified.

asparaginyl, seryl, glycyl and prolyl residues favour bends or loops.

Arginine exhibits conformational neutrality, i.e. it does not encourage the formation of an α-helix, β-conformation or a bend. Proline cannot be accommodated in an α-helix because of its pyrrolidine ring. However, the reasons why most amino acids favour a particular conformation are not understood. Comparison of predicted secondary structures with experimentally determined conformations (by X-ray diffraction studies) have shown close agreement but never identity. The disagreements usually reside in the inaccurate prediction of the residue terminating an α-helix or β-conformation.

Collagen

Collagen is one of the most abundant fibrous proteins in the vertebrate body. The importance of collagen may also be demonstrated by the consequences of over 400 mutations identified in only six types of collagen. There are at least 19 genetically distinct types of collagen, labelled Types I–XIX. The numbers reflect the chronological order of discovery. Collagen has a distinctive structure which is also found in a limited number of 'collagen-like' proteins, e.g. component C1q of the complement system, mannan-binding protein, the pulmonary surfactant proteins (SP-A and SP-D) and the conglutinin tetramer. Early electron microscopy studies suggested that collagen had a repetitive uniform structure irrespective of its source. However, this is not the case but simply appeared so because the tissues examined such as adult skin, bone, tendon, placenta and cornea contain large amounts of Type I collagen.

Collagen is recognized as a **family of molecules** based on the triple-helical structure. The collagen family is divided into several classes:

- the **fibrillar collagens**, which consist of Types I, II, III, V and XI;
- the **network-forming collagens**, which contain Types IV, VIII and X;
- the **filamentous collagen**, Type VI;
- the **anchoring collagen**, Type VII, which anchors the basement membrane;
- **FACITs** or fibril-associated collagens with interrupted triple helices, which include Types IX, XII, XIV, XVI and XIX;
- **collagens with a transmembranal domain**, namely Types XIII and XVII.

The collagens are defined as proteins of the extracellular matrix which contain at least one linear domain comprised of the repeating amino acid sequence **Gly-X-Y** where X and Y are usually other amino acids. The **fibrillar collagens**, containing about 1000 amino

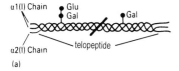

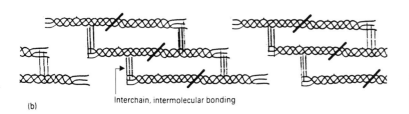

Interchain, intermolecular bonding

(b)

acid residues, illustrate the fundamental molecular structures of the triple-helical molecules:

- **Type I** is composed of two α1(I) chains and one slightly different chain called α2(I). **Type V** is produced by two α1(V) chains and one α2(V) chain.
- **Type II** comprises three α1(II) chains. **Type III** has three α1(III) chains.
- **Type XI** is formed by one α1(XI) chain, one α2(XI) and one α3 (XI) chain.

The individual chains are coiled into a left-handed helix. The three chains wind around each other to form a right-handed triple helix which creates a rope-like structure (Figure 3.7a).

The major structural features of the fibrillar collagen molecules are:

- **they contain about 330 Gly-X-Y repeats;**
- **glycine occurs as every third amino acid residue** because this position occupies a restricted space within the triple helix;
- **each triple helical domain ends in short N- and C-terminal non-helical stretches** of the polypeptide chains called **telopeptides** which remain after the removal of the propeptides.

Prolyl residues, some of which may be hydroxylated into 3-hydroxyproline, occupy about 100 of the X positions. 4-Hydroxyprolyl residues occupy about 100 of the Y positions and make important contributions to hydrogen bonding. The pyrrolidine rings of these residues cause individual collagen chains to assume an elongated helical conformation in which prolines, hydroxyprolines and interchain hydrogen bonding promote stability.

5-Hydroxylysyl residues in the Y position provide hydroxyl

Osteogenesis imperfecta (OI), also called **brittle bone disease,** is a group of hereditable disorders with an incidence of about 1 in 10,000. The severity of OI varies from mild to lethal. In the most severe forms, over 100 fractures *in utero* have been reported with resultant stillbirth.

The fundamental defect is mutation in the genes for procollagen Type I. Most of the mutations involve a single base change in the codon for glycine, resulting in the disruption of the triple helical structure. The triple helix of collagen demands that glycine occurs at every third residue. In addition to their occurence in exons, single base mutations have been located in introns thereby affecting splicing and effecting exon skipping. Deletions and insertions have also been identified.

The position of the aberration is linked to the severity of the disease. Mutations close to the C-terminus tend to be lethal whilst the severity decreases to mild the closer to the N-terminus the mutation occurs. This is because triple-helix formation commences at the C-terminus and progresses towards the N-terminus in a zipper-like fashion. The severity of the disease also depends on the properties of the amino acid which is substituted for glycine.

groups for glycosylation which involves the attachment of galacto-syl residues. Some of the galactosyl residues are modified further into glucosylgalactosyl oligosaccharide side chains. Other amino acids in the X and Y positions are clustered into regions of hydrophobicity, e.g. alanine and valine, and regions of hydrophili-city, e.g. lysine and glutamic acid. Stretches of hydrophobicity direct the assembly of collagen molecules into collagen fibrils with a characteristic longitudinal displacement called a quarter-stagger (Figure 3.7b). Each molecule is displaced by approximately one-quarter of its length relative to adjacent neighbouring molecules along the length of the fibril.

Fibrillar collagen molecules are synthesized as larger precursor molecules called **procollagens** which are processed by the loss of N- and C-terminal propeptides by **procollagen N-proteinases** and **procollagen C-proteinase** respectively. The gene for the $\alpha1(I)$ chain contains the 42 exons responsible for the triple-helical domain of collagen. Most of the exons have 54 base-pairs encoding six Gly-X-Y triplets, some have 108 or 162 base-pairs resulting in the synthesis of 12 or 18 triplets. Some 45 b.p. exons exist in the gene. Each exon commences with a codon for glycine and codes for a number of complete triplets.

Lysyl oxidase, a copper-dependent enzyme, converts some lysyl and hydroxylysyl residues, located in the telopeptides, to their aldehydic derivatives, called lysylal and hydroxylysylal respectively, by oxidative deamination. Condensation reactions between the ε-amino groups of lysyl, hydroxylysyl and glycosylated hydroxyly-syl residues and the aldehydic derivatives produce six kinds of stable mature interchain covalent crosslinks.

Tertiary structure

The **folding** of most polypeptide chains produces compact mol-ecules of maximum stability approximating in shape to elongated or oblated (orange-shaped) globes. **Globular proteins** contain repetitive stretches of secondary structure interrupted by nonrepeti-tive stretches which provide regions for the folding of the polypep-tide chain. **Folding** of the chain creates changes in its direction which are commonly achieved by the formation of a tight loop called a **β-bend,** which contains only four residues. β-Bends are stabilized by hydrogen bonding between the C=O of one residue (forming the first peptide bond) and the N–H of the fourth residue (forming the third peptide bond) along the polypeptide chain. **Proline,** whose geometry predetermines bending in a chain, is frequently the second residue, and in one form, the **Type II β-bend, glycine,** because of its small R group, is the third residue. Because of the sudden directional change between two adjacent antiparallel β-regions, the bend is termed a **hairpin bend** (Figure 3.8a).

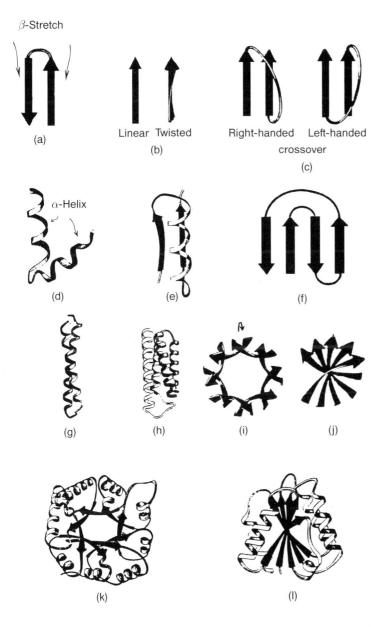

β-Stretch

(a)

Linear Twisted

(b)

Right-handed Left-handed

crossover

(c)

α-Helix

(d)   (e)   (f)

(g)   (h)   (i)   (j)

(k)   (l)

Figure 3.8 *Conformations found in proteins: (a) β-bend; (b) twisted conformation; (c) right-handed crossover; (d) helix–loop–helix motif; (e) β–α–β motif; (f) Greek key motif; (g) simple α-domain; (h) four-helix bundle domain; (i) β-barrel domain; (j) saddle domain; (k) α/β-barrel domain; (l) α/β-saddle domain*

Various combinations of secondary structures occur in the tertiary structure of proteins and are termed **supersecondary structures** or **motifs**. The most common patterns, shown as ribbon drawings, include:

- **Twisted β-conformation** (Figure 3.8b). A right-handed twist tends to occur in extended β-conformations because the light twist enhances the stability of these structures. The twist influences the relative positions of adjacent stretches of β-conformation.

- **Right-handed crossover** (Figure 3.8c). Two parallel β-stretches must be interconnected by a crossover region. In native proteins, only the right-handed conformation of the crossover has been found.

- **Helix–loop–helix motif** (Figure 3.8d) occurs in a number of calcium-binding and DNA-binding proteins. The loop constitutes the **calcium-binding site**, e.g. in calmodulin.

- **β–α–β motif** (Figure 3.8e) consists of two parallel stretches of β-conformation separated by an intervening α-helix. The carbonyl end of one β-stretch is linked by a loop (the first loop) to the N–H end of an α-helix whose C=O is connected by another loop (the second loop) to the N–H of the second stretch of β-conformation. The α-helix is approximately parallel to the β-stretches. In enzymes, the first loop frequently contributes to the formation of the active site, e.g. triose phosphate isomerase.

- **Greek key motif** (Figure 3.8f), so called because of its resemblance to a design on ancient Greek pottery. Four or more antiparallel β-stretches are linked by two hairpin loops and a longer loop connecting the outer β-regions. The Greek key motif is not associated with a specific function.

- **β-prism motif**. This contains three β-sheets that are arranged as the faces of a triangular prism.

Structural motifs may be developed into **domains**. Domains may be defined as a part of a polypeptide chain which can independently fold into a stable structure possessing a particular function. Proteins may contain a single domain or several domains, e.g. fatty acid synthase (Chapter 12).

Alpha (α)-domain structures are composed of a bundle of α-helices interconnected by loop regions. The simplest arrangement is a close pairing of adjacent helices arranged in antiparallel fashion with a short intervening loop (Figure 3.8g). The commonest α-domain structure is the four-helix bundle formed when two of the simple structures dimerize (Figure 3.8h), e.g. in cytochrome b_{562}. The intimate packing of the four helices produces a hydrophobic core by the exclusion of water. This core consists of the hydrophobic R groups contributed by each helix. The hydrophilic R groups are located on the outer surface of the bundle.

The **right-handed twisting in β-conformations** leads to an overall twist in the structure formed by multiple stretches of β-conformation. Two major alignments result:

- the **β-barrel domain** (Figure 3.8i), a cylindrical curvature promoted by a staggered hydrogen bond pattern;

- the **saddle domain** (Figure 3.8j), a centrally constricted conformation in which the upper and lower hydrogen bonds are stretched.

These structures form the core of more complex structures in which α-helices and β-conformations occur within the same polypeptide chain in some proteins.

Alpha/beta (α/β) structures are the most frequently occurring structures in which central, parallel or mixed β-stretches are surrounded by α-helices. The **α/β barrel domain** (Figures 3.8k) and **α/β saddle domain** (Figures 3.8l) are two major examples of this arrangement. Both of these structures are found in many enzymes. The substrate-binding sites differ in different examples but are mainly determined by the intra-molecular location of the loop regions which do not contribute to the structural stability. Alpha/beta structures are found in all glycolytic enzymes and in some transport proteins.

Myoglobin

Sperm whale myoglobin was the first of the globular proteins to be successfully crystallized and therefore analysed by X-ray diffraction. The structural information gained from the analysis of myoglobin served as a basis for hypotheses on tertiary structure. Myoglobin is a single polypeptide chain of molecular mass 17.5 kDa, comprises 153 amino acid residues and is an example of an α-domain structure. Myoglobin **lacks β-conformation.** There are no cysteinyl residues and therefore no disulphide bonds. However , it contains a very large proportion of α-helical structure. It also has a **haem** prosthetic group, the iron of which binds oxygen. Myoglobin functions as an oxygen-carrying protein in mammalian muscle. Sperm whale myoglobin was studied because of the large quantity of protein in the skeletal muscle of diving mammals which have a requirement for very large oxygen reserves.

The fundamental features of the structure of myoglobin (Figure 3.9) are:

- **Its dimensions** are $4.5 \times 3.5 \times 2.5$ nm.

- **The molecule is compact** and has space only for four water molecules in the interior of the convoluted chain.

- **The interior of the molecule** consists of a large proportion of hydrophobic residues and is devoid of acidic or basic amino acids.

- **Residues with a polar and non-polar part,** e.g. threonine and tyrosine, are orientated to direct the non-polar part towards the interior of the molecule.

- **Eight right-handed α-helical regions,** denoted A–H, constitute about 75% of the chain. Each amino acid residue within a helix is coded, e.g. C2 refers to the second residue of the third helix.

- **The chain contains a total of seven non-helical segments:** five between helical regions denoted according to the helices they interrupt, e.g CD, plus one at the *N*- and *C*-termini.

- **The occurrence of proline terminates an α-helix.** There are four prolyl residues in myoglobin.

Figure 3.9 *Tertiary structure of the myoglobin chain*

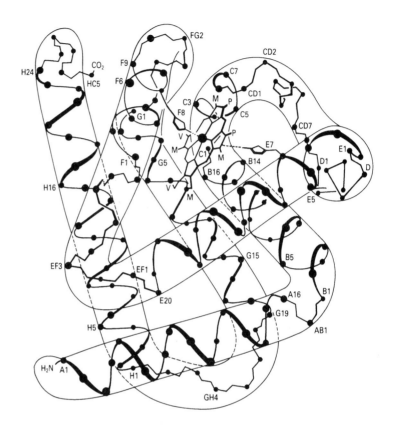

The **haem group** is located in a non-polar groove formed by the α-helices and located near the surface of the molecule. The two histidine residues which position the haem moiety are the only polar residues found in the interior of myoglobin. The hydrophobic environment of this groove does not impede the passage of the oxygen to the iron of the haem but prevents water from nullifying the oxygen-binding process. The iron of haem is bound to the nitrogen atoms of the porphyrin ring (Figure 3.10a). This arrangement occupies four of six coordination positions of iron. The histidine at F8 is bound to the iron via the fifth coordination position. The sixth position of the iron atom is vacant and available for the binding of oxygen (Figure 3.10b). Oxygenation can only occur with the iron atom in the ferrous state (Fe^{2+}) which is maintained by enzyme-catalysed redox reactions (Chapter 11). Once bound, the oxygen is stabilized by hydrogen bonding to the imidazole ring of the E7 histidine (Figure 3.9).

Quaternary Structure

Haemoglobin, the oxygen-transport protein of the blood, was the first oligomeric protein for which structural analysis was obtained by X-ray crystallography.

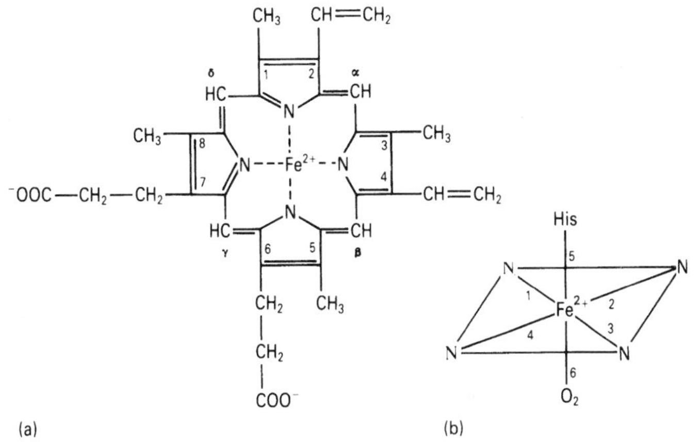

CH₃   CH=CH₂

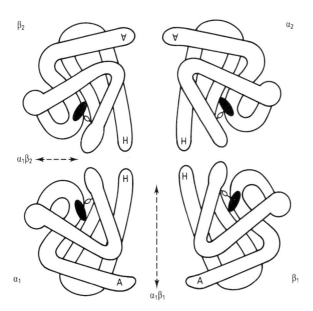

(a)

(b)

Figure 3.10   *Haem: (a) structure of haem; (b) coordination positions of haem with position 5 bonded to F8 histidine of the globin molecule*

Haemoglobin

Haemoglobin (molecular mass ~64.5 kDa) consists of four subunits. In human adult haemoglobin, the tetramer (Figure 3.11) consists of two pairs of polypeptide chains:

- **two α-subunits** of 141 amino acid residues;
- **two β-subunits** of 146 amino acid residues.

Each of the α- and β-chains carries one haem group. They share similar characteristics with each other and with myoglobin. A conformation–function relationship is thereby indicated.

The major features of the haemoglobin molecule are:

- **Between the four subunits** there is no covalent bonding although there are two cysteinyl residues per α-chain and one per β-chain.

Figure 3.11   *Tetrameric arrangement of α- and β-globin chains in haemoglobin A*

The **glycosylation of haemoglobin** occurs in **diabetes** and is exploited to monitor blood glucose control in the diabetic patient. Control is deemed to be good if HbA$_{1C}$ (glycosylated haemoglobin) levels remain within the reference range for the non-diabetic population. Above this range, progressively poorer control is assumed. However, HbA$_{1C}$ increases with age within the non-diabetic population, with the result that glucose control in older diabetics tended to be misinterpreted as worse than in reality. **Age-related reference ranges** are necessary for the accurate interpretation of HbA$_{1C}$ results.

During pregnancy, **the expectant mother's erythrocytes** supply oxygen to those of the developing foetus. This transfer of oxygen is achieved because **foetal haemoglobin (HbF)** has a higher affinity for oxygen than maternal haemoglobin and this permits the oxygen delivery. The affinity of human haemoglobin is governed by the allosteric regulatory molecule **2,3-bisphospho-glycerate (BPG)** which lowers the binding of oxygen to haemoglobin. BPG binds less successfully to foetal haemoglobin with the result that it has a higher oxygen affinity than maternal haemoglobin.

- **Between each identical subunit** there are only a few ionic and hydrogen bonds.
- **Between one α- and one β-subunit**, there are longer regions of electrostatic interactions which produce two identical dimers, $\alpha_1\beta_1$ and $\alpha_2\beta_2$, which are capable of integrated movement.
- **Between the dimers** there exists a network of ionic and hydrogen bonds which on reversible oxygenation of haemoglobin is disrupted and supplanted by the formation of new bonds. X-ray crystallography has shown that, on oxygenation, there is no change in the tertiary structure of each subunit but the α- and β-chains undergo opposite rotational and positional changes of different magnitude causing a repackaging of the subunits.

Whereas myoglobin absorbs oxygen, **haemoglobin** demonstrates a slow initial oxygen-binding which becomes progressively faster. This phenomenon is called **positive cooperativity** in which the binding of the first oxygen molecule to deoxyhaemoglobin facilitates the binding of subsequent oxygen molecules to other subunits. Conversely during deoxygenation, the loss of the first oxygen molecule from oxygenated haemoglobin promotes the dissociation of oxygen from the other subunits. In addition to changes in quaternary structure due to oxygenation/deoxygenation, other factors including the concentrations of CO_2, H^+ and **2,3-bisphosphoglycerate** (2,3-BPG, an erythrocyte metabolite) participate in the regulation of oxygen binding by haemoglobin. These substances bind to the **globin** and influence the uptake of O_2 by haem groups. This indicates that modifications at one site in the protein may vary the activity at another site. This phenomenon is called **allostery**. The allosteric behaviour of regulatory enzymes is considered to make a major contribution to the control of metabolic processes (Chapters 4 and 8).

Haemoglobinopathies

Over 300 hundred variations from the amino acid sequence of normal human adult haemoglobin (HbA) have been reported. These molecules often differ from HbA by the insertion of an incorrect amino acid into either the α- or β-chains during protein synthesis. Other variants may be due to **deletion or frameshift mutations** in which an insertion or deletion of one or more nucleotides changes the reading frame of the codons during protein synthesis (Chapter 13). Haemoglobin variants may function normally or abnormally depending on the nature and position of the substitution (Table 3.4).

Some **severe haemoglobinopathies** have been reported, e.g. HbS which causes the disease called **sickle cell anaemia** in the black population. In sickle cell anaemia, the haemoglobin (called HbS) contains normal α-chains but its β-chains contain valine instead of glutamate at residue 6. Therefore a hydrophobic amino acid

Table 3.4 *Some haemoglobin variants*

Haemoglobin type	Substitution†	Functional defect
HbS	β^6Glu → Val	Erythrocytes sickle, decreased O_2 affinity
Hb$^*_{\text{Köln}}$	β^{98}Val → Met	Unstable, increased O_2 affinity
Hb$_{\text{Torino}}$	α^{43}Phe → Val	Decreased O_2 affinity
HbG$^{**}_{\text{Honolulu}}$	α^{30}Glu → Gln	Normal oxygen affinity
Hb$_{\text{Camden}}$	β^{131}Gln → Glu	Normal oxygen affinity
Hb$_{\text{Denmark Hill}}$	α^{95}Pro → Ala	Decreased O_2 affinity

* Haemoglobins are frequently named after their place of identification.
** Hb is an abbreviation for haemoglobin; G refers to electrophoretic mobility.
† α or β refer to normal haemoglobin chains; the superscript number refers to residue number at which substitution has occurred; the substitution is recorded by first indicating the normal amino acid followed by its replacement.

replaces an acidic one. This new arrangement allows hydrophobic interaction with the β^{85}-phenylalanine and β^{88}-leucine of an adjacent deoxyHbS. This modifies the Hb conformation so that the stacking arrangement of the 280 million Hb molecules within each erythrocyte is altered by the production of fibrous aggregates of the protein. This leads to a change in the shape of the erythrocyte from a biconcave disc to a crescent or sickle shape on deoxygenation. In individuals who have two copies of the altered gene (homozygotes), the erythrocytes interact and form clumps which may occlude the capillaries reducing the normal flow of blood through the vasculature. The blockage of the microcirculation may occur anywhere in the body and may lead to damage and eventual failure of vital organs, e.g. the kidney. The life expectancy of a homozygote is less than 30 years.

The **mutation**, however, confers an important advantage on its carriers if they reside in a malaria-afflicted area of the world. *Plasmodium vivax* (one protozoon responsible for malaria) requires entry into the erythrocytes of its host during its life cycle. Sickle cells, because of their fragility, are cleared from the blood circulation by the spleen more rapidly than normal cells. The half-life of sickle cells in the blood is only 1 week compared to 1 month for normal cells. This enhanced clearance accounts for the anaemia. Any parasite contained within these cells will also be destroyed by splenic activity.

Thalassaemia

The **thalassaemias** are diseases caused by decreased synthesis of either normal α- or β-globin chains. β-Thalassaemia, common in

The most common hereditary blood disorder in man is **sickle cell disease**, the term describing any genetic aberration in which **'sickling' of erythrocytes** occurs. The most common of these conditions is **sickle cell anaemia (SCA)**. SCA afflicts black Africans or their descendants. Approximately 10% of this population are carriers of the HbS gene and 1.7% are SCA sufferers. In children, symptoms usually start after the age of 4 months and include the painful swelling of fingers and toes, and anaemia. There is a correlation with the normal decline of foetal haemoglobin F levels. HbF appears to block the effects of HbS and has potential as a therapy once its introduction into, and retention within, the erythrocyte can be adequately achieved.

SCA is associated with severe pain, lasting from a few hours to a few days. Pain management has lead to concerns over the development of patient addiction to the prescribed analgesics.

Monoclonal antibodies (MoAbs) share an absolute specificity for one antigenic determinant because each antibody molecule has an identical antigen-binding site. Traditionally, MoAbs have been produced by the **hybridoma technique**, pioneered by Köhler and Milstein in 1975. The hydridoma technique involves **spleen cells** (B lymphocytes) from an immunized mouse (a good responder) being fused with non-secretory mutant myeloma (B-cell cancer) cells. The resultant hybrid cell may be selected from the mixture of cells by a cell culture technique. The selected hybrid cell may be grown in cell culture to produce **clones** of the single cell which release monospecific antibody molecules. MoAbs can also be synthesized using micro-organism-based genetic engineering techniques which permit the production of smaller, non-immunogenic antibody fragments containing the antigen-binding amino acid sequences.

some Mediterranean countries and in malaria-infested regions of Asia, has two main varieties:

- β^+-**thalassaemia** in which a partial loss of β-chain production occurs;
- β^0-**thalassaemia** characterized by a lack of β-chain synthesis.

Immunoglobulins

Immunoglobulins, also called antibodies, are a family of extra-cellular glycoproteins which function in the body's defence against invading organisms and foreign substances. The fundamental structural features of immunoglobulins are:

- Each immunoglobulin molecule (Figure 3.12) consists of two identical heavy polypeptide chains and two identical light polypeptide chains.
- **The primary structure of their respective heavy chains**, called γ, μ, α, δ and ε chains, is the basis of classification into five classes: IgG, IgM, IgA, IgD and IgE respectively. Human IgG can be subdivided into four subclasses, i.e. IgG_1, IgG_2, IgG_3 and IgG_4, whilst IgA has two subclasses.
- **The light chains of each immunoglobulin molecule** are identical, either κ or λ chains. Natural immunoglobulins do not contain mixtures of light or heavy chains.
- **The light chains of each immunoglobulin molecule** are attached to two identical heavy chains by disulphide bonds. The two heavy

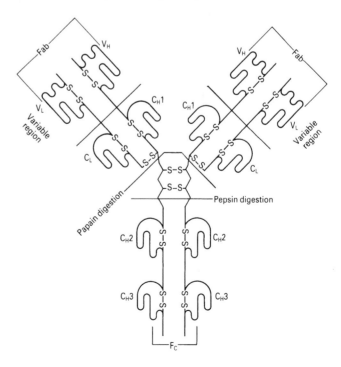

Figure 3.12 *Schematic diagram of an IgG antibody molecule illustrating heavy and light chain domains and digest fragments*

chains are also interlinked by covalent bonds. Within each chain of the molecule, intrachain disulphide bonds fold the molecule into compact globular domains.

- **Each polypeptide chain** consists of two well-defined regions, designated **V for variable** and **C for constant** amino acid sequence, within each class of antibody. The variable region of a light chain (V_L) is approximately 50% of chain length whilst the variable region of a heavy chain (V_H) is approximately 25% of chain length.

Papain digestion yields two major fragments called the F_{ab} **fragment**, which retains the antigen-binding capacity of the intact molecule, and the F_c **fragment** , which is crystallizable. Digestion by another enzyme, **pepsin**, produces a single fragment containing two linked antigen-binding sites called the $F_{(ab')2}$ **fragment**. The ability of an antibody molecule to combine specifically with a complementary antigen resides in the unique conformation and amino acid sequence of the **antigen-binding cleft** formed by the V_H and V_L regions of the molecule. Within the V_H and V_L regions, irrespective of specificity, certain positions are always occupied by the same amino acid while certain other positions exhibit only a limited variation. However, some positions display large variations in amino acid occupancy to constitute **hypervariable regions** of approximately nine to twelve residues. Hypervariability is centred around positions 31–37, 48–62, 92–101 inclusive in the V_H regions and positions 24–34, 48–60 and 89–100 inclusive in the V_L region. These hypervariable regions are juxtaposed by the foldings of the V_H and V_L regions to frame the antigen-binding sites.

The C_H regions of γ- and α-chains contain three domains whilst IgM, IgD and IgE exhibit four C_H domains. Individual domains have been associated with certain biological activities, e.g C_H2 of IgG_3 binds the complement component C1q. Blood plasma IgM is a pentamer composed of five Y-shaped structures. IgA in external secretions is a dimer. IgM and IgA contain an additional polypeptide chain called **the J chain.** Secretory IgA is associated with **a secretory component.** Oligosaccharide chains are located only in the secretory component, J chain and C_H regions. Carbohydrate is absent from light chains and V_H regions.

MoAbs are extremely useful for affinity chromatography in which a MoAb, attached to the stationary phase, may interact with a unique complementary determinant in a single protein to permit its separation from a crude mixture of proteins. MoAbs are tools in the identification of various cell surface proteins and are important in the classification of cell types and cell subsets, e.g. T_{helper} lymphocytes are CD4$^+$ whereas $T_{cytotoxic}$ cells are CD8$^+$. Modifications during the maturation of cells may be monitored by panels of MoAbs. Subtyping of micro-organisms , e.g. *Streptococcus*, and viruses, e.g. strains of influenza virus, employs MoAbs. Potential drugs may be targetted to their site of action by the use of a **monoclonal antibody–drug conjugate** which binds specifically to a unique antigen on the surface of the target cell, e.g. in the delivery of radioisotopes or cytotoxic drugs in the treatment of cancer.

Suggested further reading

Choudhury, P., Liu, Y. and Sifers, R.N. (1997). Quality control of protein folding: participation in human disease. *News in Physiological Sciences* **12**, 162–166.

Kadler, K.E., Holmes, D.F., Trotter, J.A. and Chapman, J.A. (1996). Collagen fibril formation. *Biochemistry Journal* **316**, 1–11.

Schumacher, M.A., Dixon, M.M., Kluger, R., Jones, R.T. and Brennan, R.G. (1995). Allosteric transition intermediates modelled by crosslinked haemoglobins. *Nature* **375**, 84–87.

Shimizu, T. and Morikawa, K. (1996). The β-prism: a new folding motif. *Trends in Biochemical Sciences* **21**, 3–6.

Bollag, D. and Edelstein, S.J. (1996). *Protein Methods*, 2nd edn. Chichester: Wiley.

Creighton, T.E. (1997). *Protein Structure: A Practical Approach. Protein Function: A Practical Approach*, 2nd edn. Oxford: Oxford University Press.

Self-assessment questions

1. Identify the major biological roles of the following amino acids in proteins: (a) serine; (b) threonine; (c) tyrosine; (d) asparagine; (e) glycine; (f) methionine; (g) aspartic acid; (h) lysine; (i) arginine; (j) glutamic acid.
2. In an aqueous solution of $1.0\,mol\,l^{-1}$ valine at pH 8.5, what is the percentage of molecules exhibiting a negative charge?
3. Explain why haemoglobin may be described as an allosteric protein.
4. A segment of the sense strand of a protein-coding DNA gene was sequenced by the Sanger dideoxy method and the following sequence was deduced from the autoradiograph: TTGCCATGGGCCCCGGCAAAATGC. What would be the amino acid sequence produced from this oligonucleotide during protein synthesis? Give your answer using the one-letter code.
5. Identify which amino acid functional groups may be ionized in a polypeptide chain.
6. The occurrence of which of the following amino acid residues, represented by the one-letter code, in a polypeptide chain favour a helical conformation: (a) S; (b) T; (c) Y; (d) N; (e) G; (f) M; (g) D; (h) K; (i) R; (j) E.
7. Explain how haem is attached to the globin molecule to form myoglobin.
8. Unique hydroxylated derivatives of two amino acids are found in collagen. What are their significances?
9. Draw an illustration of an α/β-barrel domain and an α/β-saddle domain.
10. Suggest why native IgE and IgG$_4$ cannot bind the complement component C1q.

Key Concepts and Facts

Proteins
- Proteins perform diverse functions.

Amino Acids
- Amino acids are found in proteins as α-amino acids of the L-series whose individual properties vary according to the nature of their R groups.
- Amino acids may be classified as non-polar or polar, the latter class being subdivided into neutral, acidic or basic amino acids depending upon their ionic properties.
- Amino acids respond to changes in their aqueous environment according to acid–base principles.

Protein Structure
- Amino acids are linked by peptide bonds to form polypeptide chains.
- The shape assumed by a polypeptide chain is governed by a variety of bonds and non-bonding interactions.
- There is a hierarchy of structural levels in proteins.

Primary and Secondary Structures
- Peptide bonds are rigid but the framework of the chain may rotate around pivotal α-carbon atoms.
- The amino acid sequence of a protein may be experimentally established from the nucleotide sequence of the corresponding gene(s).
- The α-helix and β-conformation are the two fundamental structures of protein conformation and are stabilized by hydrogen bonds.
- The most abundant fibrous protein in man is collagen which has a triple-helical structure.

Tertiary and Quaternary Structures
- The folding of most polypeptide chains produces globular domains.
- Domains are derived from a number of structural motifs.
- The analysis of myoglobin by X-ray crystallography revealed numerous structural features.
- Haemoglobin functions by regulated cooperativity between its subunits, the sequencing of which has identified a large number of variations.
- Antibodies are classified according to the primary structure of their heavy chains to which light chains are covalently attached.
- The chains of antibody molecules are folded into functional domains.

Answers to questions (Chapter 3)

1. (a) Hydrogen bonding, phosphorylation (Chapter 8), O-linkage with oligosaccharides; (b) hydrogen bonding, phosphorylation and O-linkage with oligosaccharides; (c) hydrogen bonding and phosphorylation; (d) hydrogen bonding and N-linkage with oligosaccharides; (e) occupies small spaces; (f) methyl group donor and contributes to hydrophobic interactions; (g) ionic bonding; (h) ionic bonding; (i) ionic bonding; (j) ionic bonding.

2. 7.05%.

$$
\begin{array}{ccc}
\text{CH}_3 & \text{CH}_3 & \text{CH}_3 \\
| & | & | \\
\text{CH--CH}_3 & \text{CH--CH}_3 & \text{CH--CH}_3 \\
| & | & | \\
\text{NH}_3^+\text{--CH--COOH} & \text{NH}_3^+\text{--CH--COO}^- & \text{NH}_2\text{--CH--COO}^-
\end{array}
$$

with $\text{p}K_{a1}=2.32$ between the first and second forms, and $\text{p}K_{a2}=9.62$ between the second and third forms.

Code:	A	B	C
Charge:	+1	0	−1

Relative proportion of C to B required. Given pH, $\text{p}K_a$ and relative proportions, use Henderson–Hasselbalch equation (Chapter 1):

$$
\text{pH} = \text{p}K_{a2} + \log\frac{[\text{base}]}{[\text{acid}]} \qquad \therefore 8.5 = 9.62 + \log\frac{[\text{C}]}{[\text{B}]}
$$

$$
\therefore -1.12 = \log\frac{[\text{C}]}{[\text{B}]}
$$

$\therefore$ Take antilog

$$
\therefore \frac{[\text{C}]}{[\text{B}]} = \frac{0.0758}{1}
$$

$$
\therefore \text{Relative percentage of C} = \frac{0.0758}{1.0758} \times 100 = 7.05\%
$$

3. The α- and β-chains undergo rotational and positional changes on oxygenation and reverse changes on deoxygenation causing repackaging of the subunits. Regulatory factors including 2,3-bisphosphoglycerate bind to the globin molecule and may vary the activity at a distant site where oxygen binding occurs.

4. Sense strand: TTGCCATGGGCCCCGGCAAAATGC.
    Template: AACGGTACCCGGGGCCGTTTTACG.
    mRNA: UUGCCAUGGGCCCCGGCAAAAUGC.
    Amino acid
      sequence: Leu Pro Try Ala Pro Ala Lys Cys
    One letter code: L P W A P A K C

5. The amino- and carboxy- terminal groups and all ionizable R groups, irrespective of their position in the chain.

6. (f) methionine; (h) lysine; (j) glutamic acid.

7. See Figure 3.10. The histidine at F8 is bound to the iron via the fifth coordination position.

8. Hydroxyprolines contribute to the elongated helical conformation and via their hydroxyl groups contribute to hydrogen bonding. 5-Hydroxylysine provides hydroxyl groups for glycosylation and ε-amino groups for oxidative deamination and subsequent stronger mature crosslinking.

9. See Figure 3.8k and l.

10. The primary structure of IgE does not permit the folding of the polypeptide chain into a binding site for C1q. In native IgG$_4$, the binding domain is cryptic, i.e. hidden in the structure and not naturally accessible to C1q.

Chapter 4
Enzymes

Learning objectives

After studying this chapter you should confidently be able to:

Compare the nature of enzymic reactions with that of chemical reactions.

Discuss factors which may influence the activity of an enzyme.

Discuss the nature of the catalytic site of an enzyme.

Discuss single-substrate enzymic reactions and their inhibition in terms of steady-state kinetics.

Discuss the key features of different types of enzyme inhibitors.

Describe the mechanisms of action of multisubstrate enzymic reactions.

Account for the catalytic powers of enzymes.

Discuss allosteric enzymes in terms of their kinetics and subunit cooperativity.

Describe an example of an isoenzyme in terms of subunit kinetics.

Enzymes are proteins that **accelerate the rates** of a wide variety of chemical reactions that occur in biological systems under thermodynamically unfavourable conditions (Chapter 8). Enzymes are considered to be **biological catalysts**. A catalyst is a substance that participates in a chemical reaction to enhance its rate without destruction or irreversible modification during the reaction. Intracellular enzymic reactions constitute **cellular metabolism,** the network of chemical transformations through which **cell viability** is maintained. Many enzymes are organized into **macromolecular protein complexes,** found either free in the cytosol or mitochondrial matrix or associated with cellular membranes. These complexes facilitate the coordination and control of metabolic reactions. However, it is now recognized that proteins do not have a monopoly in catalysing reactions in biological systems. Certain ribonucleic acid molecules, called **ribozymes,** may catalyse the chemical modification of RNA in the absence of protein.

Enzymes play a major role in modern **biotechnological industries** and are exploited in the laundry, food and drugs industries, the products of which make immense contributions to the quality of human life. There is nevertheless a constant demand for better, safer and more efficient products. Several important strategies are being developed to create improved enzymes. Immunoglobulin molecules, which are naturally devoid of catalytic powers, may be designed as **abzymes** to modify bound antigens. The use of gene cloning techniques permits the introduction of specific mutations into critical regions of the polypeptide chain and influences the functioning of the enzyme. This process, called **site-directed mutagenesis,** has been employed to modify the specificity of enzymic catalysis. Another advancing technique is the splicing of genes from different sources to code novel **hybrid enzymes**. Hybrid enzymes may be developed that create new specificities or enhance reaction rates.

This chapter considers the fundamentals of enzymology. The range and nature of enzymic reactions are discussed in addition to a detailed consideration of the essential features of enzyme structure. The measurement of enzymic activity, the mechanisms and kinetics of single-substrate reactions and their inhibition, and multisubstrate reactions are examined. Models of the conformational changes within the subunit structure of allosteric enzymes are described.

Enzyme classification

By the late 1950s, enzyme nomenclature was in confusion. Without a guiding authority, the increase in known enzymes had led to the assignment of misleading or inappropriate names. In many cases the same enzyme had become known by several names, while some catalytically different enzymes had been identically named. In 1961, the first Enzyme Commission reported a system for enzyme classification and the assignment of code numbers. The general principles of the current classification and nomenclature of enzymes are that:

- **enzyme names,** especially those ending in -ase, should be used only for single enzymes, i.e. single catalytic entities;
- **an enzyme is classified and named** according to the specific reaction which it catalyses;
- **enzymes be divided into groups** on the basis of the type of chemical reaction catalysed.

Each enzyme is given a four-number code, e.g. EC 3.1.3.9. The first number designates one of the six main divisions (Table 4.1), the second number indicates the subclass, the third number indicates the sub-subclass and the fourth number is the serial number of the enzyme in its sub-subclass (Table 4.2).

The word **enzyme** was introduced by Kühne in 1878 to refer to the occurrence **in yeast** of something responsible for its fermentative activity. Berzelius, some 50 years earlier, had recognized that there were naturally occurring ferments which promoted chemical reactions and had forwarded the concept of biological catalysis. Berzelius classified the ferments into 'organized' and 'unorganized' on the basis of the presence or absence of intact micro-organisms. Kühne applied the word enzyme to ferments derived from extracts of, or secretions from, yeast, i.e. the 'unorganized ferments'. In 1897, Büchner prepared by filtration of the yeast extracts the first **cell-free** enzymic extract which could catalyse fermentation.

The **chemical nature** of enzymes was controversial. In 1926, Sumner crystallized **urease** from jack bean extracts but the preparation had so little activity that other workers attributed the catalytic effect to an active contaminant rather than the protein. Willstätter, on the other hand, purified **peroxidase** with such high activity that catalysis was demonstrated in preparations which were considered protein-free. During the period from 1930 to 1936, numerous enzymes including pepsin, trypsin and chymotrypsin were crystallized and analysed leading to the acceptance that enzymes are proteins.

The **annual world enzyme production** by the biotechnological industries is currently worth some billion US dollars. The first enzyme preparation for industrial use was patented in 1884 and was a starch-degrading fungal extract from *Aspergillus oryzae*.

The use of **proteases** in detergents to enhance the removal of stains due to biological sources, e.g. blood and gravy, is one of the earliest industrial applications of enzymes. The term 'biological' on soap powder packets reflects the incorporation of a protease. Proteases are also used by restaurants to tenderize meat, by brewers to eliminate haze formation in beer, by bakers to degrade proteins in the dough to improve the texture of the bread and render it **gluten-free**, and by glove manufacturers to render hides soft.

Other enzymes also have industrial uses. For example, a **lipase** is added to washing-up liquids to degrade grease (lipid) or to some cheeses to enhance flavour development. **Pectinase** is used in the jam industry to promote maximal extraction of juice from fruits. **Amylases** may be employed to degrade the starch in certain wallpaper pastes to ease the removal of wallpaper from walls.

Enzyme-catalysed reactions

The effectiveness of enzymes may be appreciated through the comparison of spontaneous chemical reactions and enzyme-catalysed reactions. **In a chemical reaction:**

$$A + B \underset{\nu_2}{\overset{\nu_1}{\rightleftharpoons}} C + D$$

where the **rate or velocity,** ν, of the forward or reverse direction is proportional to the concentrations of the reactants, i.e. $\nu_1 = k_1[A][B]$ or $\nu_2 = k_2[C][D]$, where k_1 and k_2 are individual rate constants. **At equilibrium,** $\nu_1 = \nu_2$ and therefore $k_1[A][B] = k_2[C][D]$,

$$\therefore \frac{k_1}{k_2} = \frac{[C][D]}{[A][B]} = k_{eq}$$

where k_{eq} is the equilibrium constant. The equilibrium constant is a constant for the reaction, whether in the presence or absence of an enzyme. The presence of an enzyme, however, accelerates the attainment of the equilibrium state.

For the reaction to occur, A and B must collide in the correct orientation so that the orbital electrons can reposition to permit product formation. The closer the reactant molecules are the greater the chance of a collision, i.e. high concentrations of reactants augment the reaction. Enzymes promote the reaction by absorbing the reactants on to a polypeptide chain in close proximity and in an orientation which results in an effective concentration of the reactants frequently being present intracellularly in minute quantities.

Kinetic energy

For the reaction to occur A and B must collide with sufficient kinetic energy, i.e. energy of motion. In a solution of any molecular species, the molecules exhibit a range of kinetic energies due to fluctuations during random collisions. At a given time, only a small

Table 4.1   *The six main divisions in enzyme classification*

Number	Division	Catalytic activity
1	Oxidoreductases	Enzymes catalysing oxidoreduction reactions. The substrate is regarded as the hydrogen or electron donor
2	Transferases	Enzymes transferring a group from one compound to another compound
3	Hydrolases	Enzymes catalysing the hydrolytic cleavage of C–O, C–N, C–C plus some other bonds
4	Lyases	Enzymes cleaving C–C, C–O, C–N and other bonds by elimination, leaving double bonds or rings, or conversely adding groups to double bonds
5	Isomerases	Enzymes catalysing geometric or structural changes within one molecule
6	Ligases	Enzymes catalysing the joining together of two molecules coupled with the hydrolysis of a pyrophosphate bond in ATP or a similar triphosphate

Table 4.2 *Some examples of Enzyme Commission classification and coding*

EC No.	Explanation	Recommended name	Reaction	Basis for classification/ systematic name
1.1.1.1	With NAD^+($NADP^+$) as acceptor Acting on CH–OH group of donors Oxidoreductase	Alcohol dehydrogenase	Alcohol $+ NAD^+ =$ aldehyde $\}$ or ketone $\} + NADH$	Alcohol: NAD^+ oxidoreductase
1.2.1.2	With NAD^+($NADP^+$) as acceptor Acting on the aldehyde or oxo group of donors Oxidoreductase	Formate dehydrogenase	Formate $+ NAD^+ =$ $CO_2 + NADH$	Formate: NAD^+ oxidoreductase
2.1.3.3	Carboxyl and carbamoyltransferases Transfer of one-carbon groups Transferase	Ornithine carbamoyltransferase	Carbamoyl phospate $+$ L-ornithine $=$ orthophosphate $+$ L-citrulline	Carbamoyl phosphate: L-ornithine carbamoyltransferase
3.1.3.9	Phosphoric monoester hydrolase Acting on ester bonds Hydrolase	Glucose 6-phosphatase	D-Glucose-6-phosphate $+H_2O =$ D-Glucose $+$ orthophosphate	D-Glucose-6-phosphate phosphohydrolase

percentage of molecules will contain sufficient energy to result in the chemical reaction. The kinetic energy of the molecules can be increased by heating which causes the molecules to move faster and to collide more frequently and with greater impact. During these collisions some of the kinetic energy is converted into internal energy, causing the molecules to vibrate vigorously, enhancing bond breakage. Enzymes, being proteins, cannot exploit this mechanism because of their potential denaturation by heat (Chapter 3). The rate of chemical reaction approximately doubles for every 10°C increase in temperature. This is, however, only true for enzymic reactions within the temperature range in which the enzyme is stable. The proximity of the reactants to each other and the catalytic group on the surface of the enzyme is a positive advantage in the promotion of the reaction.

The transition-state theory

It is considered that, **in energetic terms, the reactants do not directly yield products**. According to the **transition-state theory** (based on the work of Eyring), the reaction proceeds through a high-energy

Enzymes have been employed as **therapeutic agents** in the management of a variety of diseases. **Proteases, amylases and lipases** have long been used in preparations to aid digestion.

Asparaginase has been employed in the treatment of **acute lymphocytic leukaemia** (ALL). The rationale is that normal cells are capable of synthesizing asparagine whereas certain tumour cells including those in ALL are not able to synthesize this amino acyl derivative. Intravenous administration of asparaginase destroys blood asparaginase and thereby lowers the concentration available to the tumour, thus reducing its growth.

Deoxyribonuclease (DNase) is employed in the treatment of **cystic fibrosis**. A major feature of cystic fibrosis is recurrent respiratory infections, particularly due to *Pseudomonas aeroginosa*, which results in the release of large quantities of DNA from destroyed bacteria and dead phagocytic cells of the immune system. The DNA contributes to the viscosity of the mucus which causes some of the distressing symptoms. DNase may be used to degrade the DNA and thin the mucus so that the mucus can be dislodged by the patient's ciliary action.

state called the transition state (Figure 4.1). The kinetic energy of the reactants provides the energy for their delivery to the transition state. The energy required is called the **activation energy** (E_a) which may be evaluated from an Arrhenius plot (log reaction rate versus temperature^{-1}). The transition state is a state of maximum energy not an intermediate compound. At this point, the reaction may proceed to form products or revert to initial state reactants. The concentration of the 'activated complex' at the transition state determines the rate of the chemical reaction. Enzymes achieve their reactions at relatively low temperatures by reducing the activation energy required for the reaction because of the geometry of their reversible binding of the reactants. Although activation energy is lowered, the net energetics of the reaction remains unaltered.

The **stages of an enzyme-catalysed reaction involving only one reactant** can be written as:

$$E + S \rightleftharpoons ES^* \rightleftharpoons ES \rightleftharpoons EX^* \rightleftharpoons EP \rightleftharpoons EP^* \rightleftharpoons P + E$$

where S = reactant called substrate, P = product, ES and EP = enzyme complexes and ES^*, EX^* and EP^* = 'activated complexes' at transition states. For convenience, such reactions are frequently abbreviated to:

$$E + S \rightleftharpoons ES \rightleftharpoons P + E$$

where ES = the enzyme–substrate complex. The concentrations of enzyme [E] and substrate [S] available to form ES will influence the rate of product formation and the product concentration will increase with time until an equilibrium is achieved since the reaction is reversible. Initially, the enzyme will cycle between substrate binding and product release.

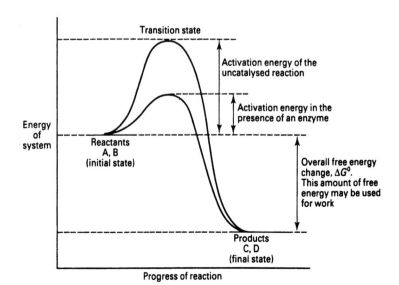

Figure 4.1   *Energy profile for uncatalysed and enzymic reactions*

Proteins as enzymes

To be **classified as an enzyme**, a protein must:

- demonstrate exceptional substrate and product specificity;
- accelerate the reaction rate;
- remain unchanged by the reaction.

The specific region of the convoluted polypeptide chain to which a substrate will bind is termed the **active or catalytic site**. The polypeptide chain may comprise several active sites. Substrates are bound to the active site by chemical bonding or interactions determined by the chemical and physical properties of the amino acids. Within the active site, there are two kinds of functional amino acid residues:

- **contact residues** which function to attract and orientate the substrate and are responsible for the specificity of the enzyme;
- **catalytic residues** which form bonds with the substrate molecule and effect catalytic change.

Assays of enzymic activity

The **catalytic activity** of an enzyme is usually **assayed** by incubating a mixture containing a known [S] and [E] at a suitable pH for an appropriate length of time. The appearance of product (or sometimes the disappearance of substrate) is estimated. A common approach is the measurement of its concentration-dependent capacity to absorb light in a **spectrophotometer** either directly or after a chemical reaction which produces a coloured solution. The activities of enzymes which utilize the coenzymes NAD or NADP in oxidized or reduced forms are generally assayed directly at a **wavelength of 340 nm** where **NAD(P)H** but not $NAD(P)^+$ exhibits an absorbance maximum. If a substrate is converted into a product by an oxidoreductase which requires $NAD(P)^+$, the resultant NAD(P)H may be measured at this wavelength. Where $NAD(P)^+ \rightleftharpoons$ NAD(P)H conversions do not apply, the product may be linked to an additional enzymic reaction which involves these coenzymes.

The activity of enzymes may be expressed in:

- **Katals**, the recommended unit of enzyme activity. One katal is the amount of activity that converts 1 mol of substrate per second. Frequently, the activities are expressed in microkatals (μkat) or nanokatals (nkat), corresponding to reaction rates of μmol s^{-1} and nmol s^{-1} respectively.
- **International units** (IU). One IU is defined as the amount of enzyme which will catalyse the transformation of 1 μmol of substrate per minute under standard conditions.

Abzymes are **catalytic antibodies**. In theory, their therapeutic potential is enormous. For example, as an antiviral vaccine, abzymes may protect hosts by targetting and hydrolysing specifically a single viral protein. An abzyme capable of the hydrolysis of blood clots may prevent heart failure. An abzyme located in plant leaves may absorb and detoxify air-borne pollutants.

The **antigen-binding sites** of antibodies and the **active sites** of enzymes bind their ligands through similar mechanisms, in that both are framed by framework amino acid residues and contain other amino acid residues in direct contact with the ligand (antigen or substrate). However, antibodies do not catalyse reactions normally in living organisms because they usually bind to low-energy structures. However, during an antigen–antibody reaction, the antibody may induce a structural modification in the ligand in which case it binds more strongly to, and stabilizes, these high-energy structures. In 1986, by the development of monoclonal antibodies to designed transition state (high energy) analogues, carboxylic esters were experimentally hydrolysed in a reaction which obeyed enzyme kinetic principles.

Abzymes have also been developed for the hydrolysis of the stronger amide bond and the peptide bond, and for certain isomerizations.

Spectrophotometry is a major technique in biochemistry. It is a powerful tool used primarily in the determination of relatively low concentrations of solutes in solutions, e.g. at nanomolar levels, and to monitor enzymic reactions by the quantification of the formation or disappearance of a light-absorbing substance per unit time.

Visible spectrophotometry utilizes light of a wavelength (λ) between 320 and 800 nm, whereas the usable **ultraviolet spectrum** consists of waves of a length between 200 and 320 nm. Spectrophotometers generate light of the desired wavelength by the use of an appropriate lamp and a diffraction grating. The light beam passes through a cuvette which holds the sample or reference solution. The emergent light is converted by a photocell into a measurable electrical signal which is manifested as a meter reading.

Other related terms are:

- **specific activity** of an enzyme preparation, expressed in $kat\,kg^{-1}$ of protein or $IU\,mg^{-1}$ of protein;
- **molar activity**, given in $kat\,mol^{-1}$ of enzyme;
- **turnover number** of an enzyme, which is the number of molecules of substrate transformed to product per active site of the enzyme per second. Because the maximum reaction rate requires high substrate concentrations to effect the occupancy of all catalytic sites, the turnover number indicates how rapidly the enzyme may convert substrate to product.

A number of **physicochemical parameters** influence the performance of an enzyme during an assay:

- **time**;
- **concentration of enzyme**;
- **concentration of substrate**;
- **pH**;
- **temperature**.

In an enzyme–substrate reaction mixture at a constant temperature, the reaction velocity decreases as a function of **time** (Figure 4.2a). This decline may occur for a number of reasons, e.g. the approach to an equilibrium and the associated influence of the reverse reaction, the depletion of the substrate leads to the reduced occupancy of active sites, the product(s) of the reaction may inhibit the enzyme or change the pH if the medium is inadequately buffered, or the enzyme may undergo progressive inactivation at the temperature or pH of the reaction. Enzymes are therefore studied within their initial velocity range, i.e. at the initial stage before these factors exert an influence on the reaction. The **initial velocity** (ν_0) may be determined from the slope of a tangent to the curve at time zero.

The **rate** of an enzyme-catalysed reaction depends directly on the **concentration of the enzyme** when the substrate is present in excess. This is because of the provision of additional catalytic sites to which the substrate may bind. This results in rate enhancement.

The **substrate concentration** also influences the initial velocity but not in a simple manner (Figure 4.2b). At a constant enzyme concentration, the hyperbolic plot obtained with different initial substrate concentrations shows that the rate is initially proportional to [S], i.e. it is **first order** with respect to substrate. (Regarding the orders of chemical reactions, a reaction is first order when its rate is proportional to the first power of the concentration of just one reactant.) At extremely high substrate concentrations, the reaction rate approaches a constant rate. This is the **maximum velocity** (V or V_{max}) attainable for this particular enzyme concentration. The available active sites of all the enzyme molecules are occupied by the substrate; the enzyme is **saturated**. To increase the rate, additional active sites must be made available by the addition of more enzyme. The **reaction rate at** V is independent of [S] and is therefore **zero order** with respect to substrate. Between the extremities, the reaction is a **mixture of zero- and first-order** kinetics. This behaviour of an enzyme led to the concept of an enzyme–substrate (ES) complex intermediate and the underpinning of modern enzyme kinetics by the Michaelis–Menten equation.

Each enzyme exhibits maximum activity at a characteristic pH called its **optimum pH** (Figure 4.3a). The bell-shaped plot illustrates that limited departures from this pH lead to a reduced enzymic performance due to changes in the ionization of contact and catalytic amino acid residues. In addition, the stability of the enzyme may be compromised by pH-induced conformational changes with loss of activity. pH changes also modify ionic substrates. If a COO^- group of an aspartate is required to bind a positively charged substrate, protonation would reduce the force of attraction and decrease the affinity of the enzyme for the substrate although it becomes more positively charged.

The **temperature** at which an enzymic reaction is measured profoundly affects v_0 (Figure 4.3b). Enzymic reactions occur slowly at $0°C$ because of the low level of molecular kinetic energy which limits substrate–enzyme collisions and the attainment of the transition state. Increasing temperature promotes both these events. The approximately two-fold rate enhancement per $10°C$ rise reflects the activation energy requirement to achieve the transition state. At higher temperatures, product formation declines due to conformational changes in the enzyme by **thermal denaturation** which reduces the effective enzyme concentration. The maximum rate of substrate conversion into product is time-dependent. As the duration of incubation is extended, the plot in Figure 4.3b is displaced to the left, i.e. the optimum temperature is lowered.

As enzymes are globular proteins, their three-dimensional conformation is governed by the bonding arrangements (Chapter 3) which fold the protein in a specific manner and may cause distal amino acid R groups to lie in close proximity. Because of the specific three-dimensional shape of the active site and the nature of the substrate–binding processes, the enzyme may only bind

Spectrophotometry is governed by the **laws of Beer and Lambert** which date from the late eighteenth century. **Lambert's law** states that 'when a ray of monochromatic light passes through an absorbing medium its intensity decreases exponentially as the length of the absorbing medium increases'. The law may be expressed mathematically as $I = I_0 \cdot e^{-k_1 l}$, where I = intensity of the emergent beam of light from the cuvette, I_0 = intensity of the incident beam of light interacting with the solution in the cuvette, I = length of absorbing solution of concentration c, and k_1 = a constant. **Beer's law** is similarly worded but relates intensity of light to the concentration of absorbing medium, i.e. $I = I_0 \cdot e^{-k_2 \cdot c}$. The two laws are combined as **Beer–Lambert's law:** $\frac{I}{I_0} \cdot e^{-k_3 cl}$.

The ratio of the intensities is called **transmittance (T)**, i.e. $T = (I \cdot e^{-k_3 cl})/I_0$, with transmittance usually expressed as a percentage, i.e. $\%T = \left(\frac{I}{I_0}\right) \times 100\%$. By the use of logarithms:

$$\log_e = \frac{I_0}{I} = k_3 cl \therefore \log_{10} \frac{I_0}{I} = 2.303 k_3 cl$$

where $\log_{10} (I_0/I)$ = **absorbance (A)** and $2.303 k_3 = \varepsilon$, **the molar absorption coefficient**, and therefore $A = \varepsilon cl$. A plot of absorbance against concentration produces a linear graph. The use of absorbance rather than transmittance improves the accuracy of readings.

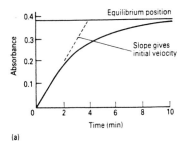

(a)

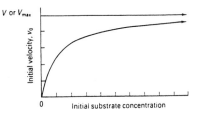

(b)

Figure 4.2 *Some influences on enzyme-catalysed reactions: (a) time; (b) initial substrate concentration*

Figure 4.3 *Some influences on the reaction rate when enzyme and substrate are incubated for a constant time: (a) pH; (b) temperature*

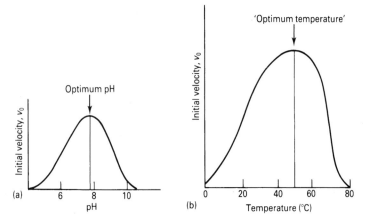

substrates with an appropriate structure. Enzymes exhibit **substrate specificity** of which there are four main classes:

- **absolute specificity** in which an enzyme binds only one biological substrate and catalyses only one of the reactions in which the substance may participate, e.g. glucose-6-phosphate dehydrogenase (Chapter 9);

- **relative (group) specificity** in which certain enzymes can act on a group of structurally similar substrates, e.g. hexokinase (Chapter 9);

- **linkage specificity** in which certain enzymes are specific for a particular type of chemical linkage, e.g. esterases only cleave ester bonds;

- **stereospecificity** in which certain enzymes can differentiate between D- and L-stereoisomers, e.g. arginase only hydrolyses L-arginine (Chapter 13).

Stereospecificity led Fischer in 1894 to propose the **lock-and-key hypothesis** (Figure 4.4a) in which substrates were considered to have a structure complementary to a rigid active site, analogous to a key fitting a lock. Although adequate to explain stereo- and absolute specificity, this model cannot account for relative and linkage specificity. In 1958, Koshland propounded a modification called **the induced-fit model** (Figure 4.4b) in which the contact residues may interact with potential substrates. Following this initial binding, the substrate induces a conformational change in a **flexible active site** to improve the enzyme–substrate fit and locate the catalytic groups.

A variety of methods have been developed to obtain information on the nature of the amino acids at the active site:

- **Identification of the intermediate form of the enzyme.** Phosphoglucomutase (Chapter 9) catalyses the conversion of glucose 1-phosphate to glucose 6-phosphate. **Phosphoserine** has

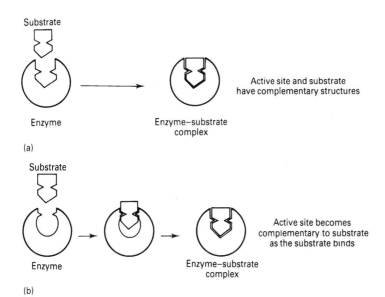

(a)

(b)

Active site and substrate
have complementary structures

Active site becomes
complementary to substrate
as the substrate binds

Figure 4.4 *Two proposed models for the binding of substrate to an enzyme: (a) Fischer's lock and key model; (b) Koshland's induced-fit model*

been identified in this enzyme to demonstrate that serine participates as the intermediate phosphate acceptor.

- **Group-specific reagents.** There are a variety of reagents which can specifically modify functional groups found in enzymes, e.g. **iodoacetate** at pH 5.5 was employed to identify the specific histidyl residues important in the catalytic activity of pancreatic **ribonuclease**. The other histidine residues in this enzyme are less reactive with iodoacetate.

- **Affinity labels.** These substances are complementary in structure to the substrate but incorporate one or more additional reactive groups. Once attached to the active site, the affinity label reacts to bond covalently to a nearby amino acid residue. These substances are designed with consideration of the mechanism of binding and catalysis and are inactive outside the active site. For example, L-1-(*p*-toluenesulphonyl)-amido-2-phenylethylchloromethyl-ketone (**TPCK**) was contrived as an affinity label for the proteolytic enzyme **chymotrypsin** which cleaves preferentially at the carbonyl end of tyrosyl, tryptophanyl, phenylalanyl and leucyl residues. The active site of chymotrypsin contains a **hydrophobic pocket** into which an aromatic residue may enter and bind to position the substrate's polypeptide chain for cleavage. The phenyl group of TPCK mimics the aromatic group of the substrate and stabilizes the enzyme–inhibitor complex by hydrogen bonding between the carbonyl (ketone) group and a seryl residue of the active site. TPCK irreversibly inactivates the enzyme. Subsequent analysis demonstrated the modification of one histidyl residue at position 57.

Proteins are not the only macromolecules capable of enzymic catalysis. In 1982, it was realized that certain RNA molecules had catalytic properties. These catalytic RNAs, called **ribozymes**, satisfied most of the criteria for enzymes. Ribozymes can cleave either the 3′- or 5′-phosphodiester bonds in themselves or other RNA molecules. The folded structure of RNA aligns the normally unreactive groups and bonds in close proximity to each other in the required orientation and stabilizes the transition state to effect the reduction of the activation energy of the reaction.

Ribozymes act in the **processing of pre-rRNA precursors** into mature ribosomal RNA. The protein component of **ribonuclease P**, which removes 5′-extranucleotides from tRNA precursors during the formation of mature tRNA, is devoid of activity *in vitro* but, under appropriate conditions, the purified RNA component may catalyse the reaction. The **peptidyl-transferase** reaction which forms peptide bonds during protein synthesis (Chapter 13) may be catalysed by 23S rRNA in the absence of ribosomal protein. In general, the catalytic rates achieved by ribosomes *in vitro* and *in vivo* are enhanced by the presence of protein. Because of ribozyme activities, it is considered that RNA evolved prior to DNA and protein.

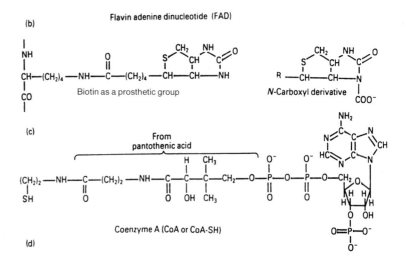

Figure 4.5 *Structures of some coenzymes: (a) nicotinamide adenine dinucleotide (NAD) and nicotinamide adenine dinucleotide phosphate (NADP); (b) flavin adenine dinucleotide (FAD); (c) biotin; (d) coenzyme A*

Cofactors

Sometimes enzyme activity results solely from the nature of the active site, e.g. pancreatic ribonuclease. However, many enzymes require an additional component called a **cofactor** for their activity. This type of enzyme is called a **conjugated enzyme or holoenzyme,** the protein component of which is termed the **apoenzyme** (apoprotein). If the cofactor is tightly bound to the protein molecule by covalent bonds it is called a **prosthetic group.** Cofactors are located in the active site along with the substrate and participate in the catalysis. The cofactor may be inorganic ions, e.g. Fe^{2+}, Zn^{2+}, Mg^{2+}, Cu^{2+}, or K^+ or complex organic molecules called **coenzymes** (Figure 4.5).

Coenzymes generally act as **acceptors or donors** of a functional group or atoms which are removed from or contributed to the substrate. They are frequently large in size in comparison with their functional group. The remainder of the molecule is responsible for their enzyme-binding properties.

All or component parts of some coenzyme molecules may not be synthesized *de novo* in man and are obtained from the diet. The required precursors are called **vitamins** (Table 4.3). The vitamin concept does not apply to photosynthetic organisms which are capable of manufacturing all necessary organic molecules from CO_2.

Steady-state enzyme kinetics

The fundamental theory of enzyme action was proposed in 1913 when Michaelis and Menten developed a mathematical expression to rationalize the hyperbolic plot of initial velocity as a function of substrate concentration.

In man, **zinc** is the second most important trace element after iron. Its earliest discovered biochemical function was as a component of the enzyme **carbonic anhydrase** but now over 100 zinc-containing enzymes are known. Within proteins, zinc may have a catalytic and/or a structural role.

In the case of **catalytic proteins**, the bonding of zinc to the protein, called **zinc coordination**, involves usually three amino acid residues, two of which are closely located and a third more distant along the polypeptide chain. Histidine (H) is the most common ligand, as in carbonic anhydrase, although some enzymes also utilize acidic amino acid residues (D and E). A water molecule which participates in the catalytic reaction is conveniently placed by occupancy of the remaining (fourth) coordination site. Where zinc aids the maintenance of the structural integrity of a protein, all coordination bonds are linked to the protein, usually through cysteinyl residues as in **alcohol dehydrogenase**.

Table 4.3 *Some coenzymes, their functions and precursor requirements*

Coenzyme	Funcion-associated enzymes	Vitamin
Nicotinamide adenine dinucleotide (NAD^+)	Hydrogen transfer (as hydride ions)–dehydrogenase	Nicotinic acid
Nicotinamide adenine dinucleotide phosphate (NAD^+	Hydrogen transfer (as hydride ions)–dehydrogenase	Nicotinic acid
Biotin	CO_2 transfer–carboxylase	Whole molecule
Coenzyme A	Acetyl group transfer–various	Pantothenic acid
Pyridoxal phosphate	Amino group transfer–transaminase	Pyridoxine
Flavin adenine dinucleotide (FAD)	Hydrogen transfer (as hydrogen atoms)–dehydrogenase	Riboflavin
Flavin mononucleotide (FMN)	Hydrogen transfer (as hydrogen atoms)–dehydrogenase	Riboflavin

Michaelis–Menten equation

The **Michaelis–Menten equation** aims to describe the interrelationship between the rate of an enzymic reaction and the concentrations of substrate and enzyme. This is accomplished using the following assumptions:

- The enzyme–substrate complex (ES) is in equilibrium with free enzyme and substrate in solution, i.e. $E + S \rightleftharpoons ES$.
- The formation of this complex is essential for product formation, i.e. $ES \rightarrow P + E$.
- The concentration of enzyme–substrate complex is constant, i.e. in a steady-state in which the formation and breakdown of ES are dynamically balanced. This assumption was incorporated by Briggs and Haldane in 1925.

The current derivation of the Michaelis–Menten equation follows. The objective is to define a general expression for ν_0, the initial velocity of the reaction. From the general equation

$$E + S \underset{k_1}{\overset{k_1}{\rightleftharpoons}} ES \underset{k_2}{\overset{k_2}{\rightleftharpoons}} P + E$$

the initial rate of product formation, $\nu_0 = k_2[ES]$. Unfortunately, k_2 and [ES] cannot be directly measured. Therefore, an alternative expression for ν_0 in measurable variables, e.g. [E] and [S], must be reasoned. This involves the consideration of the formation of ES:

$$\frac{d[ES]}{dt} = k_1[E][S]$$

As the steady state is justifiable only where $[S] > 1000 \times [E]$, the formation of ES in the reverse direction , $P + S \overset{k_{-2}}{\rightarrow} ES$ is ignored as initially it is negligible. Also, the concentrations of free and combined forms of the enzyme should be considered:

$$\frac{d[ES]}{dt} = k_1([E_t] - [ES])[S]$$

where E_t = total enzyme (free and combined forms).

When the breakdown of ES in forward and reverse directions is considered:

$$\frac{-d[ES]}{dt} = k_{-1}[ES] + k_2[ES]$$

In a steady-state, [ES] is constant, and therefore the rate of ES formation = rate of ES breakdown:

$$k_1([E_t] - [ES])[S] = k_{-1}[ES] + k_2[ES]$$

By grouping the constants:

$$\frac{([E_t] - [ES])[S]}{[ES]} = \frac{k_{-1} + k_2}{k_1}$$

The rate constant grouping is denoted by K_m, **the Michaelis constant.**

$$\therefore \frac{([E_t] - [ES])[S]}{[ES]} = K_m$$

Solving for [ES]:

$$\frac{[E_t][S]}{[ES]} - \frac{\cancel{[ES]}[S]}{\cancel{[ES]}} = K_m$$

$$\therefore \qquad \frac{[E_t][S]}{[ES]} - [S] = K_m$$

$$\therefore \qquad \frac{[E_t][S]}{[ES]} = K_m + [S]$$

$$\therefore \qquad \frac{[E_t][S]}{K_m + [S]} = [ES]$$

Since $v_0 = k_2[ES]$, substituting for [ES],

$$v_0 = \frac{k_2[E_t][S]}{K_m + [S]}$$

Also, [S] is so high that essentially all the enzyme is present as ES, i.e. the **enzyme is saturated** and the **maximum velocity, V,** is achievable and $V = k_2[E_t]$

$$\therefore v_0 = \frac{V[S]}{K_m + [S]}$$

This is the Michaelis–Menten equation.

The Michaelis–Menten equation relates the components of an enzymic reaction, [S] and [E], to velocity, initial and maximum, through a rate constant, called K_m, the Michaelis constant, where $K_m = $ (rate of breakdown of the ES complex) / (rate of formation of the ES complex). V is defined as the maximum velocity of the reaction and V is dependent upon [E] which is thereby represented in the equation. Enzyme kinetics is underpinned by this equation which allows the rate of the reaction at any substrate concentration to be calculated if K_m and V are known.

When the reaction rate is equal to 50% of maximum velocity, then $v_0 = V/2$. When substituted into

$$v_0 = \frac{V[S]}{K_m + [S]}, \qquad \frac{V}{2} = \frac{V[S]}{K_m + [S]}$$

Division by V gives:

$$\tfrac{1}{2} = \frac{[S]}{K_m + [S]}$$

and cross multiplication gives:

$$K_m + [S] = 2[S] \therefore K_m = [S]$$

K_m is an important constant because:

90   Biochemistry

Enzymes normally do not operate at saturating concentrations of substrates in cells or body fluids. The ratio of $[S]/K_m$ is likely to be within the range of 0.01–1.00. When $[S]$ is much smaller than K_m:

$$\nu_0 = \frac{V[S]}{K_m + [S]}$$

which approximates to:

$$\nu_0 \sim \frac{V[S]}{K_m} \quad \therefore \quad \nu_0 \sim \frac{K_{cat}}{K_m}[E_t][S]$$

The ratio K_{cat}/K_m is termed the **specificity constant** which provides a measure of the performance of the enzyme at low $[S]$. The specificity constant allows the comparison of the rates of catalysis of different substrates by the same enzyme.

- it is the substrate concentration at which an enzyme demonstrates 50% of its maximum velocity;
- it is the substrate concentration at which half of the active sites of the enzyme are occupied;
- it is a constant characteristic of an enzyme for its conversion of that substrate;
- the smaller the value of K_m the greater the enzyme's affinity for the substrate and the quicker the reaction.

Lineweaver–Burk plot

To estimate K_m and V, the initial rate is measured at several different substrate concentrations. However, the hyperbolic plot of initial velocity as a function of substrate concentration (Figure 4.6a) is inadequate to determine maximum velocity accurately since at a substrate concentration of $10 \times K_m$ only 90% V is achieved. At greater concentrations, additional problems such as substrate insolubility, formation of non-productive ES complexes through substrate inhibition mechanisms and salt effects may be encountered.

To obtain an accurate estimation of V and K_m, enzymologists have rearranged the Michaelis–Menten equation to produce linear plotting methods, e.g. the **Lineweaver–Burk plot** (Figure 4.6b). This popular plot is based on the Lineweaver–Burk equation deduced as follows:

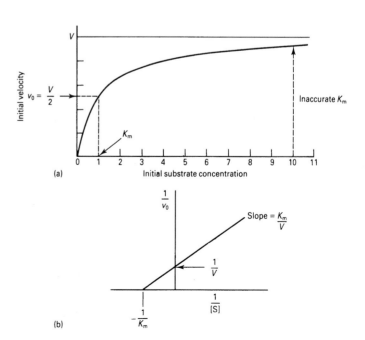

Figure 4.6 *Graphical procedures for the estimation of* V *and* K$_m$*: (a) plot of initial velocity versus substrate concentration; (b) Lineweaver–Burk plot*

$$\nu_0 = \frac{V[S]}{K_m + [S]}$$

Taking reciprocals of both sides:

$$\frac{1}{\nu_0} = \frac{K_m + [S]}{V[S]} \quad \therefore \quad \frac{1}{\nu_0} = \frac{K_m}{V[S]} + \frac{[S]}{V[S]}$$

which reduces to:

$$\frac{1}{\nu_0} = \frac{K_m}{V} \cdot \frac{1}{[S]} + \frac{1}{V}$$

This equation is employed in the plotting method as follows:

If $\dfrac{1}{\nu_0} = 0$, then $0 = \dfrac{K_m}{V} \cdot \dfrac{1}{[S]} + \dfrac{1}{V}$

$$\therefore \quad \frac{K_m}{V} \cdot \frac{1}{[S]} = -\frac{1}{V} \quad \therefore \quad \frac{1}{[S]} = -\frac{\frac{1}{V}}{\frac{K_m}{V}} \quad \therefore \quad \frac{1}{[S]} = -\frac{1}{K_m}$$

If $\dfrac{1}{[S]} = 0$, then $\dfrac{1}{\nu_0} = \dfrac{K_m}{V} \cdot 0 + \dfrac{1}{V} \quad \therefore \quad \dfrac{1}{\nu_0} = \dfrac{1}{V}$

The Lineweaver–Burk plot uses reciprocals of ν_0 and [S] and yields V and K_m as reciprocals at the intercepts of the respective axes. The use of reciprocals results in points nearest to the origin representing the highest rates at highest [S] values and emphasizes less precise measurements at low [S]. The more accurate higher rates are poorly represented. Variations from the characteristic plot may indicate contamination by activators, inhibitors or impurities. Computer packages for the plotting of kinetic data are commercially available.

Enzyme inhibition

In addition to substrate concentration, two groups of compounds alter the rate of an enzymic reaction by specific mechanisms:

- **activators** which combine with an enzyme or enzyme–substrate complex to effect an increase in activity without being modified by the enzyme;
- **inhibitors** which decrease the rate of an enzymic reaction and remain unaltered by the enzyme.

Inhibitors are divided into two categories:

- **irreversible inhibitors** which bind covalently to a functional group at the active site or elsewhere on the enzyme;
- **reversible inhibitors** which are not bound covalently to the enzyme.

Irreversible enzyme inhibitors are usually toxic substances. Irreversible inhibitors may be natural or designed synthetic substances.

The organophosphate **diisopropylfluorophosphate (DFP)** was designed to inhibit serine proteases by interaction with the hydroxyl group of the catalytic seryl residue to form a covalent adduct. DFP therefore inhibits irreversibly any enzyme whose catalytic site contains this essential seryl residue, e.g. acetylcholinesterase.

Acetylcholinesterase is crucial for nervous conduction, its inhibition resulting in the loss of motor or sensory function. Numerous insecticides and nerve gases, e.g. sarin, were based upon DFP. Sarin was employed in the terrorist attack on Tokyo underground railway system in March 1995 which resulted in ten deaths.

DFP and sarin are examples of **transition state analogues**, i.e. molecules which resemble the transition state. Other irreversible inhibitors closely resemble the substrate, e.g. **TPCK** was designed as an affinity label for chymotrypsin to allow the phenyl group to fit into a pocket in the enzyme's catalytic site.

Among the natural irreversible inhibitors are the **penicillin antibiotics** which inhibit a serine-containing enzyme responsible for linking the pentaglycine bridge to the tetrapeptide side chain during the biosynthesis of the bacterial cell wall (Chapter 5).

Irreversible inhibition

Irreversible inhibitors bind covalently to some functional group of the enzyme and permanently prevent their activity. The substrate is either hindered from entering the active site or is not converted into product and leaves the active site unchanged. In this type of inhibition, the effective concentration of the enzyme declines progressively as irreversible covalent bonding occurs. For this reason, irreversible inhibition cannot be analysed by Michaelis–Menten kinetics. This type of inhibition is frequently used to obtain information regarding the functional amino acids at the active site, e.g. in affinity labels.

Suicide inhibition is a form of irreversible inhibition in which the substrate in the first catalytic cycle is converted into a chemically reactive product which remains covalently bound to the active site, thereby rendering the enzyme permanently inactive. Such inhibitors have potential as designed therapeutic agents with minimal side-effects. For example, **difluoromethylornithine** (DFMO) is a suicide inhibitor of **ornithine decarboxylase**. In mammalian cells, ornithine decarboxylase is rapidly degraded and replaced by continuous synthesis of the enzyme. In trypanosomes, this enzyme is stable and is not subjected to rapid turnover. DFMO has proved effective against the parasitic disease, trypanosomiasis (African sleeping sickness).

Reversible inhibition

Reversible inhibition is characterized by an equilibrium between free and inhibitor-bound enzymic forms. Steady-state kinetics may therefore be applied to the analysis of these inhibitions. The inhibitor may be removed from the enzyme–inhibitor (EI) complex by simple methods, e.g. dialysis, to deliver active enzymes. Various forms of reversible inhibition have been identified through kinetic studies:

- **competitive inhibition** in which the inhibitors have an effect on the K_m but not on the V of an enzyme;
- **non-competitive inhibition** which is characterized by a change in the V but not on the K_m of an enzyme;
- **uncompetitive inhibition** which is characterized by equal effects on both V and K_m of an enzyme.

Competitive inhibitors often bear a structural similarity to the substrate and compete with the substrate for the active sites of the enzyme, e.g. malonate inhibition of succinate dehydrogenase. However, competitive inhibitors are not necessarily structurally analogous to the substrate, e.g. salicylate inhibition of 3-phosphoglycerate kinase (Chapter 9).

In competitive inhibition, the V is unchanged because the number of functional active sites is not altered but a greater substrate concentration is required to achieve the maximum utilization of the sites. Consequently, the K_m for the substrate increases. Competitive inhibition may therefore be overcome by the addition of more substrate to the enzyme reaction mixture.

Non-competitive inhibition is not reversed by additions of substrate. This type of inhibition occurs when an inhibitor binds to a site other than the active site on the free enzyme or ES complex. Non-competitive inhibitors interfere with either the formation of ES complex or its breakdown to yield product. Examples include heavy metal ions, e.g Hg^{2+} and Pb^{2+}, which bind to strategically positioned sulphydryl groups and modulate the conformation of the enzyme. This mechanism is more common in reactions involving more than one substrate.

Uncompetitive inhibitors bind only to a formed ES complex. This inhibition mechanism is rare in one-substrate reactions but may occur as a type of product inhibition in reactions with multiple substrates and products.

Figure 4.7 illustrates the mechanistic and plot differences between the above reversible inhibitions. Table 4.4 summarizes the effect of inhibitors on Lineweaver–Burk plot parameters which are modified by the factor $[1 + ([I]/K_i)]$ where K_i is the inhibition constant. The inhibition constant varies according to the type of inhibition, e.g. in competitive inhibition $K_i = ([E][I])/[EI]$. Graphical methods are available for the estimation of K_i.

Multisubstrate reactions

Most enzymes catalyse **multisubstrate**, rather than single-substrate, **reactions**. Multisubstrate reactions may proceed by different mechanisms:

- **Random substrate-binding mechanism** in which either substrate, S_1 or S_2 may be the first to bind to the enzyme (Figure 4.8a). However, usually one of the substrates is preferred for initial binding. The ES_1S_2 complex when formed generates the products, P_1 and P_2 which vacate the enzyme. Hexokinase (Chapter 9) phosphorylates glucose by this mechanism although glucose tends to bind before the ATP molecule.

- **Ordered substrate binding mechanism** in which one of the substrates, S_1 must bind to the enzyme forming an enzyme–substrate complex, ES_1 prior to significant binding of the second substrate, S_2 (Figure 4.8b). The ES_1S_2 complex creates the products, P_1 and P_2. Many dehydrogenase enzymes employing NAD^+ as coenzyme proceed by this mechanism.

- **Ping-pong mechanism** in which one substrate, S_1, is bound to the enzyme and one product, P_1, is produced and released before a second substrate, S_2, enters the catalytic site to produce a second product, P_2 (Figure 4.8c). The mechanism is so-called because of

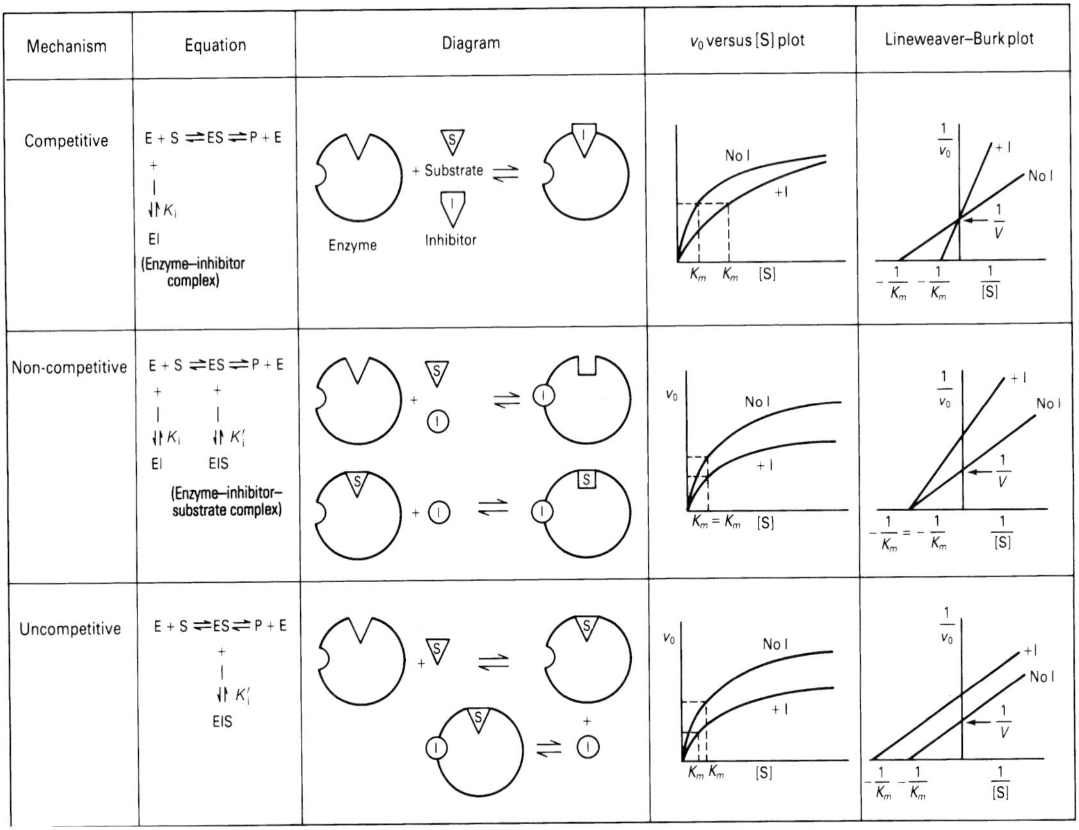

Mechanism	Equation	Diagram	v_0 versus [S] plot	Lineweaver–Burk plot
Competitive	$E + S \rightleftharpoons ES \rightleftharpoons P + E$ $+$ I $\updownarrow K_i$ EI (Enzyme–inhibitor complex)	+ Substrate $\rightleftharpoons$ Enzyme Inhibitor	No I / +I curves; axes K_m, K_m, [S]	$\frac{1}{v_0}$ axis, +I, No I; intercepts $\frac{1}{-K_m}$, $\frac{1}{K_m}$, $\frac{1}{[S]}$, $\frac{1}{V}$
Non-competitive	$E + S \rightleftharpoons ES \rightleftharpoons P + E$ $+$ $+$ I I $\updownarrow K_i$ $\updownarrow K_i'$ EI EIS (Enzyme–inhibitor–substrate complex)	$+ \rightleftharpoons$ $+ \rightleftharpoons$	v_0; No I / +I; $K_m = K_m$ [S]	$\frac{1}{v_0}$ axis, +I, No I; $-\frac{1}{K_m} = -\frac{1}{K_m}$, $\frac{1}{[S]}$, $\frac{1}{V}$
Uncompetitive	$E + S \rightleftharpoons ES \rightleftharpoons P + E$ $+$ I $\updownarrow K_i'$ EIS	$+ \rightleftharpoons$ $+ \rightleftharpoons$	v_0; No I / +I; K_m K_m [S]	$\frac{1}{v_0}$ axis, +I, No I; $-\frac{1}{K_m}$, $-\frac{1}{K_m}$, $\frac{1}{[S]}$, $\frac{1}{V}$

Figure 4.7 *Mechanisms of reversible inhibition*

Table 4.4 *Intercepts on axes of Lineweaver–Burk plot in the absence and presence of inhibitors*

	Intercept on $1/v$ axis	Intercept on $1/[S]$ axis	Slope
No inhibitor	$\dfrac{1}{V}$	$\dfrac{-1}{K_m}$	$\dfrac{K_m}{V}$
Competitive inhibitor	$\dfrac{1}{V}$	$\dfrac{-1}{K_m\left(1 + \dfrac{[I]}{K_i}\right)}$	$\dfrac{K_m}{V}\left(1 + \dfrac{[I]}{K_i}\right)$
Non-competitive* inhibitor	$\dfrac{1}{V}\left(1 + \dfrac{[I]}{K_i}\right)$	$\dfrac{-1}{K_m}$	$\dfrac{K_m}{V}\left(1 + \dfrac{[I]}{K_i}\right)$
Uncompetitive inhibitor	$\dfrac{1}{V}\left(1 + \dfrac{[I]}{K_i'}\right)$	$\dfrac{-1}{K_m\left(1 + \dfrac{[I]}{K_i'}\right)}$	$\dfrac{K_m}{V}$

* K may be K_i or K_i' depending on mechanism.

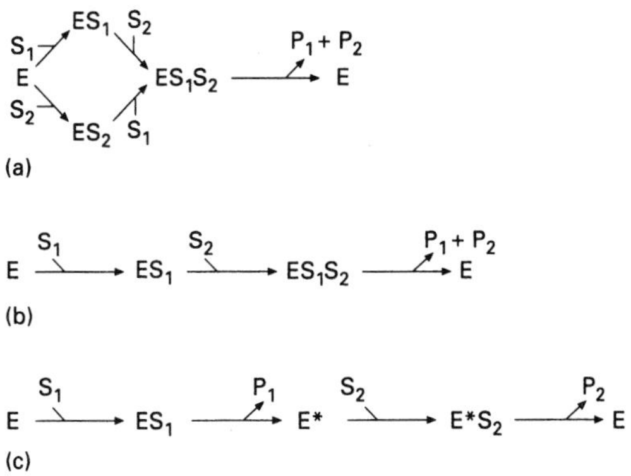

$$S_1 \nearrow \overset{ES_1 \quad S_2}{\searrow}$$
$$E \qquad \overset{}{\underset{ES_1S_2}{\longrightarrow}} \xrightarrow{P_1 + P_2} E$$
$$S_2 \searrow \underset{ES_2 \quad S_1}{\nearrow}$$

(a)

$$E \xrightarrow{S_1} ES_1 \xrightarrow{S_2} ES_1S_2 \xrightarrow{P_1 + P_2} E$$

(b)

$$E \xrightarrow{S_1} ES_1 \xrightarrow{P_1} E^* \xrightarrow{S_2} E^*S_2 \xrightarrow{P_2} E$$

(c)

Figure 4.8 *Mechanisms of enzymic reactions involving two substrates; (a) random substrate-binding mechanism; (b) ordered substrate-binding mechanism; (c) ping-pong mechanism*

the transition between enzyme and modified enzyme (E^*) which may involve the retention of a fragment of the initial substrate at the catalytic site. The reactions catalysed by UDP-glucose-1-phosphate uridylyltransferase, pyruvate carboxylase and acetyl-CoA carboxylase (Chapters 9, 10 and 12) are examples of this mechanism.

The properties of enzymes catalysing two-substrate reactions can be studied by varying the concentration of each substrate in the presence of a saturating concentration of the other substrate and employing standard graphical procedures such as the Lineweaver–Burk plot.

Mechanisms of enzyme action

The chemistry involved in substrate transformation varies among enzymes. **Four major factors** have been advanced to account for the catalytic power of enzymes:

- **Proximity and orientation effects.** Substrates may interact with the enzyme and be positioned close to each other, close to the catalytic group and accurately oriented to minimize the activation energy requirement for entry into the transition state.

- **Distortion or strain effects.** According to the induced-fit model, the substrate may induce conformational changes in the active site of the enzyme. Positional movements in the polypeptide chain may distort or stretch pertinent bonds in the substrate, contributing to the attainment of the transition state.

- **General acid–base catalysis.** The R groups of certain amino acids at the active site may donate protons to or accept protons from bound substrates. Although such mechanisms are pH-dependent, they are augmented by the internal non-aqueous environment of many enzymes which influences the acidity or basicity of amino, carboxylate, sulphydryl, imidazole and phenolic R groups. When

Figure 4.9 *Covalent catalysis: (a) nucleophilic attack by the enzyme; (b) electrophilic attack by the enzyme*

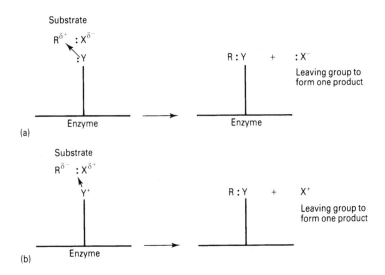

protonated, they behave as acidic catalysts and their unprotonated forms act as basic catalysts.

- **Covalent catalysis.** Substrates may bind to the enzyme by temporary unstable covalent bonds which implies a modulation of the electronic arrangement of both the substrate and the enzyme. The reactive groups involved are described as nucleophiles and electrophiles. Nucleophilic groups are electron-rich and deliver electrons to electropositive substrates (Figure 4.9a). Potential nucleophilic groups are the hydroxyls of serine and tyrosine, the carboxylates of aspartate and glutamate, the imidazole of histidine and sulphydryl of cysteine. Enzymic electrophilic groups are electron-deficient and attract electrons from the substrate (Figure 4.9b). Although there are no strongly electrophilic amino acid R groups, inorganic ionic cofactors, e.g. Mg^{2+} and Fe^{3+} or coenzymes, e.g. NAD^+, may act as an electrophile.

The mechanism of action of lysozyme employs both distortion of the polysaccharide chain and general acid–base catalysis. Lysozyme is a single polypeptide chain of 129 residues which may effect bacterial lysis through cleavage of the peptidoglycan of the cell wall (Chapter 5). Investigations with *N*-acetylglucosamine oligomers have revealed that increasing the number of residues from four to five markedly increases the rate of catalysis with further enhancement on the addition of a sixth residue. The distortion in the fourth residue is believed to reduce the activation energy which contributes to the effectiveness of the hydrolysis of the glycosidic linkage between the fourth and fifth residues. The hydrolysis is effected by general acid–base catalysis in which a glutamyl residue at position 35 acts as an acid and donates its proton to the oxygen atom of the glycosidic bond. At the end of the catalytic cycle, the same glutamyl residue receives one H^+ and is restored to its acidic form.

The **mechanism of action of the serine protease enzymes** employs both general acid–base and covalent catalyses. The serine proteases are a group of enzymes, which include chymotrypsin, trypsin, elastase, thrombin, plasmin and subtilisin, so named because their catalytic activity is dependent upon a seryl residue in the active site.

Multisubunit enzymes

Two aspects pertaining to multisubunit enzymes will be considered:

- **allosteric enzymes** are regulatory enzymes, the catalytic activity of which is determined by the non-covalent binding of a molecular modulator at a site other than the catalytic site;
- **isoenzymes** are multiple enzymic forms which catalyse the same reaction.

The two categories are not mutually exclusive; some allosteric enzymes are also isoenzymes, e.g. pyruvate kinase (Chapter 9).

Allosteric enzymes

Some enzymes, when their initial velocity is plotted as a function of substrate concentration, do not show a hyperbolic curve (Figure 4.2b) but **a sigmoidal curve** (Figure 4.10). The rate of the reaction catalysed by these enzymes at a given [S] is:

- **increased** by the addition of a specific **activator**;
- **decreased** by the addition of a specific **inhibitor**.

In the presence of an activator, the curve tends towards a hyperbola (Figure 4.10a), whilst in the presence of an inhibitor, the curve becomes more sigmoidal (Figure 4.10b).

Enzymes which exhibit this behaviour are called **allosteric enzymes** based on a concept developed earlier to explain the oxygenation/deoxygenation of haemoglobin (Chapter 3). In addition to the catalytic site, most allosteric enzymes possess other sites to which the activators or inhibitors, called **allosteric effectors,** may bind and influence catalytic events through induced conformational changes in the enzyme (Figure 4.11).

Most allosteric enzymes contain numerous subunits. In most of these enzymes, e.g. pyruvate carboxylase (Chapter 10), both catalytic and regulatory sites are located on the same polypeptide chain whilst some, e.g. aspartate carbamoyltransferase, carry the catalytic and regulatory sites on different subunits. Through the sigmoidal shape of their ν_0 against [S] plot, X-ray crystallographic and other studies, it is known that many allosteric enzymes display **cooperativity** of substrate binding even in the absence of allosteric effectors. This cooperativity may be:

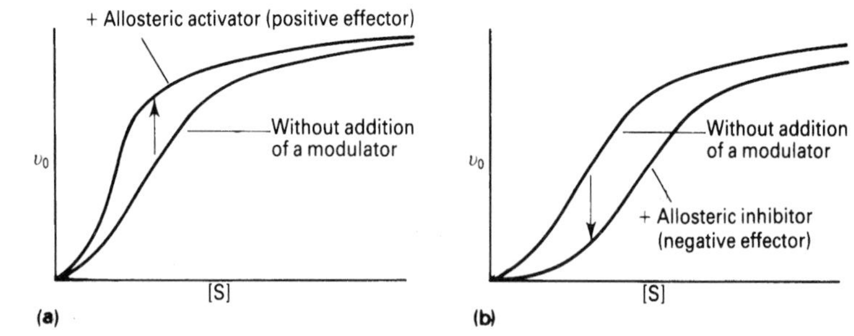

Figure 4.10 *Effect of substrate concentration on the initial velocity of an allosteric enzyme in the absence and presence of specific modulators: (a) allosteric activation; (b) allosteric inhibition*

Figure 4.11 *Induced conform-ational change in an allosteric enzyme*

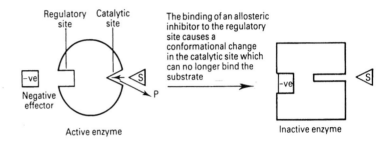

- **positive cooperativity** in which the occupancy of the first binding site facilitates the subsequent binding to other sites;
- **negative cooperativity** in which successive binding occurs with decreasing ease.

A plot of $\log v_0/(v - v_0)$ as a function of $\log$ [S], called a **Hill plot,** may be used to determine the cooperativity of an allosteric enzyme. The slope of the straight line in the central portion of the graph is known as the **Hill coefficient** (n_h). When $n_h = 1$, the enzyme is non-cooperative; when $n_h > 1$ is greater than 1 the enzyme exhibits positive cooperativity, and when $n_h < 1$ the enzyme displays negative cooperativity.

An allosteric enzyme may be termed:

- **heterotropic** where the effector and the substrate are different ligands;
- **homotropic** where the substrate creates a positive cooperative effect by binding to the catalytic sites rather than to distinct allosteric sites.

Homotropic cooperativity is advantageous in the utilization of accumulated substrate and may also be useful because it enables larger rate changes for smaller changes in the substrate concentration. The structure of the allosteric enzyme is therefore particularly suited to a role in the regulation of metabolic pathways.

Two main models form the basis of approaches to explain the sigmoidal relationship between ν_0 and [S] (Figure 4.10) in molecular terms:

- **the concerted (or symmetry) model** of Monod, Wyman and Changeux (MWC) cannot account for negative cooperativity.
- **the sequential model** of Koshland, Némethy and Filmer (KNF) may account for negative cooperativity.

Although most allosteric enzymes are composed of at least four subunits, for simplicity the principles of the **KNF model** will be outlined employing a dimer. The sequential model (Figure 4.12) is an extension of the principle of induced fit (Figure 4.4b). The effectors modify subunit conformation directly and not through a shift in an assumed equilibrium between two forms. This model proposed that **ligand-binding sites** within analogous conformations may have differing affinities for the same ligand. The binding of an effector to its allosteric site in one subunit induces conformational changes within that subunit which then induces conformational changes in the other subunit.

If the effector is an **activator** (Figure 4.12a), its binding to the first subunit effects a conformational change that enhances substrate binding to the same subunit and which induces a conformational change in the second subunit to increase its affinity initially for the activator and then for substrate. **Inhibitors** function by lowering the affinity of the active sites for the substrate through conformational changes in both subunits (Figure 4.12b).

Isoenzymes

Isoenzymes (also called isozymes or isotypes) are families of enzymes which catalyse the same reaction but differences in their amino acid composition modify the rate at which each molecular species transforms the substrate. Most isoenzymes are oligomeric proteins. Isoenzymes may be divided into:

- **primary isoenzymes** which are the products of multiple gene loci which code for distinct protein molecules or the products of multiple alleles at a single gene locus (and are called alloenzymes);
- **secondary isoenzymes** which are derived by post-translational modifications including glycosylation.

Primary isoenzymes may be detected by differences in their electrophoretic mobility because variations in their primary structure are reflected in their ionic character.

Lactate dehydrogenase (LDH) is a primary isoenzyme which catalyses reversibly the oxidation of lactate to pyruvate. Five major tetrameric isoenzymes of human LDH have been identified. Two chains, A and B, form two homogeneous and three hetero-

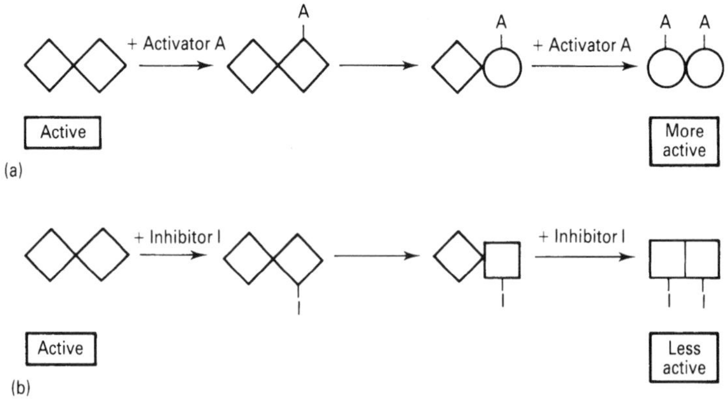

Figure 4.12 *The sequential model of Koshland, Némethy and Filmer (KNF). Allosteric effect of: (a) an activator; and (b) an inhibitor*

geneous types which are denoted as LDH_1 (A_4), LDH_2 (A_3B), LDH_3 (A_2B_2), LDH_4 (AB_3) and LDH_5(B_4), the subunit composition being shown in parentheses. LDH_1 and LDH_5 predominate in heart muscle and liver respectively. The A_4 type has the lowest K_m for pyruvate as substrate whilst the B_4 type has the highest K_m for pyruvate. The other isoenzymes exhibit kinetics relative to the proportions of each type of subunit. The tissue distribution of LDH isoenzymes, however, demonstrates major variations from species to species which makes a rational kinetic-based explanation of the physiological roles of these isoenzymes difficult. Rather than variations in enzymic kinetics, other biological advantages such as differential binding to subcellular organelles or differential rates of protein degradation may be important.

Suggested further reading

Marino, A. and Fedriani, J.R. (1996). Enzeduc 1.0: a user-friendly software package for computation of hyperbolic enzyme kinetic data in biochemical education. *Computer Methods and Programs in Biomedicine* 49, 131–135.

Scott, W.G. and Klug, A. (1996). Ribozymes: structures and mechanisms in RNA catalysis. *Trends in Biochemical Sciences* 21, 220–224.

Wagg, J. and Sellers, P.H. (1996). Enzyme kinetics: thermodynamic constraints on assignment of rate coefficients to kinetic models. *Annals of New York Academy of Science* 779, 272–278.

Cornish-Bowden, A. (1995). *Fundamentals of Enzyme Kinetics.* Colchester: Portland Press.

Webb, E.C. (1992). *Enzyme Nomenclature: Recommendations of the Nomenclature Committee of the International Union of Biochemistry and Molecular Biology on the Nomenclature and Classification of Enzymes.* San Diego: Academic Press.

Isoenzyme levels may be employed in the **diagnosis of clinical disorders**. In man, most organs demonstrate different isoenzyme patterns. Since **LDH_1** is a cytoplasmic isoenzyme and predominates in cardiac muscle, its levels increase significantly in the blood circulation after a heart attack because of its release from damaged cells. However, LDH_1 peaks at 3 days and remains elevated for at least 10 days.

   Creatine kinase (CK) is also released during myocardial infarction. The **myocardial-bound (MB) isoenzyme** of CK is specific for cardiac muscle damage and has the advantage of peaking within 24 h. It normally returns to baseline level within 48 h. This profile of release renders the MB isoenzyme useful in the early detection of heart attacks. The quantity of isoenzyme release correlates with the severity of the infarction.

Gutfreund, H. (1995). *Kinetics for Life Sciences*. Cambridge: Cambridge University Press.

Self-assessment questions

1. List four differences between enzymic and chemical catalysts.
2. Distinguish between competitive and non-competitive reversible inhibition in terms of inhibitor binding to the enzyme.
3. The molar absorption coefficient for ATP is 1.54×10^4 litre mol^{-1} cm^{-1} at a wavelength of 259 nm. Calculate the concentration of ATP in a solution which gives an absorbance reading of 0.154 at $\lambda_{259\,nm}$.
4. The initial velocity of an enzyme-catalysed reaction was measured at various substrate concentrations in the presence and absence of an inhibitor. From the following experimental data, using a suitable plot, determine: (a) the type of inhibition; (b) K_m of the enzyme; (c) V of the reaction.

Substrate concentration (mM)	Product (mg min^{-1})	
	No inhibitor	1 mM inhibitor
0.5	0.775	0.510
0.3	0.637	0.420
0.2	0.526	0.341
0.125	0.388	0.256
0.083	0.293	0.191

5. (a) Draw the structure of NADH. (b) How may NADH as a coenzyme be exploited in the assays of dehydrogenases?
6. With reference to allosteric enzymes, explain what is meant by positive and negative cooperativity.
7. In an assay of lactate dehydrogenase (LDH) activity, 0.38 ml of Tris buffer (0.1 mol l^{-1}, pH 7.4) containing 0.0035 mol l^{-1} NADH were added to two acrylic microcuvettes and followed by the addition of 0.1 ml sodium pyruvate (0.021 mol l^{-1}). After equilibration at 25°C, 20 µl of a prewarmed LDH solution were added to one microcuvette (an equal volume of Tris buffer without NADH was added to the other microcuvette) and both microcuvettes were incubated for 10 min before the reaction was stopped. The absorbances were read spectrophotometrically at $\lambda_{340\ nm}$ against a reference solution containing buffer, pyruvate and LDH but devoid of NADH. The absorbance of the solution lacking LDH was 0.80 and the reading of that containing LDH was 0.66. (a) What is the substrate in this reaction? (b) The molar absorption coefficient for NADH at 340 nm is 6.22×10^3 litre mol^{-1} cm^{-1}. Calculate how many nanomoles of lactate were produced in the LDH-containing microcuvette?

8. Malonate, oxaloacetate and pyrophosphate are inhibitors of succinate dehydrogenase. Draw the structures of the reactant, product and inhibitors (Figures 8.2, 10.4 and 12.6 will assist.) By what kind of mechanisms do they inhibit the enzyme? Explain the logic applied in developing your answer.

9. What is the relationship between vitamins and coenzymes?

10. Derive the Michaelis–Menten equation from the equation:

$$\text{E} + \text{S} \underset{k_1}{\overset{k_1}{\rightleftharpoons}} \text{ES} \underset{k_2}{\overset{k_2}{\rightleftharpoons}} \text{P} + \text{E}.$$

Key Concepts and Facts

Enzymic Reactions
- Enzymes are proteins which accelerate the rates of reactions in biological systems.

- There is an international system of enzyme classification and assignment of code numbers.

- The equilibrium constant is constant for the reaction in the absence or presence of an enzyme.

- An enzyme reaction proceeds through a high-energy transition state and the formation of an enzyme–substrate complex.

- Enzymic activity is often measured spectrophotometrically.

- Enzymic activity may be influenced by a number of physico-chemical parameters.

- Enzymes may demonstrate absolute, relative, stereo- or linkage specificity.

- Many enzymes require an additional cofactor for activity.

Steady-State Enzyme Kinetics
- Enzyme kinetics is based upon the Michaelis–Menten equation.

- K_m and V may be determined using the Lineweaver–Burk plot.

- Reversible enzyme inhibitors can be classified according to their influence on K_m and V of a reaction into competitive, non-competitive and uncompetitive inhibitors.

- Most reactions in biological systems involve more than one substrate.

Enzyme Catalysis
- The catalytic power of enzymes may be ascribed to proximity and orientation effects, distortion, general acid–base principles and covalent catalyses.

Multisubunit Enzymes
- The catalytic activity of an allosteric enzyme is modulated by conformational changes in the constituent polypeptide chain(s).

- Allosteric effectors may bind to a site other than the catalytic site.

- Allosteric enzymes produce a sigmoid curve on plotting ν_0 against [S].

- Isoenzymes are families of structurally different enzymes which catalyse the same reaction.

Answers to questions (Chapter 4)

1. Enzymes absorb the reactants on to a polypeptide chain; enzymes will denature on heating, enzymes reduce the activation energy; enzymes form an ES complex.
2. In competitive inhibition, I normally competes with S for the active site. In non-competitive inhibition, I binds to a site other than the active site.
3. $10 \, \mu mol \, l^{-1}$:

$$A = \varepsilon cl \quad \therefore \quad c = \frac{A}{\varepsilon l} = \frac{0.154}{1.54 \times 10^4 \times 1 \, litre \, mol^{-1} \, cm^{-1} \, cm}$$

$$= \frac{0.154}{1.54 \times 10^4} \, mol \, l^{-1}$$

$$\therefore \quad c = 1 \times 10^{-5} \, mol \, l^{-1} = 10 \, \mu mol \, l^{-1}$$

4. Using the Lineweaver–Burk plot, put [S] and ν_0 into reciprocals:

$1/[S] \, (mM^{-1})$	2.00	3.33	5.00	8.00	12.00
$1/\nu_0$ minus inhhibition $(min \, mg^{-1})$	1.29	1.57	1.90	2.58	3.41
$1/\nu_0$ with inhibition $(min \, mg^{-1})$	1.96	2.38	2.93	3.90	5.24

Plot graph and extrapolate to cut the $1/\nu_0$ axis and meet the $1/[S]$ axis.
(a) Inhibition is non-competitive (compare with Figure 4.6).
(b) Intercept on the $1/[S]$ axis: $-1/K_m = -3.9 \, mM^{-1}$ $\therefore \; K_m = 1/3.9 \, mM = 2.56 \times 10^{-4} \, mol \, l^{-1}$.
(c) Using the intercept on the $1/\nu_0$ axis of uninhibited plot: $1/V = 0.83 \, min \, mg^{-1} \; \therefore \; V = 1/0.83 \, min \, mg^{-1} = 1.2 \, mg \, min^{-1}$.
5. (a) See Figure 4.5a. (b) NADH absorbs light at 340nm whereas at this wavelength the oxidized form, NAD^+, does not. When NADH is oxidized, the spectrophotometric reading will decrease. If NADH is produced, the reading will increase.
6. Positive cooperativity is the phenomenon in which ligand or substrate binding to one subunit assists binding to another subunit; negative cooperativity is the phenomenon in which ligand or substrate binding to one subunit impedes binding to another subunit.
7. (a) Pyruvate. (b) 11.25 nmol:

$$A = \varepsilon cl \quad \therefore \quad c = \frac{A}{\varepsilon l} = \frac{0.80 - 0.66}{6.22 \times 10^3 \times 1 \, litre \, mol^{-1} \, cm^{-1} \, cm}$$

$$= \frac{0.14}{6.22 \times 10^3} \, mol \, l^{-1}$$

$$\therefore \quad c = 0.0225 \times 10^{-3} \, mol \, l^{-1} = 2.25 \times 10^{-5} \, mol \, l^{-1}$$

But volume in a tube $= 0.5 \, ml$

$$\therefore \quad c = 2.25 \times 10^{-5} \times 10^{9} \times \frac{0.5}{1000} \text{ nmol} \quad (\text{mol} \rightarrow \text{nmol} = 10^{9})$$

$$= 11.25 \text{ nmol}$$

8.

| succinate | | fumarate | malonate | oxaloacetate | pyrophosphate |

They are all competitive inhibitors of succinate dehydrogenase. The inhibitors all achieve their effects by ionic bonding to the contact amino acid residues.

9. Vitamins provide structures which cannot be biosynthesized by the organism but are necessary for the synthesis of coenzymes.

10. See text.

Chapter 5
Carbohydrates

Learning objectives

After studying this chapter you should confidently be able to:

Identify important carbohydrates as monosaccharides, oligosaccharides and polysaccharides.

Construct a series of monosaccharides from simpler sugars.

Discuss the cyclization of pentoses and hexoses.

Describe oligosaccharides and polysaccharides in terms of monomers and glycosidic bonds.

Describe the impact of the nature of the glycosidic bond on the shape of polysaccharides.

Describe the major features of important homoglycans.

Describe the salient features of the glycosaminoglycans of the extracellular matrix.

Discuss the structures of the peptidoglycans of Gram-positive and Gram-negative bacterial cell walls.

Carbohydrates are substances containing carbon, hydrogen and oxygen which conform to the empirical formula, $C_x(H_2O)_y$, where x and y equal 3 or more. One of the carbon atoms forms a carbonyl (aldehyde or ketone) group whilst the other carbon atoms exhibit hydroxyl groups. The term carbohydrate is used to describe those substances which are more accurately defined as **polyhydroxyaldehydes or polyhydroxyketones** with the definition extended to include their derivatives and the products of their polymerization by condensation reactions.

Carbohydrates may be divided into **monosaccharides, oligosaccharides and polysaccharides** (Chapter 1). Polysaccharides may be subdivided into various **homopolysaccharides** and **heteropolysaccharides** on the basis of whether their structure yields on hydrolysis one or more type(s) of monosaccharide(s).

This chapter considers the structures and properties of major monosaccharides, oligosaccharides, polysaccharides, glycosaminoglycans and the peptidoglycans of bacterial cell walls.

Monosaccharides

Monosacharides are the simplest carbohydrates; they conform to the general chemical formula $(CH_2O)_x$ and are termed simple sugars.

The open-chain structures of monosaccharides

The **major aspects** of the commonly occurring open-chain monosaccharides are that:

- **They comprise three to six carbon atoms** in an **unbranched** single-bonded chain.
- **A monosaccharide containing an aldehyde group** is referred to as an **aldose.**
- **A monosaccharide containing a ketone group** is termed a **ketose.**
- **A three-carbon sugar** is called a **triose.** The term **aldotriose** or **ketotriose** identifies the functional group. Sugars with four, five or six carbon atoms are termed **tetroses, pentoses** or **hexoses** respectively.
- **Monosaccharides are water soluble** and are insoluble in nonpolar solvents.

Glyceraldehyde (Figure 1.6) **and glycerone (dihydroxyacetone)** are considered to be the simplest aldose and ketose respectively. From these trioses, the **homologous series** of the monosaccharides may be constructed. Glyceraldehyde exists in two stereoisomeric forms D and L (Chapter 1), which serve as the precursors from which the D- and L-series of aldoses arise. Each aldose series may be chemically constructed or dismantled in a stepwise manner:

- the **Kiliani–Fischer nitrile synthesis** introduces a chiral carbon (H–C–OH or HO–C–H) at position 2 in the carbon chain (C-2);
- the **Wohl degradation** removes a chiral carbon at C-2 in the carbon chain.

Since in biological systems, the D-forms of sugars predominate, the D-series of aldoses is presented in Figure 5.1 using **Fischer projection formulae.** The configuration of the penultimate carbon from the carbonyl carbon atom determines the series to which the sugar belongs.

D-Glucose is the most abundant monosaccharide. D-Galactose, D-mannose and D-fructose are also of major biological importance. The syllable **-ul-** in the names of some ketoses allows distinction from the corresponding aldose, e.g. D-ribulose from D-ribose.

L-Monosaccharides are the **mirror image** (i.e. enantiomers, Chapter 1) of the corresponding D-sugar. The term **diastereoisomer** refers to sugars of the same series and which contain the same number of carbon atoms. Diastereoisomers that differ in the configuration of the –OH group on one specific chiral carbon

In the **empirical formula for carbohydrates**, hydrogen and oxygen are present in the same proportions as in water. It was therefore believed that this group of compounds could be chemically described as **hydrates of carbon**. With the passage of time, it became clear that this representation did not adequately fit the facts. For example, $C_3H_6O_3$ is also the formula of lactic acid which has a different chemistry to that of a carbohydrate whilst $C_5H_{10}O_4$, namely 2-deoxyribose, is chemically a carbohydrate. In addition, some carbohydrates contain the elements nitrogen and sulphur.

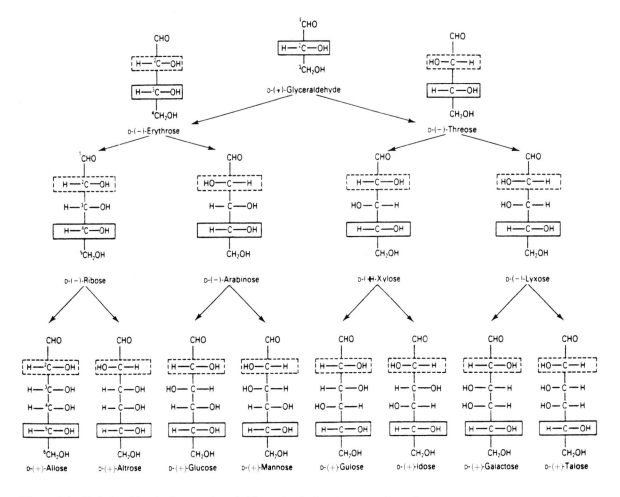

Figure 5.1 *Relationships in the D-series of aldoses (optical activity is indicated)*

atom are referred to as **epimers**. D-Glucose is an epimer of both D-galactose (different only at C-4) and D-mannose (different only at C-2) but D-galactose and D-mannose are not epimers.

The ring structures of monosaccharides

The monosaccharides have been presented as **open-chain compounds** (Figure 5.1). However, in solution, only the trioses and tetroses exist in appreciable quantities in this form. Pentoses and hexoses undergo **cyclization**, i.e. they form ring structures. The projection formulae disregard:

• possible rotation around carbon–carbon single bonds;
• bond angles of 109.5°.

Certain hydroxyl groups and the carbonyl carbon may lie close

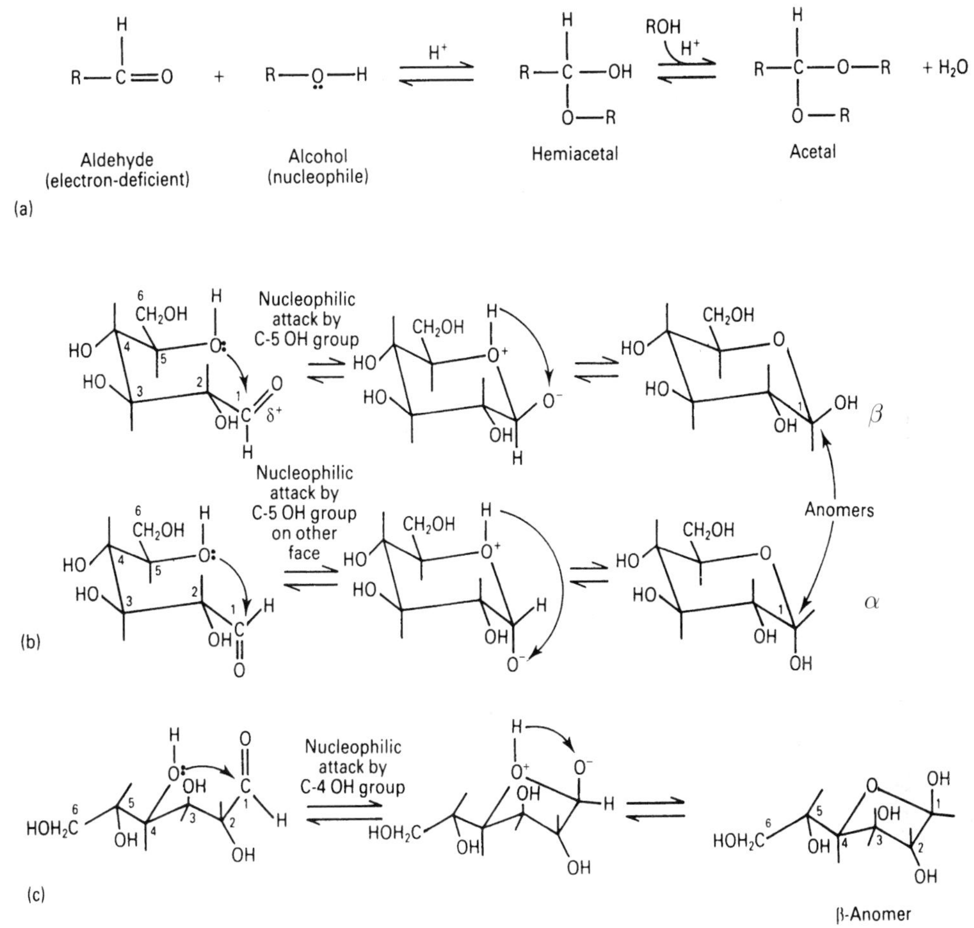

Figure 5.2 *The ring structures of monosaccharides: (a) the formation of a hemiacetal and acetal; (b) the formation of ring structures through nucleophilic attack by the electrons of an alcoholic hydroxyl group at position C-5; (c) the formation of ring structures through nucleophilic attack by the electrons of an alcoholic hydroxyl group at position C-4*

together enabling electrons of the oxygen atom of the hydroxyl group to subject the electron-deficient carbonyl group to **nucleophilic attack**. Nucleophilic groups or reagents seek to replenish the electronic complement of atomic orbitals.

When one aldehyde molecule reacts with one alcohol molecule in the presence of acid, the product is a **hemiacetal** since the reaction of one aldehyde and two alcohol molecules yields an **acetal** (Figure 5.2a). Similarly, ketones may form **hemiketals and ketals**. Therefore, if the carbonyl carbon atom and a hydroxyl group are positioned in the same monosaccharide molecule so as to permit their interaction to form a five- or six-membered ring, a cyclic hemiacetal or hemiketal will be produced.

The hydroxyl substituent on C-5 may attack an aldehyde group at C-1 to create a six-membered ring structure (Figure 5.2b). Depending on the orientation of the C-1 group, two hemiacetal products are possible. These products differ only in the configuration of the hydroxyl group on C-1 and so they are epimers. To emphasize the positional importance, they are referred to as **anomers** with C-1 being termed the **anomeric carbon atom**.

When the OH group of the anomeric carbon atom of a D-monosaccharide is:

- **below the plane of the ring,** the compound is termed the α-anomer;
- **above the plane of the ring,** the compound is termed the β-anomer.

When the OH group of the anomeric carbon atom of a L-monosaccharide is:

- **below the plane of the ring,** the compound is termed the β-anomer;
- **above the plane of the ring,** the compound is termed the α-anomer.

Therefore, the terminology for the L-series is reversed.

Ring structures may similarly be formed by the interaction of the hydroxyl group at C-4 with the carbonyl carbon atom. This type of reaction produces a five-membered ring structure again based upon hemiacetal formation (Figure 5.2c). The conformation adopted by the newly formed ring will be its most stable conformation.

When monosaccharides are placed in an aqueous environment, the stable ring systems which can be formed are the five- or six-membered rings which contain four or five carbon atoms respectively and one oxygen atom (Figure 5.2b,c). As a result of their resemblance to **furan** and **pyran**, the ring structures of the monosaccharides are named as their derivatives, i.e. α-D-**glucofuranose**, β-D-**glucofuranose**, α-D-**glucopyranose** and β-D-**glucopyranose**, and represented using Haworth projection formulae (Figure 5.3). (Ketoses similarly form furanose and pyranose ring structures of varying stability.)

Since the hemiacetal (and hemiketal) reaction is reversible, the ring structures may revert to their open-chain structure. An aqueous solution of glucose therefore contains both glucopyranose anomers and both glucofuranose anomers in equilibrium with a small percentage of the open-chain form. Whilst in the open-chain form, the carbonyl oxygen can donate one or more electrons to a number of substances, thereby effecting their **reduction**. Sugars which may decyclize are therefore referred to as **reducing sugars**. Glucose can reduce cupric ions (Cu^{2+}) to cuprous ions (Cu^{+}) and is a reducing sugar.

Intracellular environments are essentially aqueous and so pentoses and hexoses in metabolic pathways are usually denoted

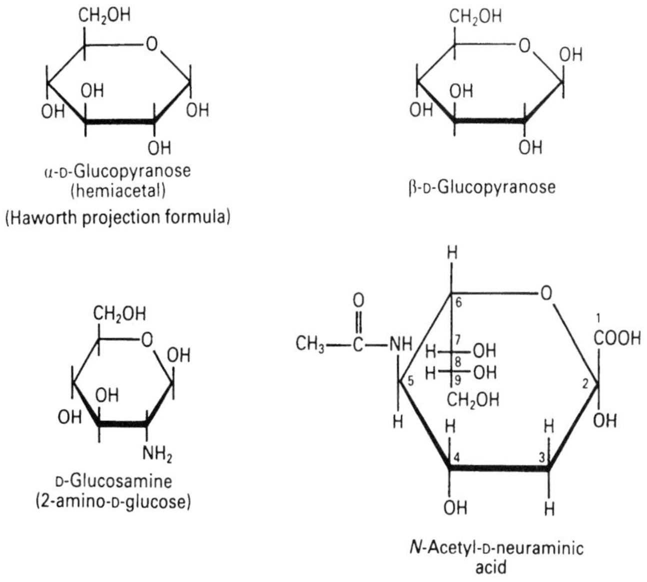

Figure 5.3 *Structures of α-D-glycopyranose, β-D-glycopyranose, D-glucosamine and N-acetylneuraminic acid*

by the major ring form. Also, the condensation of monosaccharides into oligosaccharides and polysaccharides involves the development of chains comprising the major ring conformation of the monomer.

Derivatives of monosaccharides

The monosaccharides may be **oxidized** under various conditions to yield different sugar acids:

- at C-1 to yield aldonic acids, e.g. gluconic acid;
- at C-6 to yield alduronic acids, e.g. glucuronic acid;
- at both C-1 and C-6 to yield aldaric acids, e.g. glucaric acid.

Phosphorylated monosaccharides play important roles in cellular metabolism, e.g. glucose 6-phosphate (Chapter 9). 6-Phosphogluconate, a derivative of gluconic acid, is an intermediate in the pentose phosphate pathway (Chapter 9). Phosphorylation involves the interaction of an alcoholic hydroxyl group and phosphoric acid to form an ester linkage. Substitution of monosaccharides at the anomeric carbon atom, e.g. glucose 1-phosphate, prevents reversion to an open-chain structure and so such derivatives are non-reducing.

Deoxy sugars are monosaccharides in which one (or more) hydroxyl group(s) has been replaced by one (or more) hydrogen atom(s) (Figure 2.2). The most abundant of the naturally occurring derivatives is **2-deoxy-D-ribose** which is found in DNA in the furanose form. Other important deoxy sugars include L-**rhamnose** and L-**fucose**. L-Fucose appears in the oligosaccharide moieties of some animal and human glycoproteins and glycolipids, e.g. in ABO blood group antigens.

The suffix -**itol** added to the root of a monosaccharide's name indicates an alcoholic derivative. These substances are often termed **sugar alcohols**. The **alditols** are in the form of a straight chain with an alcoholic group at C-1, the result of reduction of the aldehydic group. D-**Sorbitol** (D-glucitol) and D-**xylitol** taste sweet and are widely employed to sweeten jams, gums and sweets. Sorbitol is implicated in cataract formation in diabetics in whose eyes this alcoholic derivative accumulates. D-**Ribitol**, from ribose, is a constituent of riboflavin, a structural component of flavin coenzymes (Figure 4.5b).

L-**Ascorbic acid**, known as **vitamin C**, is a derivative of an aldonic acid (L-gulonic acid). Ascorbate is an essential cofactor in the **hydroxylation reactions** in which 4-hydroxyprolyl, 3-hydroxyprolyl and 5-hydroxylysyl derivatives are formed from prolyl and lysyl residues by the action of prolyl-4-hydroxylase, prolyl-3-hydroxylase and lysyl-5-hydroxylase respectively in the biosynthesis of collagen. Vitamin C may be synthesized from glucose by plants and most animals, excluding man, primates and the guinea-pig.

Prolonged deficiency of ascorbic acid in man results in the disease called **scurvy,** a condition characterized by swollen and bleeding gums, loosening of teeth, spontaneous bruising and haemorrhage, and failure of wound healing. This condition was prevalent among sailors on long voyages before the 1770s when limes were introduced into their diet as a source of vitamin C. In the UK today, vitamin C deficiency is restricted to babies fed on boiled milk, people whose diet is devoid of vegetables, Asians subsisting on a diet of rice and chapatis and followers of certain food fashions.

The hydroxyl group on C-2 of some monosaccharides may be substituted by an amino group to produce **amino sugars** (Figure 5.3). Amino derivatives of hexoses, e.g. D-**glucosamine** or D-**galactosamine**, are the most common. This amino group may be **acetylated** or **sulphonated** to form *N*-**acetyl** or *N*-**sulphate** derivatives, e.g. *N*-**acetylglucosamine**. These derivatives are abundant in polysaccharides and proteoglycans.

These amino sugars are also constituents of more complex structures. *N*-Acetylneuraminic acid (Figure 5.3) is a major component of the oligosaccharide chains of the glycoproteins and glycolipids found on the membrane surfaces of animal and human cells. Neuraminic acid derivatives are known as sialic acids.

Oligosaccharides

The term **oligosaccharide** describes short polymeric structures that contain up to 10 monosaccharide units linked by **glycosidic bonds.** A glycosidic bond is produced by the formation of an **ether linkage** between two monomeric units, the condensation reaction involving the most reactive hydroxyl group of the monosaccharide, i.e. the one attached to the anomeric carbon atom. In oligosaccharides:

- the monosaccharide residues may be present as **a pyranose or furanose ring;**
- the monosaccharide residues may be in either **an α- or β-anomeric form;**
- each glycosidic bond will be **in one of a variety of possible positions.** The glycosidic bond may involve the hemiacetal hydroxyl group of one unit with any stereochemically permissible hydroxyl group on the other unit.

These three factors result in numerous possible permutations involving the same monomeric units. Biological processes, e.g. enzyme activity, limit the variety of oligosaccharides of natural occurrence. Oligosaccharides may contain:

- only one type of monosaccharide unit and be termed **homo-oligosaccharides.** Maltose, isomaltose, cellobiose and trehalose are glucose-containing homodisaccharides which contain an α-$(1 \rightarrow 4)$, an α-$(1 \rightarrow 6)$, a β-$(1 \rightarrow 4)$ and an α-$(1 \rightarrow 1)$ glycosidic bond respectively (Figure 5.4a).
- **more than one type** of monosaccharide unit and be termed **hetero-oligosaccharides.** Lactose and sucrose are glucose-containing heterodisaccharides (Figure 5.4b).

The glycosidic linkage prevents reversion to the open-chain structure of the unit which has donated the hydroxyl group of its anomeric carbon atom. The moiety is no longer able to reduce substances and is termed the non-reducing end. Disaccharides that

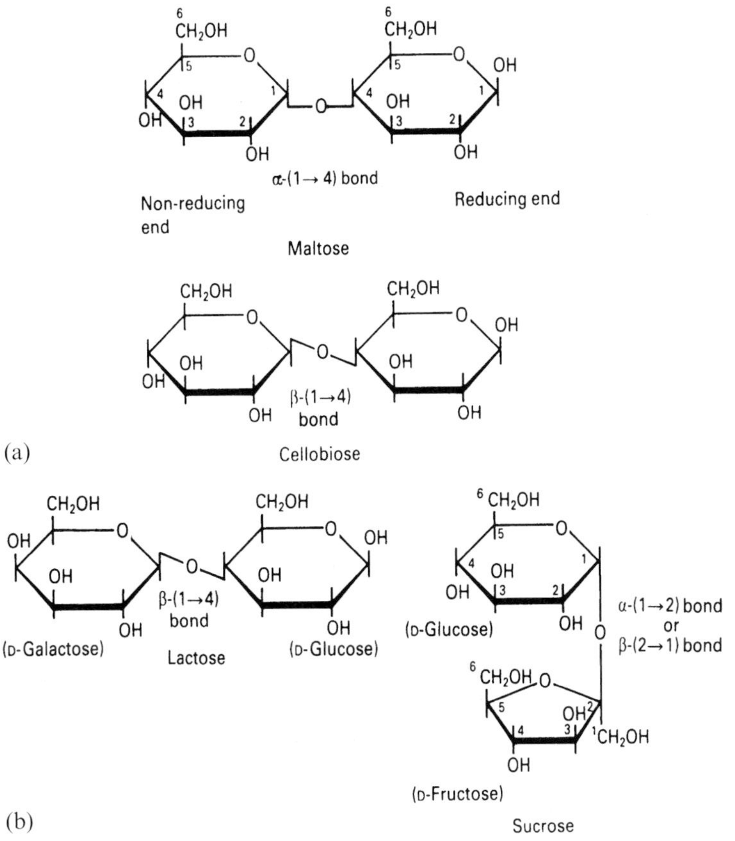

(a)

(b)

Figure 5.4 *Structures of some glucose-containing disaccharides: (a) homodisaccharides; (b) heterodisaccharides*

have a free anomeric carbon atom may act as reducing sugars because they retain the ring-opening potential whereas disaccharides such as sucrose are non-reducing. Glycosidic bond position is determined from the **non-reducing end** of the oligosaccharide to its reducing end. **Maltose** therefore contains an α-$(1 \rightarrow 4)$ bond and not an α-$(4 \rightarrow 1)$ bond. In **sucrose** the anomeric carbon atoms of different monomeric units are involved in the linkage. Accordingly, the glycosidic bond of sucrose is α-$(1 \rightarrow 2)$ when considered from glucose but β-$(2 \rightarrow 1)$ when considered from fructose. In addition to their trivial names, systematic nomenclature may be employed, e.g. maltose is O-α-D-glucopyranosyl-$(1 \rightarrow 4)$-β-D-glucopyranoside and sucrose is either O-α-D-glucopyranosyl-$(1 \rightarrow 2)$-β-D-fructofuranoside or O-β-D-fructofuranosyl-$(2 \rightarrow 1)$-α-D-glucopyranoside.

Polysaccharides

Polysaccharides, like oligosaccharides, are long polymers of monosaccharide residues held together by glycosidic linkages. The polysaccharides may be subdivided into:

Glycosides are the **acetal** or **ketal product** of the reaction of the hemiacetal or hemiketal form of the monosaccharide with an alcohol to form a glycosidic bond. The non-carbohydrate moiety of a glycoside is termed the **aglycone**.

Several natural glycosides serve as therapeutic agents. An example is **Streptomycin**, a member of the **aminoglycoside group** of antibiotics. Its systematic chemical name is O-2-deoxy-2-methylamino-α-L-glucopyranosyl-$(1 \rightarrow 2)$-O-5-deoxy-3-C-formyl-α-L-lyxofuranosyl-$(1 \rightarrow 4)$-N^3,N^3-diamidino-D-streptamine. Streptomycin was first isolated from a strain of *Streptomyces griseus* in 1944 and was the first aminoglycoside antibiotic marketed.

Streptomycin is particularly active against *Mycobacterium tuberculosis* as well as having activity against many Gram-negative organisms. Today its use is restricted to the treatment of **tuberculosis** in which it is employed in combination with other drugs due to the rapid development of resistance by the micro-organisms. Streptomycin also suffers from the major side-effect of **ototoxicity** and, like other aminoglycosides, necessitates monitoring of blood levels to maintain a therapeutic dose without risking deafness in the patient. Other aminoglycoside antibiotics include **kanamycin**, **gentamycin** and **tobramycin**.

Table 5.1 *Homoglycan subgroups.*

Nomenclature	Major monomeric unit
Glucans	Glucose
Fructans	Fructose
Mannans	Mannose
Xylans	Xylose
Arabans	Arabinose
Galactans	Galactose
Chitin	N-Acetylglucosamine
Glycuronans	Glycuronic acids

> **Man and most animals** can metabolize polysaccharides such as starch and glycogen but fail to degrade cellulose which remains undigested as 'fibre'. Cellulose is extremely resistant to acid hydrolysis and its degradation requires **cellulase**, the endohydrolytic β-glucosidase capable of cleaving the β-$(1 \rightarrow 4)$ glycosidic linkages of cellulose.
>
> **Cattle, sheep, deer** and a few other animals have a multichambered stomach, the first section of which is called the **rumen**. Bacteria which produce cellulase flourish in the rumens of these **ruminants**. Cellulase degrades cellulose and cellobiose to glucose, enabling the ruminants to obtain energy by the consumption of cellulose-rich plants, e.g. grass. The digestion of grass is a slow process because the hydrogen-bonded glucan chains are tightly packed which reduces the access of cellulase to the glycosidic bonds. The rumen also permits regurgitation of partially degraded grass for mastication (i.e. chewing the cud) to enhance the degradative process.
>
> **Termites** destroy wood because they have cellulase-producing bacteria in their digestive tracts. Again, the degradation of cellulose is slow.

- **homoglycans** which contain a **single type** of monosaccharide monomer;
- **heteroglycans** which contain **more than one type** of monosaccharide unit.

Homoglycans

Although by definition homoglycans contain a single type of monosaccharide monomer, in actuality homoglycans frequently contain a low percentage of other monosaccharides. Homoglycans can be classified on the basis of the nature of the monosaccharide unit (Table 5.1).

Glucans have both structural and nutritional functions. **Cellulose** is the most abundant of the naturally occurring macromolecular compounds. It is the main structural component of plants, constituting 20–30% of their primary cell walls. It comprises up to 14 000 D-glucose residues joined only by β-$(1 \rightarrow 4)$ glycosidic linkages which are responsible for cellulose being a long, straight, unbranched polymer (Figure 5.5a). Cellulose contains intra-molecular hydrogen bonds between the hydroxyl at C-3 and the ring oxygen of the adjacent monosaccharide and inter-molecular hydrogen bonds which crosslink individual chains to form a fibrous and insoluble structure (Figure 5.5b). The hydrogen bonding contributes to the strength required to support large trees.

Starch, unlike cellulose, can be readily hydrolysed to its monosaccharide units and is therefore utilized as an energy reserve by plants. Starch consists of two components, **amylose and amylopectin** which are complexed together approximately in a 1:3 ratio to form discrete **starch granules**. Both molecules contain only α-glycosidic linkages. Amylose contains only α-$(1 \rightarrow 4)$ glycosidic linkages but amylopectin contains additional α-$(1 \rightarrow 6)$ glycosidic bonds which give rise to its branched structure (Figure 5.6a). The nature of the α-glycosidic linkage confers a helical conformation to the molecule (Figure 5.6b) in contrast to cellulose. **Glycogen**

(a)

(b)

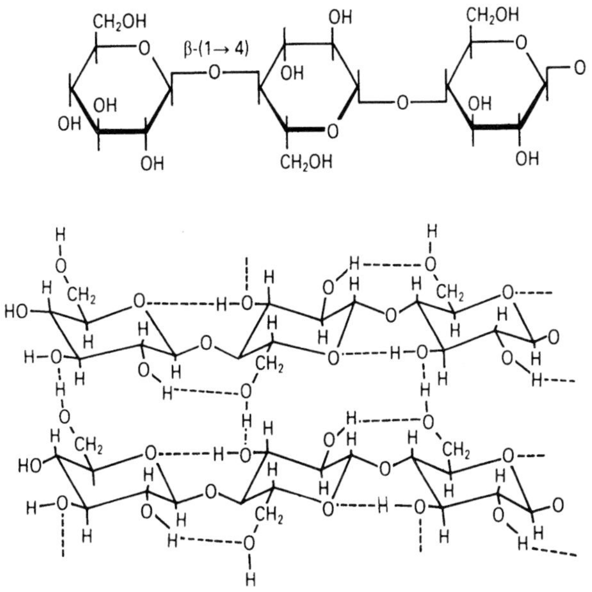

Figure 5.5 *Structures of cellulose: (a) representation by Haworth projection formula; (b) intramolecular and intermolecular hydrogen bonding in cellulose*

(Figure 5.6c), the animal storage glucan (Chapter 9) is equivalent to the starch of plants and has a similar structure to amylopectin but is more highly branched (Table 5.2).

The **galactan** called **agarose** is the major polysaccharide of **agar**, employed by microbiologists as a gel medium for the culture of micro-organisms. Agarose consists of alternating D-galactose and a derivative of L-galactose called 3,6-anhydro-L-galactose. Two types of glycosidic linkages, α-(1 → 3) and α-(1 → 4) bonds, create a double helical structure in which the anhydromonosaccharide enhances stability.

Glycosaminoglycans

Heteroglycans contain more than one type of monosaccharide. An important class of heteroglycans are the **glycosaminoglycans.** Glycosaminoglycans may be considered structurally as polysaccharides composed of **repeating disaccharide units** in which the

Table 5.2 *Comparison of amylose, amylopectin and glycogen*

	Amylose	Amylopectin	Glycogen
Monomeric unit	D-Glucose	D-Glucose	D-Glucose
Molecular weight	$4000 \rightarrow 500\,000$	$50\,000 \rightarrow 16 \times 10^6$	$50\,000 \rightarrow n \times 10^6$
Type of polymer	Linear	Branched	Branched
Distance between branches	–	20–25 Glucose units	8–12 Glucose units
Glycosidic bonds	α-(1 → 4)	α-(1 → 4), α-(1 → 6)	α-(1 → 4), α-(1 → 6)

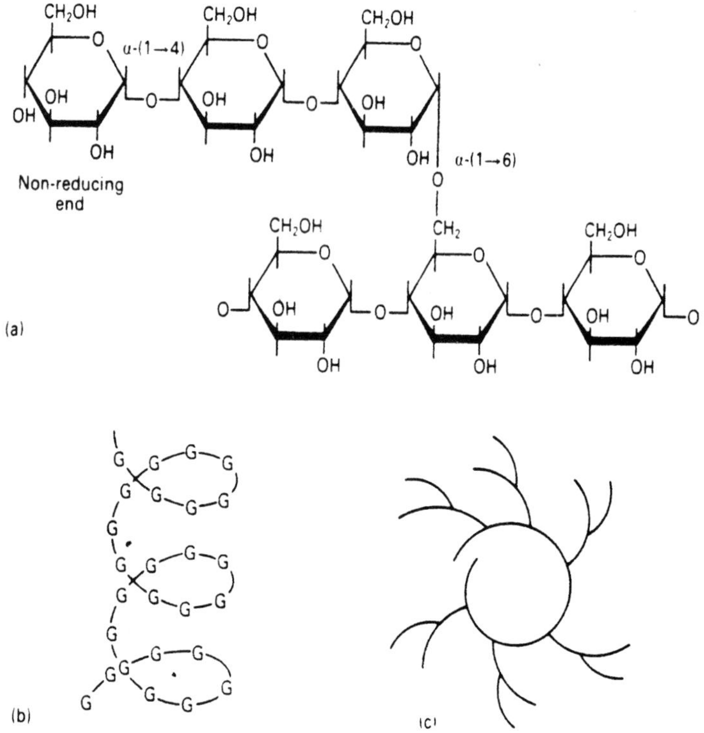

Figure 5.6 *Part structures of some glucans: (a) a branch point in amylopectin or glycogen; (b) helical conformation of amylose; (c) a segment of glycogen*

Glucans of medical and industrial importance include the **dextrans**. The dextrans differ in chain length and the degree of branching. Their backbones have α-(1 → 6) linkages with branching via α-(1 → 3) or α-(1 → 4) bonds.

Dextrans may be employed to expand the volume of circulating blood in patients suffering from shock as an aid in the restoration of cardiac output and blood pressure. Dextran 40 (mol. mass 40 000 Da) has a powerful osmotic effect (Chapter 1) and draws fluid into the intravascular compartment from the extracellular fluid compartment. This process may increase the circulating volume by as much as twice the existent volume. The **viscosity** of the blood is concomitantly reduced but there are compensatory physiological mechanisms. There are, however, three disadvantages to the use of Dextran 40: it coats the plasma membranes of erythrocytes so that if a blood transfusion may be required, a blood sample must be obtained for ABO blood group crossmatching prior to dextran administration; it forms a complex with fibrinogen to interfere with blood coagulation; it is rapidly removed by kidney filtration. The loss of dextran can be reduced by the use of Dextran 70 which has a longer half-life in the blood.

constituent monosaccharide residues are different. The class name reflects their high content of **amino sugars**. Table 5.3 shows the major repeating disaccharides in some glycosaminoglycans but it should be noted that the chains may be **copolymeric**, i.e. contain several different disaccharides.

The general features of the repeat disaccharides of glycosaminoglycans are:

- **the configuration of the glycosidic linkage** between repeating disaccharides frequently differs from that of internal linkage comprising the disaccharide;
- **an amino sugar** is one of the monosaccharide residues;
- **a uronic acid** is the second monosaccharide residue;
- **sulphation** of either monomer may occur although the amino sugar is the principal target;
- **they form highly anionic polymeric chains.**

All known **glycosaminoglycans**, except hyaluronate, are progressively synthesized from a **core protein** as carbohydrate side chains. By weight, the core protein is the **minor component**, the carbohydrate eventually accounting for up to 95% of these hybrid molecules, which are called **proteoglycans**. Proteoglycans are therefore composed of long glycosaminoglycan chains covalently linked to

Table 5.3 *The structure of the major repeating disaccharides of some important glycosaminoglycans of the extracellular matrix*

Glycosaminoglycan	Major repeating disaccharide			Glycosidic bond between adjacent dimers
	Component 1	*Glycosidic bond*	*Component 2*	
Hyaluronate	D-Glucuronate	β-(1 → 3)	N-Acetylglucosamine	β-(1 → 4)
Chondroitin sulphate	D-Glucuronate	β-(1 → 3)	N-Acetylgalactosamine*	β-(1 → 4)
Dermatan sulphate	L-Iduronate†	α-(1 → 3)	N-Acetylgalactosamine*	β-(1 → 4)
Keratan sulphate	D-Galactose‡	β-(1 → 4)	N-Acetylglucosamine‡	β-(1 → 3)

*May be sulphated at C-4 and/or C-6.
†May be sulphated at C-2.
‡May be sulphated at C-6.

the core protein. Some proteoglycans are important constituents of the **extracellular matrix**, a shock-absorbing gel (reinforced by various fibrils, e.g. collagen) which supports and interacts with cells (Chapter 7).

Sulphation involves specific **sulphotransferase** enzyme activities which utilize **3′-phosphoadenosine 5′-phosphosulphate (PAPS)** as sulphate donor. The biosynthesis of chondroitin sulphate involves the action of two sulphotransferases on available disaccharide sequences:

- **chondroitin-4-sulphotransferase** functions at C-4 of the amino sugar to produce stretches of 4-sulphate derivatives;
- **chondroitin-6-sulphotransferase** acts at C-6 of the amino sugar to produce stretches of 6-sulphate derivatives.

In a given chain, not all the disaccharides are sulphated and disulphated disaccharides may also be produced.

The carboxyl group on C-6 of glucuronate, e.g. in dermatan sulphate, may be enzymatically epimerized from an equatorial to an axial configuration. D-Glucuronate is thereby converted to L-**iduronate** since C-5 determines the stereospecificity of the monosaccharide. By convention, the glycosidic bond changes from β-(1 → 3) to α-(1 → 3). On production, L-iduronate may be sulphated at C-2 which prevents enzymatic reversion to D-glucuronate.

One of the most thoroughly studied proteoglycan molecules is **the aggregate of cartilage**. The core protein is **aggrecan** which contains 2024 amino acid residues. Aggrecan is folded into three globular domains. Approximately 100 chondroitin sulphate chains and about 50 keratin sulphate chains covalently bond via serine or threonine residues as O-glycosidic linkages in the intervening non-folded regions. Aggrecan at its N-terminal end interacts with hyaluronate, the interaction being stabilized by another protein called the **link protein**. The proteoglycan aggregate of cartilage is

Heparin, a natural anticoagulant, is a highly sulphated glycosaminoglycan (GAG). It is composed mainly of two repeat disaccharides, L-iduronate-2-sulphate linked by an α-(1 → 4) glycosidic linkage to N-sulpho-D-glucosamine-6-sulphate or D-glucuronate linked by an β-(1 → 4) glycosidic linkage to N-sulpho-D-glucosamine-6-sulphate. The repeat disaccharides are bonded by α-(1 → 4) glycosidic linkages. The degree of sulphation varies between heparin molecules depending on the duration of action of two sulphation enzymes, one for N-sulphates and the other for O-sulphates. On average, each disaccharide repeat of heparin has two or three sulphate groups which render the GAG highly anionic and lead to it being surrounded by aligned water molecules.

Unlike most GAGs, heparin is not a constituent of the **extracellular matrix**. It is found within the granules of mast cells which line the blood vessel walls of especially the liver, lungs, gastrointestinal tract and skin. The release of heparin during tissue injury prevents excessive blood coagulation. In medicine, heparin is employed to prevent blood clotting within the vasculature, e.g. in post-surgical patients.

A related GAG, **heparan sulphate**, differs in structure from heparin in that it has less sulphate groups and retains more N-acetylglucosamine residues. In contrast to heparin, heparan sulphate is a common cell-surface component as well as an extracellular substance in blood vessel walls.

therefore a huge structure which may exceed a molecular mass of 2 million daltons.

Peptidoglycans

The **cell walls of bacteria** contain substances called **peptidoglycans**, formerly called mureins. Bacteria are classified according to their staining characteristics with Gram stain into:

- **Gram-positive bacteria**, e.g. *Staphylococcus aureus*, which have a thick cell wall (~25 nm) consisting of multiple layers of peptidoglycan which surround the bacterial plasma membrane;
- **Gram-negative bacteria**, e.g. *Escherichia coli*, which have a thin cell wall (~ 2 – 3 nm) consisting of a single layer of peptidoglycan which is inserted between the inner and outer lipid membranes.

In both cases, the peptidoglycan is a continuous crosslinked single molecule which encompasses the bacterial cell.

The polymeric backbone of peptidoglycans is composed of **N-acetyl-D-glucosamine** and its 3-lactyl derivative, **N-acetylmuramic acid**, which are linked together by β-(1 → 4) bonds (Figure 5.7a). Chains of this structure are covalently crosslinked to each other through a tetrapeptide side chain composed of alternating D- and L-amino acid residues (L-alanyl- D-isoglutamyl-L-lysyl-D-alanine; **iso-** indicates that the γ-carboxyl group of D-glutamate forms the peptide bond with L-lysine). The tetrapeptide is attached to the backbone through the lactic acid moiety of the N-acetylmuramic acid. In Gram-positive bacteria, the carboxyl group of the terminal D-alanine of the tetrapeptide chain is joined to the first residue of a **pentaglycine bridge**. The terminal glycyl residue of this bridge is connected to the ε-amino group of L-lysine of the tetrapeptide of another chain (Figure 5.7b). The cell walls of Gram-negative bacteria lack the pentaglycine bridges; the L-lysyl ε-amino group forms a peptide bond directly with the carboxyl group of the D-alanine.

Within this framework, which is responsible for the rigidity of the bacterial cell wall, variations may occur in:

- **The amino acyl residues of the tetrapeptide**, e.g. some D-alanyl residues may be replaced to provide attachment via hydrophobic proteins to the outer membrane of Gram-negative cells.
- **The substitution of glycine in the pentaglycine bridge**, e.g. in some Gram-positive bacteria L-alanine or L-serine may substitute for a glycine residue.
- **The frequency and nature of crosslinking**, e.g. in Gram-positive cells D-alanine of the peptidoglycan layer is sometimes found in ester linkage to teichoic acids. Teichoic acids may account for up to 50% of the dry weight of the Gram-positive cell wall.

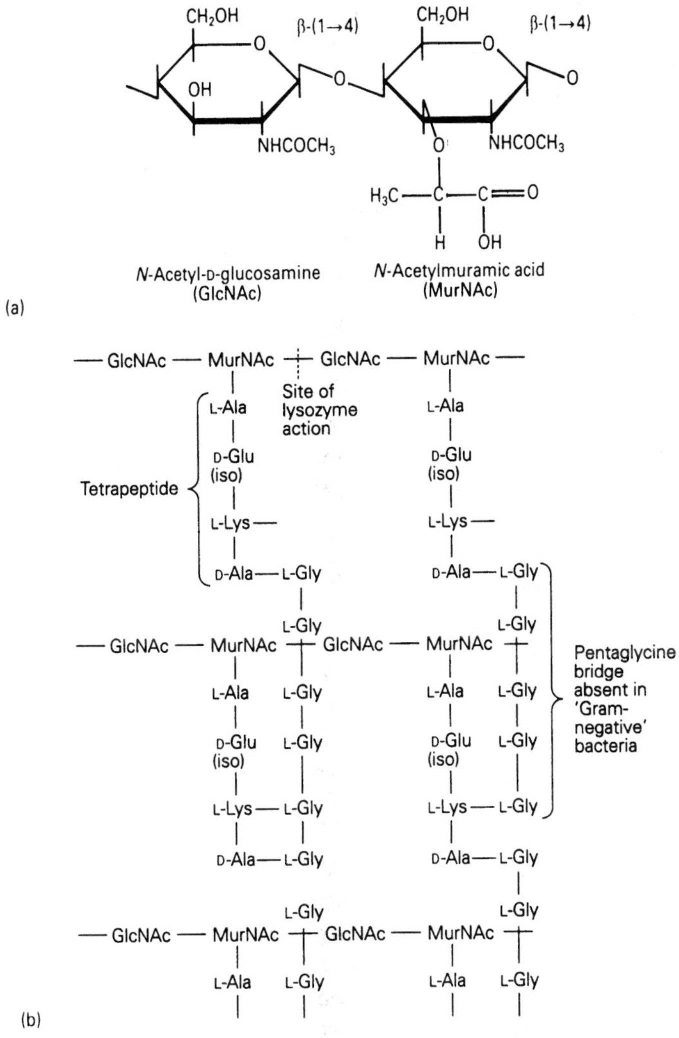

Figure 5.7 *Bacterial cell wall: (a) repeating disaccharide of peptidoglycan; (b) structure of the peptidoglycan of* Staphylococcus aureus

The enzyme lysozyme (Chapter 4) may weaken the cell wall by the hydrolysis of the glycosidic bonds between repeating disaccharides.

Suggested further reading

Fischer, D.-C., Henning, A., Winkler, M., Rath, W. and Hanbeck, H.-D. (1996). Evidence for the presence of a large keratan sulphate proteoglycan in human uterine cervix. *Biochemical Journal* **320**, 393–399.

Glaudemans, C.P.J., Kovac, P. and Nashed, E.M. (1994). Mapping of hydrogen bonding between saccharides and proteins in solution. *Methods in Enzymology* **247**, 305–325.

Nelson, R.M., Venot, A., Bevilacqua, M.P., Linhardt, R.J. and Stamenkovic, I. (1995). Carbohydrate–protein interactions in vascular biology. *Annual Review of Cell and Developmental Biology* **11**, 601–631.

Weis, W.I. and Drickamer, K. (1996). Structural basis of lectin – carbohydrate recognition. *Annual Review of Biochemistry* **65**, 441–473.

Barton, D. and Ollis, W.D. (1979). *Comprehensive Organic Chemistry: The Synthesis and Reactions of Organic Compounds*, Vol. 5. *Biological Compounds*, ed. E. Haslam. Oxford: Pergamon.

Collins, P.M. and Ferrier, R.J. (1995). *Monosaccharides. Their Chemistry and Their Roles in Natural Products*. New York: Wiley.

Self-assessment questions

1. From Figure 5.1, identify two sugars which are diastereoisomers.
2. The resilience of cartilage is accomplished through structural glycosaminoglycans. What feature of glycosaminoglycans is paramount in establishing the property of resiliency?
3. Why are D-galactose and D-mannose not epimers?
4. Which monosaccharide derivative is an essential cofactor for some biological hydroxylation reactions?
5. What is the major structural difference between chondroitin sulphate and dermatan sulphate?
6. Cellulose and glycogen are both homopolymers of glucose and yet chains of cellulose, but not those of glycogen, have great strength. Explain.
7. Why is sucrose not a reducing sugar?
8. Identify a major difference between the structures of peptidoglycans of the cell wall of Gram-positive bacteria and those of Gram-negative bacteria.
9. Alditols have an alcoholic group at C-1. Why does this group result in a linear structure?
10. Draw the structure of N-acetylneuraminic acid as represented by the Fischer projection formula.

Key Concepts and Facts

Carbohydrates
- Carbohydrates may be classified as monosaccharides, oligo-saccharides and polysaccharides.

Monosaccharides
- Glyceraldehyde and glycerone are the simplest aldose and ketose respectively.

- Monosaccharides containing five or more carbon atoms may exist as open-chain or ring structures.

- The stereochemistry of the penultimate carbon atom determines whether the monosaccharide belongs to the D- or L-series.

- Epimers differ in the configuration of the -OH group on one specific chiral carbon atom.

- Nucleophilic attack on electron-deficient carbonyl groups results in cyclization of the monosaccharide.

- A solution of glucose will comprise various ring forms and the open-chain form in equilibrium.

- Monosaccharides may be substituted to produce derivatives of biological importance.

Oligosaccharides
- Oligosaccharides contain up to 10 monosaccharide residues and may be classified as disaccharides etc. according to the numbers of residues.

- The nature of the glycosidic bonds may differentiate between homo-oligosaccharides.

- Glycosidic bonds are named from the non-reducing end of the chain.

Polysaccharides
- Polysaccharides are long polymers of monosaccharide residues and may be subdivided into homo- and heteroglycans.

- Glucans are of major biological importance, the glycosidic linkages determining their roles.

- Glycosaminoglycans are composed of repeating disaccharide units, frequently containing alternating monosaccharide derivatives.

- Proteoglycans comprise glycosaminoglycans synthesized as side chains from core proteins.

- Peptidoglycans are the continuous crosslinked single molecules which comprise the cell wall of different bacteria.

Answers to questions (Chapter 5)

1. D-Glucose and D-mannose are examples of six-carbon diastereoisomers; D-ribose and D-arabinose are examples of five-carbon diastereoisomers.

2. The GAGs of cartilage are highly charged polymeric chains. These have the ability to attract water molecules through their many electronegative charges, creating multiple layers of water molecules along the GAG chain. Proteoglycan aggregates bind large amounts of water. When pressure is applied to cartilage, water is displaced from sulphate and carboxyl groups. Compression may continue until the repulsive forces of the negative charges prevent further compression. When the pressure is released, water returns to the charge domains.

3. They differ at two chiral carbon atoms (C-2 and C-4).

4. L-Ascorbic acid.

5. Chondroitin sulphate contains D-glucuronate whereas dermatan sulphate contains the product of enzymatic epimerization, L-iduronate, within the repeating disaccharide unit.

6. The β-$(1 \rightarrow 4)$ glycosidic bond confers linearity to the unbranched cellulose chain and hydrogen bonding, particularly between parallel chains, confers strength. Glycogen has α-bonds and is branched.

7. Because its anomeric carbon atoms participate in the formation of the glycosidic bond. The disaccharide has therefore lost its potential to revert to an open-chain structure.

8. The presence of the pentaglycine bridge in Gram-positive cells.

9. Electron deficiency at C-1 is absent and nucleophilic attack cannot occur, thus cyclization is prevented.

10.

Chapter 6
Lipids

Learning objectives

After studying this chapter you should confidently be able to:

Identify the major classes of lipid.

Discuss the important features of each class.

Assign biological functions, based on chemical and physical properties, to each class.

Describe the fundamental nature of biological membranes and their lipid components.

Identify the classes of products from arachidonate metabolism and describe their biological roles.

Discuss the important features of the steroid ring system.

Identify the major biological functions of steroid hormones.

Discuss the nature and biological roles of the different lipoproteins.

Lipids are a structurally and functionally diverse group of substances which have the common feature of being essentially non-polar molecules. They are insoluble in water but soluble in the **'lipid solvents'**. 'Lipid solvents' are a variety of non-polar solvents including chloroform, methanol, hexane and ether either used singly or as cocktails. Lipids can be classified into the following major groups: fatty acids, waxes, acylglycerols, phosphoacylglycerols, plasmalogens, sphingolipids, eicosanoids, terpenes and steroids.

This chapter considers the chemical structures, physical properties and biological significance of the classes of lipids. The chapter also includes a discussion on lipoproteins.

The classes of lipids

Numerous classes of lipids contain fatty acid residues or are derived from fatty acids. Terpenes and steroids do not contain fatty acids.

Fatty acids

Fatty acids are **carboxylic acids** originally isolated from fats. Fatty acids have the following distinctive features:

- **A hydrocarbon tail** terminating in a carboxyl group.
- **They may be either saturated**, i.e. contain no double bonds, or **unsaturated**, i.e. contain double bonds. A **monounsaturated** fatty acid contains one double bond whilst a **polyunsaturated** fatty acid contains two or more double bonds. The double bonds of polyunsaturated fatty acids are rarely conjugated but tend to occur between sequences of three carbon atoms.
- **The saturated fatty acids conform to the general formula** of $CH_3-(CH_2)_n-COOH$. At physiological pH, they exist in an ionized form (Table 6.1).
- **Natural fatty acids often have an even number of carbon atoms.** They generally contain between 12 and 20 carbon atoms, i.e. $C_{12}-C_{20}$ fatty acids, although shorter and longer fatty acids do exist. Branched, cyclic and odd-numbered fatty acids also occur, particularly in micro-organisms.

It is not possible to write a general formula for unsaturated fatty acids because of the variable position of the double bonds. Each double bond introduces rigidity into the structure (Chapter 1). In most naturally occurring unsaturated fatty acids, the double bond is of the *cis* configuration (Figure 6.1) which creates a rigid 30°

Table 6.1   *Some important naturally occurring fatty acids*

	Abbrevation	Name		Structure
		Common	Systematic	
Saturated fatty acids (acylates)	12:0	Laurate	n-Dodecanoate	$CH_3(CH_2)_{10}COO^-$
	14:0	Myristate	n-Tetradecanoate	$CH_3(CH_2)_{12}COO^-$
	16:0	Palmitate	n-Hexadecanoate	$CH_3(CH_2)_{14}COO^-$
	18:0	Stearate	n-Octadecanoate	$CH_3(CH_2)_{16}COO^-$
	20:0	Arachidate	n-Eicosanoate	$CH_3(CH_2)_{18}COO^-$
Unsaturated fatty acids (acylates)	$16:1^{\Delta 9}$	Palmitoleate	*cis*-9-Hexadecenoate	$CH_3(CH_2)_5CH = CH(CH_2)_7COO^-$
	$18:1^{\Delta 9}$	Oleate	*cis*-9-Octadecenoate	$CH_3(CH_2)_7CH = CH(CH_2)_7COO^-$
	$18:2^{\Delta 9,12}$	Linoleate	*cis,cis*-9,12-Octadecenoate	$CH_3(CH_2)_4(CH = CHCH_2)_2(CH_2)_6COO^-$
	$18:3^{\Delta 9,12,15}$	Linolenate	all-*cis*-9,12,15-Octadecenoate	$CH_3CH_2(CH = CHCH_2)_3(CH_2)_6COO^-$
	$20:4^{\Delta 5,8,11,14}$	Arachidonate	all-*cis*-5,8,11,14-Eicosatetraenoate	$CH_3(CH_2)_4(CH = CHCH_2)_4(CH_2)_2COO^-$

Saturated fatty acids under systematic nomenclature contain the syllable '-an-' while unsaturated fatty acids contain the syllable '-en-'.

Δ denotes double bond.

Δ^9 denotes the double bond position, i.e. between C-9 and C-10 on numbering from the carboxyl carbon atom.

Δ^5 denotes double bond position, i.e. between C-5 and C-6.

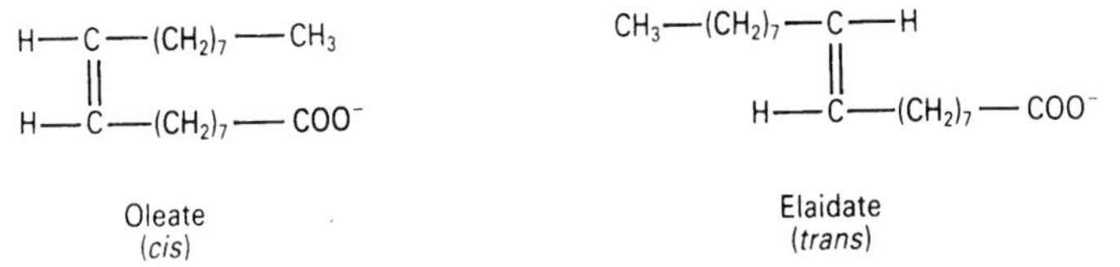

Figure 6.1   *An example of* cis–trans *isomerism in unsaturated fatty acids*

bend in the long aliphatic chains and renders them sensitive to oxidation.

The **carboxylate** (COO^-) **group** is normally water soluble but the long hydrocarbon chain repels water (hydrophobic) rendering the entire molecule water insoluble. Since fatty acids have both hydrophobic and hydrophilic regions they are referred to as amphipathic (Greek *amphi* = both) molecules. In a polar environment, because of their amphipathic properties, fatty acids organize themselves into spherical **micelles** in which the hydrocarbon chains are directed towards the interior of the structure with the carboxylate groups on the outside in contact with the polar solvent. The structure is held together by weak non-covalent attractive forces called **van der Waals' forces** between the hydrocarbon chains. Micelle fluidity increases with the degree of unsaturation of the component fatty acids.

Acylglycerols

Acylglycerols, also called **glycerides**, are fatty acid esters of the alcohol, glycerol. The two CH_2OH groups of glycerol cause difficulties for the D and L system of nomenclature (Chapter 1). The remedy was the introduction of **stereospecific *numbering***, indicated by the prefix *sn*, and based on the designation of L-glycerol 3-phosphate as *sn*-glycerol 3-phosphate (Figure 6.2). The *sn* system allows accurate description of the structures of mixed triacylglycerols in which:

- the *sn*-1 position is frequently occupied by a saturated fatty acid;
- the *sn*-2 position is often occupied by an unsaturated fatty acid.

Esterification of the glycerol by fatty acids, a process called acylation, yields a:

- **monoacylglycerol** when acylation involves only one of the alcoholic groups;
- **diacylglycerol** when acylation engages two of the alcoholic groups;
- **triacylglycerol** when all three alcoholic groups participate in the reaction (Figure 6.3a).

Only a small amount of **free fatty acids** is found in tissue, the bulk of the fatty acids being stored as triacylglycerols in specialized animal cells called **adipocytes**. This energy reserve molecule is rich

Vitamin E is considered to be a major **non-enzymic antioxidant**. Vitamin E is located in cell membranes where its biological function is to protect polyunsaturated fatty acids from oxidation. Degradation of membranous polyunsaturated fats by a combination of light and oxygen results in leakiness of membranes.

The **membranes of the retina** (the light-receptive tissue at the rear of the eye) have amongst the highest known levels of polyunsaturated fats of any human tissue. During vitamin E deficiency, exposure of the retina to bright light may cause cellular damage. The **lens** (the tissue at the front of the eye through which light passes) may also incur damage from the same combination of factors. There is evidence that cataract (opacity of the lens) development may be retarded by regular dietary supplements of vitamin E together with other antioxidants such as **vitamin C** and β-**carotene**. Animals reared in the light synthesize much more retinal vitamin E than those raised in the dark. Exposure of the skin to ultraviolet light reduces its antioxidant levels.

Figure 6.2 *Nomenclature of glycerol derivatives indicating* D, L *and stereospecific conventions*

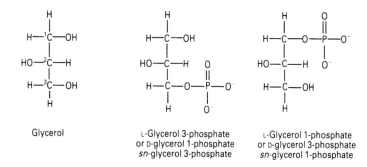

Glycerol

L-Glycerol 3-phosphate
or D-glycerol 1-phosphate
sn-glycerol 3-phosphate

L-Glycerol 1-phosphate
or D-glycerol 3-phosphate
sn-glycerol 1-phosphate

in reduced carbons and has the potential to yield large amounts of energy during oxidative cellular metabolism (Chapter 12). Below the skin of animals which live in cold climates, there are layers of adipocytes which, because of their lipid content, serve as thermal insulation.

Triacylglycerols may be composed of only one fatty acid, either saturated (e.g. tripalmitin) or unsaturated (e.g. triolein), or a mixture of saturated or unsaturated fatty acids. Since acyl groups lose their negative charge during esterification, they are electrically

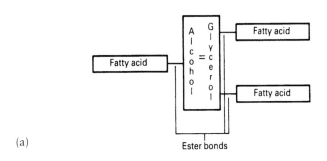

(a)

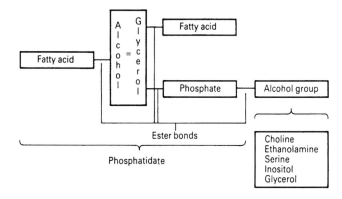

Figure 6.3 *General structure of (a) triacylglycerols and (b) phosphoacylglycerols*

(b)

neutral and so the triacylglycerols they comprise are termed **neutral fats**. Most neutral fats, e.g. butter or olive oil, are complex mixtures of simple and mixed triacylglycerols containing a variety of fatty acids differing in chain length and degree of saturation. In general, animal triacylglycerols are composed of long-chain saturated fatty acids and tend to be solid at room temperature, i.e. fats. Plant triacylglycerols, however, tend to contain unsaturated fatty acids, are liquid at 20°C and are called oils.

Phosphoacylglycerols

Phosphoacylglycerols, also called **phosphoglycerides**, are composed of glycerol in which the *sn*-1 and *sn*-2 alcoholic groups are esterified with fatty acids and the *sn*-3 alcoholic group is esterified with phosphoric acid. This pattern of esterification derives the parent compound, phosphatidate (Figure 6.3b), which is the simplest phosphoacylglycerol. Only a small amount of phosphatidate is present in cellular membranes but it serves as an intermediate in the synthesis of the major membranous phosphoacylglycerols. The phosphate group is further esterified by the alcoholic hydroxyl group of a variety of reactants to form the major phosphoacylglycerol groups. When this alcoholic group is supplied by **choline**, the product is a **phosphatidylcholine** (formerly called a lecithin). Similarly, **ethanolamine, serine, glycerol** and **inositol** derive **phosphatidylethanolamine** (formerly called a cephalin), **phosphatidylserine, phosphatidylglycerol** and **phosphatidylinositol** respectively.

Structurally similar to phosphoacylglycerols are the **plasmalogens**, a class of lipids abundant in nerve and muscle cell membranes. In plasmalogens, a **2,3-unsaturated alcohol** is substituted by an ether linkage at the *sn*-1 (or *sn*-2) carbon atom, rather than a fatty acid in ester linkage, and the alcoholic group is provided only by choline, ethanolamine and serine.

The ester bonds of phospholipids may be cleaved enzymically at different positions by members of the phospholipase family:

- phospholipase A_1 cleaves at position *sn*-1 to release the saturated fatty acid;
- phospholipase A_2 cleaves at position *sn*-2 to release the unsaturated fatty acid;
- phospholipase C cleaves the first phosphodiester bond at position *sn*-3 to release a phosphorylated alcoholic moiety, e.g. phosphocholine from phosphatidylcholine;
- phospholipase D cleaves the **second phosphodiester bond** to release phosphatidate and an alcoholic moiety, e.g. choline from phosphatidylcholine.

In aqueous media, the phosphoacylglycerols (and also plasmalogens and sphingomyelins) assume a characteristic shape

The **desire for chocolate** amongst some members of western societies, so-called 'chocoholics', is still not explainable in biochemical terms. This craving appears to be dependent upon sensory components of the nervous system. Attention has focused upon the **methylxanthines** (purines) which are believed to be competitive antagonists operating at brain adenosine receptors, and **N-arachidonoylethanolamine (anandamide)** which binds to cannabinoid receptors in the brain.

Analysis of cocoa powder and chocolate has revealed the presence of three **N-acylethanolamine derivatives**: *N*-oleoylethanolamine, *N*-linoleoylethanolamine and anandamide, each of which is not detectable in white chocolate. *N*-Oleoylethanolamine and *N*-linoleoylethanolamine do not activate the cannabinoid receptors but anandamide, a natural brain lipid, binds to these receptors with high affinity. However, both of the other unsaturated *N*-acylethanolamines inhibit the degradation of anandamide by **anandamide amidohydrolase** in rat brain microsomes.

It has been speculated that anandamide plays an important role in the craving for chocolate due to its increased level in the brain as a result of its absorption from chocolate or the inhibition, by other unsaturated *N*-acylethanolamines, of its breakdown.

Figure 6.4 *Amphipathic phosphoacylglycerols: (a) structural representation; (b) the formation of a lipid bilayer*

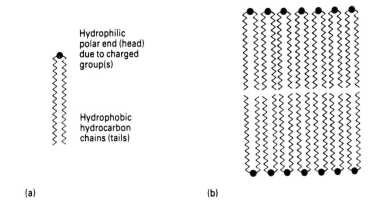

(a)　　　　　　　　　　　(b)

Hydrophilic polar end (head) due to charged group(s)

Hydrophobic hydrocarbon chains (tails)

Phosphatidyl choline
(PtdCho) is the principal class of phospholipid in mammalian cells, in which it may constitute as much as 50% of the total cellular phospholipid content. In PtdCho, the fatty acids at positions C-1 and C-2 are normally **saturated** and **unsaturated** respectively. The major form of PtdCho in most cells consists of **1,2-diacyl-*sn*-glycero-3-phosphocholine** which contains mainly oleic and linoleic acids at C-2 and is relatively deficient in arachidonic acid. However, **1-*O*-alkyl-2-acyl-*sn*-glycero-3-phosphocholine** is the predominant form in myeloid cells and is rich in arachidonic acid, the metabolism of which is of major importance in neutrophils.

Cleavage of membranous arachidonate from 1-*O*-alkyl-2-acyl-*sn*-glycero-3-phosphocholine is catalysed by **phospholipase A$_2$**, an enzyme whose activity is controlled by the cytoplasmic calcium ion (Ca^{2+}) concentration. The arachidonate is processed in neutrophils by the **lipoxygenase system** to leukotriene B$_4$ (LTB$_4$). LTB$_4$ is released from these cells and attracts other neutrophils to the site of discharge. LTB$_4$ also acts directly on the plasma membrane to increase membrane permeability to Ca^{2+} to enhance further Ca^{2+}-dependent functions such as microfilament and microtubule assembly.

(Figure 6.4a). The long hydrocarbon chains of the fatty acids are non-polar and hydrophobic whilst the charged groups, e.g. phosphate, create a polar, hydrophilic end. In a polar environment these amphipathic molecules can, like fatty acids, form micelles. However, they preferentially assume a **bilayer formation** (Figure 6.4b) which serves as the fundamental structure of cellular membranes. Bilayer formation is a spontaneous event due to the hydrophobicity of the hydrocarbon chains reinforced by van der Waals' forces which favour close packing of these chains to such an extent that, on disruption, the bilayer may re-form. Additional stability emanates from interactions between the polar groups and the polar solvent (Chapter 1).

Sphingolipids

Sphingolipids are common constituents of membranes and are similar in structure to phosphoacylglycerols except that:

- The alcohol moiety is **sphingosine** (or dihydrosphingosine) which is an amino alcohol (Figure 6.5a).
- The **linkage is an amide linkage** to give a parent compound called a **ceramide** (Figure 6.5b). Ceramides are therefore N-acyl derivatives of sphingosine or dihydrosphingosine.

Phosphorylation of a ceramide followed by a second esterification yields a **sphingomyelin** (Figure 6.5c). Brain and nervous tissue are rich in sphingomyelins.

Another class of derivatives of ceramides called **cerebrosides** are abundant in brain membranes (but are also found in other tissues). Cerebrosides lack phosphate groups and are glycosylated ceramides, containing a single D-glucose or D-galactose at position C-1 of the ceramide moiety. Cerebrosides are therefore glycolipids. In some **galactocerebrosides**, position C-3′ of the sugar is sulphated, giving the compound an anionic nature. If the glycosylation of the ceramides involves an oligosaccharide chain, the products are called

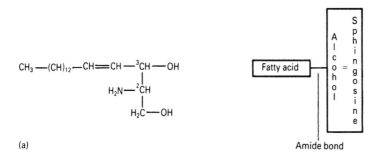

Figure 6.5 *General structures of sphingolipids: (a) sphingosine; (b) ceramides; (c) sphingomyelins*

(a)

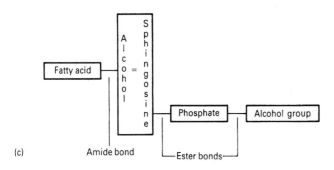

(c)

gangliosides. Gangliosides are the most complex group of sphingoglycolipids and include at least one N-acetylneuraminic acid residue among their sugar moieties which create very large polar heads. Fifteen different gangliosides have been identified in the membranes of the brain but their functions remain to be elucidated. The structures of over 60 gangliosides are known. A system of nomenclature has been developed in which gangliosides are identified as G_{M1}, G_{M2} etc. Gangliosides act as receptors for some pituitary hormones and some bacterial protein toxins, e.g. cholera toxin.

Eicosanoids

The **eicosanoids** are four families of highly active biological molecules (Figure 6.6) which are oxygenated derivatives of polyunsaturated C_{20} fatty acids (the eicosaenoic acids). The families are **prostaglandins** (PGs), **thromboxanes** (TXs), **leukotrienes** (LTs) and **lipoxins** (LXs). Other eicosanoids include the hydroxyeicosaenoic acids (HETES) and hydroperoxyeicosaenoic acids (HPETES), the latter being metabolic intermediates in the biosynthesis of the leukotrienes. The prostaglandins and thromboxanes comprise the **prostanoids**. The general features of the eicosanoids include:

- **they act as local hormones,** i.e. close to the cells responsible for their synthesis (Chapter 8);
- **they act at very low concentrations,** normally below $10^{-9}\,\mathrm{mol\,l^{-1}}$;

- **they bind to cell-surface receptors** (Chapter 7) and their actions are mediated by G proteins and cyclic AMP (Chapter 8);
- **they have short half-lives,** in some cases less than 2 min, most being metabolized during a single pass of the circulatory system;
- **different members of a family are identified by a letter** of the modern Roman alphabet;
- **a given subscript number** denotes the number of double bonds in their structure, e.g. PG_2;
- **arachidonate is a major precursor molecule** for some families.

Prostaglandins (Figure 6.6a), so named because it was thought that they originated from the prostate gland, can be synthesized by a variety of mammalian tissues. The first prostaglandins extracted from human semen were named in accordance with their solubility characteristics, i.e. PGE is *ether* soluble and PGF is soluble in phosphate buffer (*fosfat* in Swedish, the language of the disco-

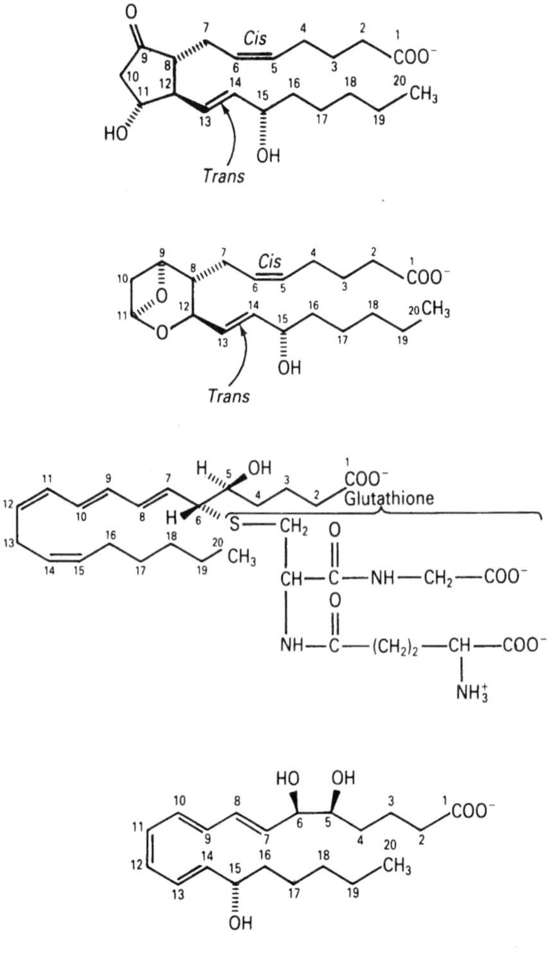

Figure 6.6 *Example structures from eicosanoid families: (a) prostaglandin E_2 (PGE$_2$); (b) thromboxane A$_2$ (TXA$_2$); (c) leukotriene C$_4$ (LTC$_4$); (d) lipoxin A$_4$ (LXA$_4$)*

verers). **Arachidonate** ($\Delta^{5,8,11,14}$-eicosatrienoic acid) derives the major human prostaglandins, the PG_2s. PG_1s and PG_3s are synthesized from $\Delta^{8,11,14}$-eicosatrienoic acid and $\Delta^{5,8,11,14,17}$-eicosapentaenoic acid respectively. Structurally, they are a group of C_{20} monocarboxylic acids which contain an internal cyclopentane ring. All prostaglandins (except PGG) have an α-hydroxy group at C-15 but differ in the position of ring-substituent carbonyl and hydroxyl groups.

The **prostaglandins** have a wide variety of physiological roles in different tissues including modulation of the following: smooth muscle contraction, the inflammatory response including pain development, wound healing, ovulation, uterine implantation and embryo development, glomerular filtration and water balance, bone development, and transmission of nervous impulses. PGE_2 may be employed in obstetrics to induce labour. Frequently the action of one prostaglandin is antagonistic to that of another. They are degraded rapidly upon their delivery to lung tissue.

Thromboxanes (Figure 6.6b) are produced from PGH_2 by the action of **thromboxane synthase**. The thromboxanes are so named because they were originally isolated from thrombocytes (blood platelets). Thromboxane synthesis also occurs in the lungs and kidneys. Thromboxanes differ from prostaglandins because of a six-membered ring system which contains an ether linkage. Their biological function involves the promotion of blood coagulation through platelet aggregation and vasoconstriction to reduce the flow of blood to the site of the clot. These effects of TXA_2 are counteracted by PGI_2. Hydrolysis of TXA_2 produces TXB_2.

Leukotrienes (Figure 6.6c) are so named because they are synthesized by leukocytes (white blood cells) and contain three conjugated double bonds. The leukotrienes of biological interest have four double bonds, e.g LTC_4. Although their biological effects especially the constriction of the bronchioles had been observed in the late 1930s, the elucidation of leukotrienes as the causative agents was not reported until 1979. LTC_4 and LTD_4 are potent contractors of smooth muscle, being especially effective as bronchoconstrictors, vasoconstrictors and constrictors of intestinal smooth muscle, as well as increasing mucus secretion. LTC_4 and LTD_4 have been implicated in the pathophysiology of asthma. LTB_4 is active in the modulation of the function of neutrophils, e.g. chemotaxis, aggregation, degranulation and adherence to vascular endothelium.

Lipoxins (Figure 6.6d) were first reported in 1984. These substances contain four conjugated double bonds and are synthesized from LTA_4 by leukocytes. LXA_4 provokes slow-onset but long-lasting contractions in lung tissue and inhibits the activity of certain leukocytes. LXB_4 stimulates protein kinase C activity (Chapter 8).

Terpenes

Terpenes are polymers of **2-methyl-1,3-butadiene**, more commonly called **isoprene** (Figure 6.7a). An isoprene unit contains five carbon atoms (C_5) and two or more isoprene units constitute a terpene. A **monoterpene** (C_{10}), e.g. menthol, consists of two isoprene units, whilst squalene and lanosterol, precursors in the biosynthesis of cholesterol and other steroids (Chapter 12), are **triterpenes** (C_{30}).

Isoprenoid compounds or their derivatives are found as constituents of a variety of biological substances, e.g. **vitamin A** (important in vision), **vitamin E** (an antioxidant), **vitamin K** (a blood clotting factor), **chlorophylls** (the light-absorbing molecules of green plants) and the mitochondrial electron carrier, **ubiquinone** (Figure 6.7b; Chapter 11).

Steroids

The **steroids** are an important class of lipid because of their wide range of biological activities, often at picomolar concentrations (i.e. 10^{-12} mol l^{-1}) although plasma levels are normally in the nanomolar (10^{-9} mol l^{-1}) range. Structurally, they consist of four fused hydrocarbon rings, labelled A, B, C and D (Figure 6.8a). Rings A, B and C are six-membered cyclohexane rings while ring D is cyclopentane. Chemically, the arrangement is called a **perhydrocyclopentanophenanthrene** ring system which has a characteristic numbering convention for its carbon atoms. The properties of the individual steroids are determined by the substituent groups attached to the ring system. The nature and position of these groups determine with which intracellular nuclear receptor molecules the steroid hormone can interact. The presence, and occupancy, of a receptor determines which cells can be influenced by that steroid. The steroid–receptor complex may modify the expression of genes and consequently the array of proteins synthesized in the cell.

Many steroids have an alcohol group and strictly should be referred to as **sterols**. The most abundant sterol is **cholesterol** which is an important membrane constituent either in free (Figure 6.8b) or esterified form. Cholesterol possesses a planar steroid ring system, a polar 3β-hydroxyl group and a hydrophobic tail which makes the molecule amphipathic in character, enabling orientation of the hydroxyl group towards aqueous media whilst the rings and tail penetrate the hydrophobic regions of membranes. Cholesterol is also a precursor for the synthesis of **steroid hormones** (Figure 12.8), **vitamin D** and **bile salts** (Figure 6.8c).

There are five major classes of steroids in man:

- **Androgens**, e.g. **testosterone**, synthesized principally by the testes, is responsible for the sexual development and the promotion and maintenance of sex characteristics in the male.

Vitamin A, together with vitamins D, E and K, belongs to the family of **fat-soluble vitamins**. Vitamin A was originally observed to be an essential dietary factor in experimental animals and was subsequently extracted from fish-liver oils. Today it is recognized that man synthesizes vitamin A from dietary β-carotene, originating in green leafy vegetables. **Deficiency of vitamin A** has multiple clinical features in man including impaired dark adaptation followed by night blindness, dry skin and dryness of the conjunctiva and the cornea of the eyes as a result of keratinization. This may result in corneal ulceration and eventual blindness.

Vitamin A is **retinol** which may be oxidized to **11-cis-retinal**. Retinal interacts with the protein, opsin, to comprise **rhodopsin**, the visual pigment located in the rod cells of the retina. On activation by light, the 11-cis double bond of retinal isomerizes to a trans double bond forming **all-trans-retinal**. This double bond shift causes the retinal to be released from the opsin, a process which initiates the nervous impulse for transmission to the brain.

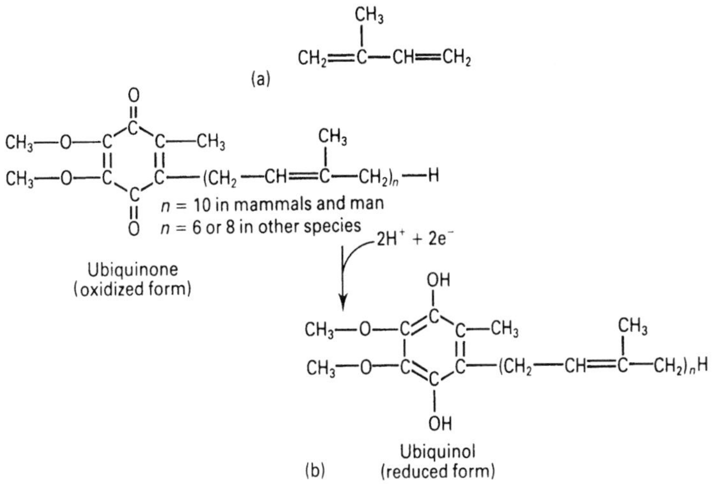

Figure 6.7 *Structures of some isoprenoid compounds: (a) an isoprene unit; (b) ubiquinone and ubiquinol (oxidized and reduced Q)*

- **Oestrogens**, e.g. **oestradiol**, synthesized by the ovaries, functions similarly in the female.
- **Progestins**, e.g. **progesterone** is a precursor of other steroids and in the female prepares the uterus for implantation of the ovum as well as preventing ovulation during pregnancy. **Oestradiol and progesterone** together are largely responsible for the regulation of the menstrual cycle. Combinations of synthetic progestins and oestrogens are employed in contraceptive pills for females to prevent pregnancy by the suppression of the maturation of the ovarian follicle and consequently ovulation, or to regulate menstruation.

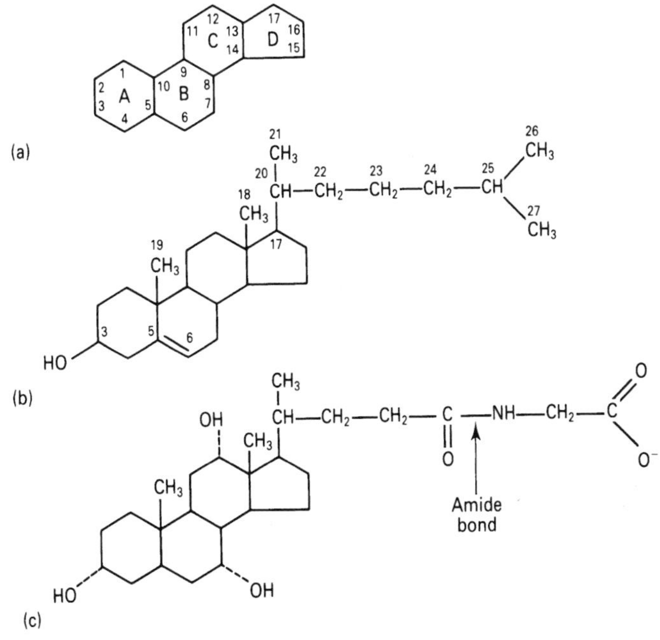

Figure 6.8 *Structures of steroids: (a) the steroid ring system; (b) cholesterol; (c) a bile salt, glycocholate (choloylglycine)*

Although the **illegal use of testosterone** had been well known, the first scientific study into its capacity to improve athleticism was reported in 1996. Healthy male volunteers were administered either weekly injections of testosterone (600 mg) or a placebo over a 10-week period. Athletes who received testosterone significantly increased both limb muscle mass and strength whereas those given the placebo showed no significant difference in these parameters.

Another illicit practice in athletics to increase stamina and muscle mass is the use of **insulin-like growth factor-1 (IGF-1)**, a peptide required for normal cell growth. However, there is long-term consequential damage following its administration.

- **Glucocorticoids**, e.g. **cortisol**, synthesized by the adrenal cortex, has an important role in the regulation of cellular metabolism, especially of carbohydrates, but it also influences that of fatty acids and proteins. It also exhibits anti-inflammatory properties by inhibiting the degranulation of tissue mast cells. Cortisol plasma levels vary significantly depending on the time of day of sampling.
- **Mineralocorticoids**, e.g. **aldosterone** functions in the maintenance of the ionic balance of the body by promoting reabsorption of Na^+, Cl^- and HCO_3^- in the kidney.

Bile salts, e.g. **sodium or potassium glycocholate**, are salts of derivatives of **cholic acid** which contain an amide linkage to an amino acid (Figure 6.8c). Note that the prefix in glycocholate does not refer to a carbohydrate moiety but to the amino acid, glycine. Bile salts have amphipathic properties and act in the emulsification of fats in the small intestine to aid absorption of dietary fat. Minor bile acids differ from cholic acid by virtue of their loss of at least one substituent hydroxyl group at position 3, 7 or 12, e.g. deoxycholate (Chapter 11) has no hydroxyl group at position 7. The conversion to bile salts in the liver is the major route of cholesterol excretion from the body.

Circulatory lipid complexes

Cholesterol, triacylglycerols and phospholipids are transported in the body as lipid–protein complexes, most of which are called **lipoproteins**.

The nature of lipoproteins

The lipoprotein complexes contain spheroid micelle structures which have a non-polar core of triacylglycerols and cholesteryl esters encompassed by an amphipathic layer of protein, phospholipid and cholesterol. The protein moiety is composed of **apolipoproteins**. Some of the apolipoproteins are unique to one class of lipoprotein, e.g. apoB-48 is found only in chylomicrons and apoD only in high-density lipoproteins, but others, e.g. apoC-II and apoC-III, are found in various lipoproteins.

Four main classes of lipoproteins have been described:

- **Chylomicrons** are composed mainly of triacylglycerols (85%) but have small amounts of phospholipid (9%), cholesterol (4%) and protein (2%). The major apolipoproteins are A-I, A-II, B-48, C-I, C-II, C-III and E. They are the largest of the lipoprotein complexes and have the lowest density because of their triacylglycerol and protein concentration. They are synthesized by the epithelial cells of the small intestine and provide the principal form of transport for dietary fat from the small intestine to adipose tissue, skeletal and cardiac muscle.

- **Very-low-density lipoproteins (VLDL)** are composed mainly of triacylglycerols (**50%**) but have significant amounts of phospholipid (18%), cholesterol (15%) and some protein (10%). The major apolipoproteins are B-100, C-I, C-II, C-III and E. They are synthesized mainly in the liver and transport endogenous (synthesized by the liver) triacylglycerols from the liver to the above peripheral tissues.

- **Low-density lipoproteins (LDL)** are composed mainly of cholesterol (45%) but have sizeable quantities of protein (23%) and phospholipid (20%) and some triacylglycerol (10%). The major apolipoprotein is B-100. LDLs are the major cholesterol-carrying lipoprotein in the blood.

- **High-density lipoproteins (HDL)** are composed mainly of protein (55%) and also contain phospholipid (25%), cholesterol (16%) and a little triacylglycerol (4%). The major apolipoproteins are A-I, A-II, C-I, C-II, C-III, D and E. HDLs also contain on their surface the enzyme **cholesterol acyltransferase** which catalyses the formation of cholesteryl esters. They are synthesized by both liver and intestine. HDLs carry endogenous cholesterol and phospholipids from peripheral tissues back to the liver.

The lipid cycles

Chylomicrons and VLDL function in the delivery of triacylglycerols from dietary (exogenous) and endogenous sources respectively to peripheral tissues. The routes of transport constitute the lipid cycles and are:

- the **exogenous cycle** which involves the chylomicrons;
- the **endogenous cycle** which utilizes VLDL, LDL and HDL.

On synthesis, chylomicrons are secreted into the lymphatic system and enter the blood circulation via the thoracic duct. On arrival at tissues which may employ fats as an energy source, the chylomicrons adhere to capillary walls from which an extracellular enzyme, **lipoprotein lipase**, frees the fatty acids from the triacylglycerols for entry into tissue cells, e.g. adipocytes. The chylomicrons shrink progressively as the triacylglycerols are hydrolysed and become in essence cholesterol-containing **chylomicron remnants** which are then released from the wall and re-enter the circulation. These remnants are removed by the liver.

VLDL is also delipidated by capillary lipoprotein lipase. Initially formed is **intermediate-density lipoprotein (IDL)** which progresses to LDL on further delipidation. Most of the LDL binds to specific high-affinity plasma-membrane receptors present on all cells and located within regions called **coated pits** (Chapter 7). The receptors

Oestrogen is believed to influence powerfully behaviour, mood and mental state in women. The role of oestrogen in depression and mania is suggested by the association between menopausal (and post-natal) depression and a large drop in plasma oestrogen concentrations. Indeed, oestrogen is an effective treatment for depression in some women.

Oestrogen significantly increases the binding of a synthetic, highly selective ligand for **5-hydroxytryptamine$_{2A}$ receptors** in the higher centres of the forebrain responsible for emotion, mental state and mood. It is believed that the effect of oestrogen on these receptors may be a major mechanism by which oestrogen levels affect behaviour.

Atherosclerosis is a chronic disease of the vascular system in which changes occur in the **tunica intima** (the innermost of the three layers of a blood vessel) of medium-sized arteries, resulting in **atherosclerotic plaques**. These plaques are the result of focal accumulation of lipids (cholesterol being a major component) surrounded by smooth muscle cells and fibrous tissue. The accumulation may be the result of inflammation or damage to the intima, resulting in blood platelet aggregation at the affected site.

Atherosclerosis is rarely present in early childhood but is often detectable in 20–30-year-old men and is almost universal in the elderly in the west. It is one of the most common causes of death. A high blood level of cholesterol has been established as **a risk factor** for this condition. However, more recently it has been realized that a distinction should be made between the levels of plasma HDL cholesterol and plasma LDL cholesterol. LDLs transport cholesterol from the liver to body cells whilst HDLs convey excess cholesterol from body cells, including those in arterial walls, to the liver. HDLs thus serve to guard the body from developing atherosclerosis. Factors such as exercise and moderate amounts of alcohol, which tend to raise HDL cholesterol levels with a concomitant reduction in LDL cholesterol, are deemed to be beneficial with respect to protection against atherosclerosis.

recognize apoB-100. The receptor–LDL complex undergoes **endocytosis** during which it is encompassed by the plasma membrane and internalized as a **vesicle**. The vesicle makes contact and fuses with **lysosomes** containing a variety of hydrolytic enzymes including proteases and esterases which release amino acids and cholesterol from the complex. The number of receptors influence the level of circulating LDL. When the cell has sufficient cholesterol, the intracellular concentration prevents the replenishment of the receptors and so their numbers decrease thereby inhibiting LDL uptake by the cell. When intracellular cholesterol levels are depleted, receptor numbers are increased (i.e. upregulation).

On synthesis **HDL** is released into the blood circulation where it gathers cholesterol from other lipoproteins. Its **cholesterol acyltransferase** produces cholesteryl esters which penetrate the core of the HDL initiating a change of shape from discoid to spheroid. Spheroid HDL transports this cholesterol from peripheral tissues back to the liver where excess cholesterol is converted to bile salts for excretion.

The **free cholesterol** may be employed in membrane biosynthesis or re-esterified for intracellular storage, mainly as cholesteryl oleate or cholesteryl palmitoleate. Free cholesterol also inhibits the activation and synthesis of the enzyme **hydroxymethylglutaryl-CoA reductase** which controls the rate of cholesterol biosynthesis (Chapter 12). By these means, dietary cholesterol may suppress endogenous cholesterol synthesis.

Suggested further reading

Alaupovic, P. (1996). Significance of apolipoproteins for structure, function and classification of plasma lipoproteins. *Methods in Enzymology* **263**, 32–62.

DeWitt, D. and Smith, W.L. (1995). Yes, but do they still get headaches? *Cell* **83**, 345–348.

Herschman, H.R., Xie, W. and Reddy, S. (1995). Inflammation, reproduction, cancer and all that. ... The regulation and role of the inducible prostaglandin synthase. *Bioessays* **17**, 1031–1037.

Singer, S.J. and Nicholson, G.L. (1972). The fluid mosaic model of the structure of cell membranes. *Science* **175**, 720–731.

Gurr, M.I. and Harwood, J.L. (1991). *Lipid Biochemistry – An Introduction*, 4th edn., London: Chapman and Hall.

Papa, S. and Tager, J.M. (1995). *The Biochemistry of Cell Membranes*. Boston: Birkhäuser.

Self assessment questions

1. How would you define a substance as a lipid?
2. Draw the structures of, and identify, three steroid hormones by

starting from the structure of cholesterol and following the following clues: (a) at position C-17, substitute the tail by an acetyl group, at C-3 dehydrogenate and shift the double bond to Δ^4; (b) at position C-17, substitute the tail by a hydroxyl group, make ring A aromatic, hydrogenate Δ^5 and remove the methyl group at C-19; (c) at position C-17, substitute the tail by a hydroxyl group, at C-3 dehydrogenate and shift the double bond to Δ^4.

3. Which location in man would you expect to be the site of synthesis of aldosterone?

4. Some lipids are amphipathic. Identify the hydrophilic component parts of the following: (a) cholesterol; (b) ganglioside; (c) phosphatidylcholine; (d) sphingomyelin.

5. Draw a cleavage map for the action of phospholipases.

6. Which fatty acid is a precursor of PGE_2?

7. From which of the classes of lipoproteins is intermediate-density lipoprotein formed?

8. What is the difference between a sterol and a steroid? Give a hormonal example of each.

9. Why are neutral lipids non-polar?

10. Distinguish between the structures of a plasmalogen and a phosphoglyceride.

The diterpenes **cafestol** and **kahweol** are known to raise the serum levels of LDL cholesterol and alanine transaminase of liver origin in humans. These diterpenes occur in filtered coffee brews at levels of less than 1 mg l^{-1} but are present in cafetière and Turkish coffee at a much higher level (about 40 times that of filtered coffee). The diterpenes are released from ground beans by hot water. However, the diterpenes are retained by commercial filter papers during filtration.

The consumption of cafetière coffee raised serum concentrations of LDL cholesterol and alanine transaminase in volunteers. Filtered coffee was without effect on these parameters. The increase in alanine transaminase may be unimportant but the elevated cholesterol levels may increase the risk of coronary disease. It may be advisable for patients at risk and young people to drink filtered coffee.

Key Concepts and Facts

Lipids
- Lipids are a diverse group of compounds in terms of structure and function.

- Lipids are generally non-polar and insoluble in water but soluble in 'lipid solvents'.

Fatty Acids
- Fatty acids are carboxylic acids with a long hydrocarbon tail which may be saturated or unsaturated.

- The major fatty acids found in man have an even number of carbon atoms.

- Fatty acids exhibit amphipathic properties in polar solvents.

- The important eicosanoids are the products of arachidonate metabolism.

Acylglycerols and Phosphoacylglycerols
- Acylglycerols are fatty acid esters of the alcohol, glycerol.

- The *sn*-1 position of an acylglycerol is usually occupied by a saturated fatty acid whilst the *sn*-2 position is usually occupied by an unsaturated fatty acid.

- Triacylglycerols are storage molecules for fatty acids destined to be employed as fuel molecules.

- Phosphoacylglycerols are derived from the parent compound phosphatidate which is esterified by a variety of reactants containing an alcoholic hydroxyl group.

- Phosphoacylglycerols may be cleaved by phospholipases.

- Phosphoacylglycerols may associate to form a bilayer, the fundamental structure of membranes.

Sphingolipids
- Sphingolipids are common membrane constituents which contain the amino alcohol, sphingosine.

Steroids
- Steroids consist of four fused hydrocarbon rings to which are attached substituent groups.

- Five classes of steroids function as hormones.

Circulatory Lipid Complexes
- There are four main classes of lipoprotein.

- Chylomicrons are synthesized from dietary lipids and function in the exogenous lipid cycle whilst VLDL, LDL and HDL are components of the endogenous lipid cycle.

Answers to questions (Chapter 6)

1. A water-insoluble substance which is soluble in 'lipid solvents'.
2. Refer to Figure 12.8: (a) progesterone; (b) oestradiol; (c) testosterone.
3. Aldosterone is a mineralo**corticoid** and, as its name suggests, it is synthesized in the cortex of the adrenal glands which are located adjacent to the kidneys.
4. (a) 3β-Hydroxyl group; (b) oligosaccharide chain; (c) phospho-choline; (d) phosphate residue and second alcoholic group, e.g. phosphocholine.

5.

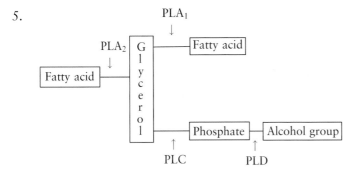

6. Arachidonate.
7. IDL is produced by the action of lipoprotein lipase on VLDL.
8. The presence of an alcoholic hydroxyl group gives a sterol. Oestradi**ol** and testoster**one**.
9. The acyl groups lose their negative charge during esterification.
10. At *sn*-1, plasmalogens have an 2,3-unsaturated alcohol in an ether linkage. Phoshoglycerides (phosphoacylglycerols) have a fatty acid in ester linkage.

Chapter 7
Mammalian cellular organization

Learning objectives

After studying this chapter you should confidently be able to:

Relate subcellular structures to different cellular functions.

Describe the salient features of each organelle.

Identify adjacent organelles with continuous membranes.

Outline the nature of chromatin.

Identify the proteasome as the complex responsible for intracellular protein degadation.

Describe the structural features of the cytoskeleton.

Describe the various mechanisms by which molecules gain entry to the cell.

Classify cellular adhesion molecules.

Describe the structures and functions of components of the extracellular matrix.

Mammalian cells belong to the class of cells called **eukaryotes**. The major physical characteristics of **prokaryotic** and **eukaryotic cells** were identified in Chapter 1. Most mammalian cells are found aggregated into tissues, although in some cases the cells function in a unicellular manner, e.g blood leukocytes and erythrocytes. Mammalian cells are surrounded by a **plasma membrane**. Being eukaryotic in nature, they contain a variety of intracellular **membrane-bound organelles**. Some organelles are present in multiple copies, e.g. mitochondria, but others are single copy organelles, e.g. endoplasmic reticulum. Indeed, the membrane (Chapter 6) is the fundamental structure of mammalian cells. Although a prokaryotic cell is encompassed by a plasma membrane, its internal molecular structures are not confined or compartmentalized by membranes.

The contents of a eukaryotic cell excluding the nuclear region are collectively called the **cytoplasm**. A membrane called the **nuclear envelope** separates the **nucleus** from the cytoplasm. The nuclear envelope, a double structure, is continuous with a highly coiled and twisted membraneous structure called the **endoplasmic reticulum**. Some **ribosomes**, organelles which lack an integral membrane, may be found attached to the endoplasmic reticulum. The cytoplasm also contains stacks of membranous vesicles called the **Golgi complex or apparatus**. Vesicles are sacs filled with dissolved solutes. Non-complexed vesicles such as calciosomes also exist in the cytoplasm.

The aqueous phase of the cytoplasm is termed the **cytosol**. Numerous intracellular **granules** are present within the cytoplasm. Membrane-bound organelles include **mitochondria, lysosomes** and **peroxisomes**. The mitochondrion is enclosed by a double membrane whereas the lysosome and peroxisome have a single membrane. A three-dimensional cytoplasmic proteinaceous framework called the **cytoskeleton** supports the plasma membrane. The cytoskeleton dictates cell shape and the position of organelles within the cytoplasm. The intracellular cytoskeleton is in contact with molecules external to the cell, called the **extracellular matrix**, via molecular systems which traverse the plasma membrane. The extracellular matrix is a network of macromolecules which helps to consolidate the cells into tissues.

This chapter considers the organization of mammalian cells from the centre of the cell to its periphery and beyond to the extracellular matrix. The essential aspects of the structure and functions of the nucleus, nuclear envelope, cytoplasm, mitochondria, ribosomes, endoplasmic reticulum, Golgi complex, lysosomes, peroxisomes, cytoskeleton, plasma membrane and extracellular matrix are briefly reviewed.

Nucleus

The **nucleus** of the cell is the largest subcellular organelle (Figure 7.1), measuring approximately 4–10 μm in diameter. All mammalian cells, except erythrocytes, contain at least one nucleus. Although muscle cells are multinucleate, most cells have a single nucleus. The nucleus houses the larger part of the **genome** which orders and coordinates all cellular activities. The nucleus is the cellular compartment in which almost all of the cellular DNA is stored and the syntheses of DNA and RNA occur. It is surrounded by the nuclear envelope which segregates nuclear material from the cytoplasm.

Figure 7.1 *Schamatic diagram of a mammalian cell*

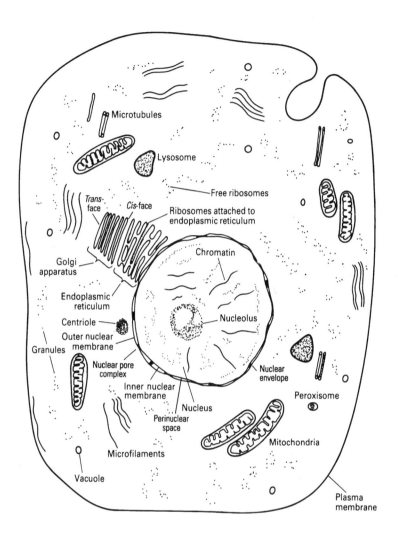

Nucleolus

The **nuclear envelope** encloses a semi-fluid particulate mass, called the **nucleoplasm,** which is, in part, organized into one or more spherical bodies called **nucleoli**. A nucleolus, like the nucleus, is mainly composed of **chromatin** but it also has a high content of RNA. Unlike the nucleus, the nucleolus is not enveloped by a membrane. The role of the nucleolus is in the synthesis of ribosomal RNA molecules for which it contains multiple copies of rRNA-specifying DNA sequences. Cells active in protein synthesis require the synthesis of ribosome subunits. These cells display enlarged nucleoli whereas cells conducting minimum protein synthesis have reduced, frequently crescent-shaped, nucleoli.

Chromatin and chromosomes

Most of the DNA is dispersed throughout the nucleoplasm as

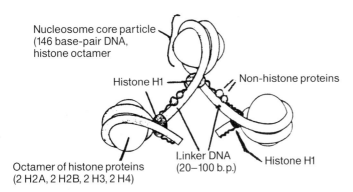

Figure 7.2 *Structure of chromatin*

chromatin fibres which stain with basic dyes. The chromatin is not evenly dispersed and near to the inner nuclear membrane it may be clumped into darker staining regions referred to as **heterochromatin**. Between the peripheral chromatin and the nucleolar chromatin lie lightly staining regions called **euchromatin**. During an early stage in cell division, the chromatin becomes packaged into **chromosomes** which are readily stained structures.

Chromatin is a nucleoprotein complex. DNA binds two classes of proteins:

- **histones** are abundant, small arginine- and lysine-rich structural proteins which package the DNA into **nucleosomes**;

- **non-histone chromosomal proteins,** each of which is present as a few molecules, may be nuclear enzymes, hormone receptor proteins or regulatory proteins.

Histones are cationic and may form ionic bonds with the negatively charged phosphate groups of DNA. Five types of histones have been classified: H1, H2A, H2B, H3 and H4, each with a different ratio of lysine to arginine and different molecular masses. Pairs of histones H2A–H4 associate to form an octameric structure (from which H1 is absent) around which duplex DNA is wound to form the nucleosome (Figure 7.2). This arrangement permits the large amount of human nuclear DNA (>2 m in length) to be stored in the limited space within the nucleus. Histone H1 binds to the DNA outside the nucleosome and serves to orientate the DNA correctly on the octamer.

The particulate appearance of chromatin arises from the large numbers of nucleosomes attached to a single strand of duplex DNA like 'beads on a string'. During cell division, a suprastructure may be created by the association of these nucleosomes. Nucleosomes coil in the form of a helix to form structures of six nucleosomes per turn of DNA. These solenoid structures form loops of DNA of variable length. Eighteen such loops are arranged radially around the circumference of a single turn of DNA to form the basic unit of a chromosome called a **miniband**. A **chromosome** is a stack containing millions of miniband units.

The cell-division cycle describes the series of events which occurs when a resting eukaryotic cell is activated to divide into two daughter cells. The four phases of the cell cycle, in sequence, from the resting or intermitotic phase (G_0) are the **pre-DNA synthetic** or the first gap **phase** (G_1), the **DNA synthetic phase** (S), the **pre-mitotic** or second gap **phase** (G_2) and **mitotic phase** (M). The daughter cells may continue in the cell cycle, exit from the cycle to differentiate or enter the resting phase.

In G_1, cells prepare for cell division by numerous changes in gene expression and enzyme activity. **In S**, the nuclear DNA strands separate and replicate. DNA repair, to prevent the generation of errors, and histone synthesis also occur. **In G_2**, reorganizational and further synthetic events proceed. DNA and chromatin proteins are packaged into sister chromosomes. Intertwined chromosomes are untangled by topoisomerases. **In M**, the nuclear membrane disperses and chromosomes become visible and align on the mitotic spindle formed by the reorganization of microtubules. Segregation occurs by movement towards the opposite poles of the spindle where intact nuclei are reformed. Division of the cell through the process of **cytokinesis** follows and marks the end of mitosis.

Nuclear envelope

The **nuclear envelope** defines the nucleus (Figure 7.1). In mammalian cells, it is a double membrane which contains several thousand **nuclear pore complexes**. The inner and outer nuclear membranes are generally separated by 2 nm forming the **perinuclear space** which is continuous with the cisternae of the endoplasmic reticulum. The inner nuclear membrane contains specific proteins which bind to the meshwork of the supportive **nuclear lamina**. The inner nuclear membrane is continuous with the outer membrane which is biochemically similar to the membrane of the endoplasmic reticulum. The outer surface of outer membrane is overlaid with ribosomes. Proteins formed on these ribosomes enter the perinuclear space.

The **nuclear pore complexes** regulate the export of large molecular complexes, e.g. ribosome precursors and mRNA, from the nucleus. They also control the import of proteins, e.g. histones, which are synthesized on free ribosomes. The nuclear pore complex is composed of over 100 different proteins in the characteristic arrangement of octagonal symmetry.

Each complex has at least one open aqueous channel through which small molecules (< 5 kDa) may passively diffuse unrestricted. A 60 kDa globular protein cannot enter the nucleus while proteins of an intermediate size may gain access, the time for entry being size-dependent. However, the nucleus may selectively import and export very large structures e.g. polymerase enzymes and ribosomal subunits. These proteins have a variable short sequence (four to eight residues) called a **nuclear localization signal** which contains lysyl, arginyl and usually prolyl residues. These sequences allow different proteins to bind to different specific receptor proteins, located in the pore complex. After binding, the proteins are driven through the pore by **active transport**.

Cytoplasm

The **cytosol** is the highly viscous aqueous phase of the cytoplasm. It contains many proteins, including metabolic enzymes, cytoskeletal proteins and intracellular transport proteins. The cytosol holds many small organic molecules, e.g. amino acids and nucleotides, which are involved in metabolic processes, coenzymes, cations e.g. Mg^{2+} and Ca^{2+}, and anions, e.g. HCO_3^- and HPO_4^{2-}. In aerobic cells, oxygen is detectable in the cytosol.

Numerous **vesicles** have been identified in the cytoplasm. For example, the **calciosome** functions as a specialized intracellular storage vesicle for Ca^{2+} ions. These ions are released from the calciosome in response to inositol trisphosphate, a secondary messenger in signal transduction (Chapter 8). **Cytoplasmic granules** may contain reserve fuel molecules such as glycogen (Chapter 5) and the enzymes concerned with its synthesis or degradation.

The **proteasome** is a multisubunit, multicatalytic protease complex present in both the cytosol and nucleus of all eukaryotic cells. It is the site of degradation of most cellular proteins and therefore is important in diverse cellular activities such as the regulation of the cell cycle, signal transduction, the removal of abnormal proteins and DNA repair. Proteasomes may be isolated as **20S and 26S particles**, the 20S particle being the enzymically active core of the 26S complex. The 20S particle is barrel-shaped, being made up of four stacked rings each comprising seven α- or β-polypeptide chains. In mammalian proteasomes, the β-chains are polymorphic and are responsible for the variety of proteolytic specificities. Additional polypeptides found in the 26S particle are required for the regulation of proteasome activity.

Proteasomes may efficiently degrade small peptides but require folded proteins destined for degradation to be tagged by the energy-requiring covalent attachment of a small protein called **ubiquitin**. To enter the barrel, ubiquitinated proteins must be unfolded and threaded through its entrance before accessing the catalytic sites associated with β-chains located deep within the barrel. This arrangement protects cellular proteins from undesirable degradation. It is believed that ATP is also required for the proteolytic activity of the proteases.

Mitochondria

The **mitochondrion** (Figure 7.1) is an organelle enclosed by a double membrane (Figure 7.3). This organelle functions in the oxygen-requiring process called **oxidative phosphorylation** (Chapter 11) in which energy contained within electrons is conserved in a form of energy usable by the cell, i.e. as the nucleotide **adenosine triphosphate** (ATP). For this reason, the mitochondria may be described as the power houses of the cell. Mitochondria are considered to be the evolutionary descendents of bacteria which colonized early eukaryotic cells because of similarities in key features such as size, structure, metabolism, circular DNA and lipid composition.

Cell culture is the growing of cells *in vitro*. Cells are disaggregated from embryonic or adult tissues by either mechanical, enzymic or chemical means. The cells are then placed in a sterile vessel containing a supplemented culture medium and maintained in an appropriate atmosphere at an appropriate temperature. Under optimal conditions, cells may survive unchanged for up to 50 cell divisions. **Culture media** are usually mixtures of inorganic salts (to regulate membrane integrity and pH), energy sources, e.g. glucose, micronutrients, amino acids, nucleotides and vitamins. Although glutamine and cysteine are non-essential amino acids *in vivo* in rat and man (Chapter 13), they are required for the growth of mammalian cells cultured *in vitro*.

Culture media are frequently supplemented by **serum** which provides proteins (including growth factors, transport proteins and attachment factors, e.g. fibronectin), steroid and thyroid hormones, other lipids and minerals (which may be required for enzyme activation). Serum has numerous disadvantages in cell culture (e.g. batch-to-batch variations resulting in insufficient levels of cell-specific growth factors) which, together with cost, has stimulated the development of **low-serum** and **serum-free culture systems**. **Antibiotics** are employed to prevent bacterial, mycoplasma and fungal growth which destroy cells in culture.

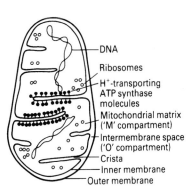

Figure 7.3   *Schematic diagram of a mitochondrion*

Various shapes have been recorded for mitochondria, e.g. oval, round and cylindrical, but they are commonly observed as oval organelles about 1–2 μm long and 0.5–1 μm wide. Their numbers and distribution are closely related to the capacity of the cell for aerobic energy production, e.g. the human hepatocyte may contain between 800 and 2500 mitochondria whereas the erythrocyte is devoid of mitochondria since this cell type does not produce ATP through oxidative phosphorylation. However, hepatocytes have a relatively low rate of ATP production and utilization compared with cells of cardiac muscle. Liver mitochondria consequently have fewer cristae than cardiac myocytes.

All mitochondria have two separate membranes which are chemically and functionally distinct. The major features of the structure of the mitochondrion are:

- the outer membrane;
- the intermembrane space (or 'O' compartment);
- the inner membrane;
- the matrix (or 'M' compartment).

The **outer membrane** maintains the shape of the organelle. It contains, in essence, open pores created by the transmembrane protein called **porin** which render the membrane freely permeable to molecules with a molecular mass of < 6000 Da and ions. Porins are also found in the membranes of Gram-negative bacteria, cyanobacteria and plant chloroplasts. The mitochondrial porin (molecular mass 35 kDa) contains one α-chain and 12 β-chains which traverse the membrane. The diameter of the pore may be adjusted by either positive or negative voltages across the outer membrane, i.e. the channel of mitochondrial porin is **voltage gated**. The outer membrane contains relatively few enzymic activities, e.g. acyl-CoA synthase (Chapter 12), but more than the intermembrane space.

The **'O' compartment** separates the outer and inner membranes. It is filled with a fluid in which very few enzymic activities have been detected, e.g. adenylate kinase (Chapter 8) which maintains the relative concentrations of the different adenine nucleotides.

The **inner membrane** exhibits numerous folds, called **cristae**, which invaginate into the matrix. The **cristae** increase the length of the inner membrane thus enabling this membrane to house large numbers of **electron-transport complexes** and associated ATP-synthesizing enzymes. It is estimated that the inner membrane of a single liver mitochondrion may contain from 2600 to 15 600 electron-transport complexes. The passage of electrons over the redox carriers (Chapter 11) comprising these complexes releases the energy used to phosphorylate ADP in the production of ATP. This membrane is relatively rich in enzymes, e.g. succinate dehydrogenase and enzymes associated with the electron-transport complexes. During periods of high activity in oxidative phosphorylation, the intermembrane space appears to expand with concomitant shrinkage of the matrix.

The **'M' compartment** is surrounded by the inner membrane. The matrix is aqueous and gel-like in nature and accommodates most of the enzymes associated with **aerobic oxidative processes**, e.g. the tricarboxylic acid cycle (Chapter 10) and β-oxidation of fatty acids (Chapter 12). Proteins synthesized on cytoplasmic ribosomes are imported into the mitochondrial matrix at thousands of sites where the outer and inner membranes make contact. The other enzymes necessary for these pathways are either integral membrane proteins or associated with the inner membrane.

The matrix contains discrete double-helical strands of circular DNA and ribosomes. The DNA constitutes the mitochondrial genome. Unlike nuclear DNA, mitochondrial DNA (mDNA) is not complexed with protein. The synthesis of the majority of mitochondrial proteins is, however, directed by nuclear DNA. The mDNA contains the code for its 22 unique tRNA molecules, two rRNA molecules of its own ribosomes and mRNA. The mRNA provides the template from which only 11 subunits of three enzymes of the inner-membrane electron-transport complexes are translated. Two subunits of ATP synthase (Chapter 11) are also encoded by mDNA. The primary structure of these proteins is determined by a genetic code which, although triplet in character, reads differently from that pertaining to prokaryotes and the eukaryotic nucleus. The matrix also serves as an important reservoir of Ca^{2+} ions (Chapter 8).

Ribosomes

The **ribosome**, endoplasmic reticulum and Golgi complex (Figure 7.1) are the three organelles associated with the synthesis of protein and its subsequent modification. Ribosomes, the number of which may exceed 10 000 per cell, may be found:

- **Free in the cytoplasm.** Free ribosomes participate in the synthesis of proteins which will be located and function within the cytosolic milieu. During protein synthesis, numerous ribosomes may become bound to mRNA to form **polyribosomes**.
- **Attached to subcellular structures.** Ribosomes attached to the membranes of the endoplasmic reticulum synthesize proteins destined for lysosomes or the cell surface as components of membranes or secretions. Substantial evidence suggests that ribosomes also adhere to components of the cytoskeleton.

Whether they are attached or not, the function of the ribosomes is the same (Chapter 13). Their structure is shown in Figure 2.14. Mammalian ribosomes are 80S structures composed of a large subunit (60S) and a small subunit (40S).

The **human mitochondrial genome** encodes, in addition to some mitochondrial ribosomal proteins, 13 proteins which are constituents of the membrane complexes (Chapter 11) involved in oxidative phosphorylation. Most of the mitochondrial proteins are encoded from the nucleus but mutations in mDNA may have severe consequences for the individual. Defects in these proteins tend to be evidenced in tissues with high energy requirements, e.g. brain and nervous tissues and cardiac and skeletal muscle. **In spermatozoa**, the energy for motility is generated from densely packed clusters of mitochondria located at the base of the flagellum. Mutation in mDNA may result in significant reductions in energy production which may be manifested as reduced sperm motility and consequently poor fertility.

mDNA is inherited from the mother and as a consequence mitochondrial genetic disorders are transmitted by females although the disorders may be expressed in both male and female progeny. **Leber's disease**, which affects predominantly males, is characterized by a loss of central vision whilst peripheral vision is maintained. This condition is correlated to various mutations in **complex I**. Because of maternal transmission of its DNA, the mitochondria provide an important source of DNA for anthropological studies on human ancestry and origins.

Cell death occurs by two major processes, **necrosis** and **apoptosis**. **Necrosis** is passive and does not involve the synthesis of macromolecules. *In vivo*, necrosis results mainly from **hypoxia** and **nutrient insufficiency** which disrupts the functioning of energy-dependent ion channels with a consequential increase in cell volume (Chapter 1), loss of membrane integrity and cell lysis.

Apoptosis, also termed **programmed cell death** or suicide, is a normal process which occurs in cell development and morphogenesis, e.g. during thymic maturation of T-lymphocytes. Apoptosis is characterized morphologically by cell shrinkage, blebbing of the plasma membrane, chromatin condensation and extensive fragmentation of nuclear DNA into ~ 200-base-pair fragments through the action of endogenous nucleases. The resultant membrane-bound cell remnants, called **apoptotic bodies**, are ingested by neighbouring macrophages. Apoptosis is triggered by the interaction of certain ligands with their cell-surface receptors, e.g. **Fas receptor** and **tumour necrosis factor receptor 1 (TNFR1)**. The binding of the Fas ligand (FasL) or TNF generates biochemical signals within the cell which lead to the activation of numerous genes, e.g. the interleukin-1 converting enzyme (ICE) family of genes, *Fas*, *p53*, *myc* and *WAF1*, the products of which contribute to the mechanism of apoptosis.

Endoplasmic reticulum

The **endoplasmic reticulum** (ER, Figure 7.1) is single-copy organelle which is continuous from the outer nuclear membrane. It is an extensive network (or reticulum) of continuous folded membranes with a complex shape. Cells active in protein synthesis frequently display an enlarged ER. The ER membrane separates the cytosol from the inner aqueous cavities created by its folds called **cisternae**. Molecules and ions transfer selectively between these two compartments. The ER is specialized for the sequestration of Ca^{2+} ions from the cytosol and their storage. Rapid release mechanisms liberate the Ca^{2+} ions in response to extracellular signals mediated through signal transduction (Chapter 8) and for the contraction of skeletal muscle.

The ER may be described as **rough** (RER) or **smooth** (SER) depending on the attachment to its cytosolic face of a large number of ribosomes which give a rough appearance to the structure. **SER**, which lacks ribosomes, is generally tubular whereas **RER** is composed of flattened membrane. Polypeptides assembled on RER are synthesized with an additional section of variable length called a **signal** or **leader sequence** at their N-termini. This extension facilitates the insertion of the growing polypeptide chain into the ER membrane via the interaction between the signal peptide with its **signal recognition particle** (SRP) on the ribosome. Upon fulfilling its function, the leader sequence is cleaved from the chain by a **signal peptidase** associated with the ER membrane.

Co- and **post-translational modifications** of proteins are catalysed by enzymes within the cisternae which occupy over 10% of the total cell volume. Cotranslational processing may be defined as enzymic modification of the growing polypeptide chain whilst it is attached to the ribosome. Post-translational changes occur following the release of the polypeptide from the ribosome. An example of cotranslational processing is hydroxylation whereas glycosylation may commence whilst the polypeptide remains attached to the ribosome but continues after its release. Indeed, glycosylation is frequently completed in the Golgi complex to where the protein is transported by specialized vesicles. The folding of proteins into their tertiary structures also occurs in part in the RER, a process which is assisted by **chaperone proteins**, e.g. some members of the hsp 70 family of heat-shock proteins.

SER contains enzymes involved in lipid and phospholipid syntheses and **cytochrome P-450 isoenzymes** which also function in **drug detoxification** (Chapter 9). SER is particularly abundant in cells which specialize in steroid metabolism since additional SER is required to house the enzymes necessary for cholesterol biosynthesis and its subsequent conversion into steroid hormones (Chapter 12).

Golgi complex

The **Golgi apparatus** (Figure 7.1), discovered by Camillo Golgi in 1898, is another single-copy organelle, located between the endoplasmic reticulum and the plasma membrane. This complex appears in electron micrographs as a stack of several distinct sets of flattened membranes, some of which are connected by tubules. Each set of membranes is disc-shaped and encloses a fluid-filled **cisterna**. The role of the Golgi complex is to sort proteins for delivery to different intracellular locations, e.g. lysosomes and plasma membrane, or for export in secretions.

The Golgi complex receives newly synthesized and partly modified proteins from the endoplasmic reticulum encased within **coated vesicles**. These small vesicles are formed by budding from the membrane of the endoplasmic reticulum with the assistance of a non-glycosylated protein called **clathrin** which provides the external framework for their formation.

The Golgi complex is highly ordered, being composed of three distinct compartments which hold different collections of enzymes required for glycoprotein processing:

- *Cis* **compartment** (*cis*-Golgi). Clathrin-coated vesicles deliver their contents to the cytoplasmic surface of this sector opposite to the endoplasmic reticulum, called the ***cis*-face**. This compartment contains a mannosidase, *N*-acetylglucosaminyl phosphotransferase and *N*-acetylglucosamine-1-phosphodiester *N*-acetylglucosaminidase. This sector is also concerned with the recycling of proteins back to the endoplasmic reticulum and protein folding.

- **Medial compartment**. Another mannosidase, *N*-acetylglucosaminyltransferases and fucosyltransferase function within this compartment.

- *Trans* **compartment** (*trans*-Golgi). The enzymes within this location include galactosyltransferases, sialyltransferases and sulphatases. The *trans*-Golgi is responsible for sending the glycoproteins to their correct destinations, e.g. glycoproteins destined for lysosomes display mannose 6-phosphate residues which are recognized by lysosomal mannose 6-phosphate receptors. The sorting process is believed to be pH-dependent, an acidic environment favouring sorting. Sorted proteins are transported to the cell surface also by clathrin-coated vesicles, the generation of which is facilitated by enzymic modification of the membrane phospholipids of the ***trans*-face**.

As a protein progresses through the stack from the *cis*-face to the *trans*-face, transport between the sectors of the Golgi complex also involves vesicles. These **shuttle vesicles** possess another type of coat consisting of four types of **coat proteins (COPs)** called α-, β- γ- and δ-COP with molecular masses of 160, 110, 98 and 61 kDa respectively. During the journey, residues of mannose are pruned

Lysosomal storage disorders
are due to deficiencies in enzymes
which normally function in the
lysosomal degradation of
macromolecules. Over 30
disorders have been identified,
most of which result from the
failure to synthesize some
functional enzyme. The
predominantly affected tissues are
those in which an uncatalysed
substrate accumulates, frequently
the central nervous system, joints,
bones, liver and spleen.

Mucopolysaccharidoses are
conditions in which
glycosaminoglycans (Chapter 5)
accumulate, e.g. **Hurler's
syndrome** which is characterized
by excessive dermatan sulphate
and heparan sulphate due to a
deficiency in α-L-**iduronidase**.
Lipidoses result in sphingolipid
(Chapter 6) accumulation, e.g.
Gaucher's disease involves a
glucocerebrosidase deficiency
resulting in abnormal storage of
cerebrosides in motile and tissue-
fixed macrophages. The defect in
Niemann–Pick disease is a
sphingomyelinase which
normally hydrolyses
phosphorylcholine from
sphingomyelin. Niemann–Pick
disease does not involve joints and
bones. **Glycoproteinoses** are
characterized by excessive
amounts of glycoproteins, e.g.
α-**mannosidosis** (Chapter 5) is
caused by a deficiency in
α-**mannosidase**.

There are other disorders which
are not classified according to an
undigested macromolecule, e.g.
Pompe's disease, due to an
α-**1,4-glucosidase**, affects
tissues such as cardiac muscle,
skeletal muscle and liver in which
glycogenolysis (Chapter 9) is
important.

and those of N-glucosamine, fucose, galactose, neuraminidic acid and possibly sulphate are added to complete the processing of the glycoprotein. Indeed, the core proteins of proteoglycans (Chapter 5) are subjected to the largest amount of glycosylation of any protein.

The Golgi complex may lose its well-defined compact structure, e.g. during cell division and certain drug treatments such as by brefeldin A. During mitosis, the Golgi complex disassembles thus blocking transport to and through the Golgi complex. Disassembly results in Golgi remnants from which the Golgi complex may reassemble.

Lysosomes and peroxisomes

Lysosomes and **peroxisomes** (Figure 7.1) are small single-membrane organelles of about $0.5\,\mu m$ in diameter. Each type of organelle possesses a discrete series of enzymes. Lysosomes may be formed from the vesicles which bud from the Golgi complex whereas peroxisomes are formed by budding from the smooth endoplasmic reticulum.

Lysosomes contain a wide variety of hydrolases which, at acidic pH (optimum pH ∼ 5.5), are capable of the degradation of carbohydrates, lipids, nucleic acids and proteins. The requirement for enzymic activation through the metabolic acidification of the lysosomal milieu serves to protect the cell from **autolysis**, i.e the destruction of cells by their own enzymes. Lysosomes function to degrade molecules taken into the cell from the exterior by the process called **endocytosis**. Endocytic vesicles fuse with lysosomes to deliver their contents to the degradative enzymes.

Peroxisomes, also called **microbodies** in the context of animal cells, contain non-digestive enzymes which produce or degrade toxic hydrogen peroxide. The compartmentalization of peroxide-generating reactions within a specialized organelle serves to protect the remainder of the cell from subsequent potentially damaging reactions involving toxic by-products of the cell's metabolism.

Cytoskeleton

The **cytoskeleton** is the remaining fibrous framework following the treatment of eukaryotic cells with non-ionic detergents under conditions in which most of the cellular proteins are extracted. The cytoskeleton consists of three distinct cytoplasmic systems of aggregated proteins identifiable by the dimensions of their fibres:

- **microfilaments** are 5–7 nm in diameter;
- **microtubules** are hollow cylinders of about 25 nm in diameter;
- **intermediate filaments** are 8–10 nm in diameter.

Microfilaments and **microtubules** (Figure 7.1) undergo carefully regulated disassembly to and reassembly from their globular monomeric component molecules of **actin** and **tubulin** respectively. These processes may be influenced by certain drugs. **Cytochalasins** and **colchicine** inhibit the polymerization of actin and tubulin respectively. Contrarily, **phalloidins** and **taxol** promote the polymerization of actin and tubulin respectively through polymer stabilization.

Microfilaments have a role in cell locomotion, cell adhesion, cell division, endocytosis and in the migration of some vesicles within the cell. The structural status of microfilaments may be modulated by over 30 different proteins some of which, e.g. **ankyrin, spectrin** and **vinculin**, may directly or indirectly connect microfilaments to the integral proteins of the plasma membrane. These connections limit the lateral movement of the constituent proteins of this membrane.

Microtubules may serve as cables along which some organelles and some vesicles move and are positioned in the cytoplasm. They are important structural elements of centrioles and the mitotic spindle to which chromosomes attach during cell division. A variety of **microtubule-associated proteins** (MAPs) have been identified.

Intermediate filaments are elongated fibrous molecules. They are found in most but not all animal cells. They are considered to provide internal mechanical support for the cells. The intermediate filaments are classified into four groups, one of which is nuclear in location, the others being found in the cell cytoplasm:

- **Lamin filaments** form the meshwork which lines the inside of the nuclear membrane. Lamin filaments may also disassemble and reassemble.
- **Vimentin filaments** are found in fibroblasts, endothelial cells and leucocytes and are also expressed in other cells during cellular development. There are a number of vimentin-related proteins, e.g. **desmin filaments** position the Z-discs of striated muscle and **glial filaments** are found in the astrocytes of the central nervous system.
- **Cytokeratin filaments** provide covalently crosslinked lattices in certain epithelial cells, e.g in the tongue, liver and skin.
- **Neurofilaments** provide rigidity to the axons of neurones.

Plasma membrane

The **plasma membrane** (Figure 7.1) encapsulates the cell and physically separates the cytoplasm from the external environment. All substances which enter or leave the cell must pass through the plasma membrane which plays an important role in the selective uptake of nutrients from the extracellular medium and the discharge of waste products of metabolism from the cell. The plasma

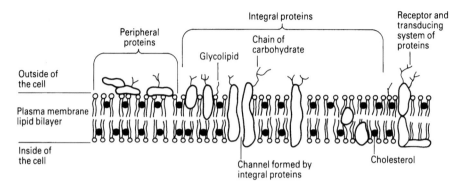

Figure 7.4   *The fluid mosaic model of membrane structure*

membrane is the most extensively researched and best understood of all cell membranes and its properties have led to the development of models of membrane structure from the fundamental lipid bilayer composed of amphipathic phospholipids (Chapter 6) to the currently most widely accepted model called the **fluid mosaic model**.

Structure

According to the fluid mosaic model (Figure 7.4), the plasma membrane is a phospholipid bilayer which incorporates various proteins and cholesterol. In mammalian cells, all plasma membrane proteins expose at least one oligosaccharide chain to the outside, but never to the inside, of the cell. Two terms are used to describe the position of plasma membrane proteins:

- **Peripheral proteins** are glycoproteins which bind loosely and externally to polar groups of membranous phospholipids. Although they are displaced easily from the membrane, i.e. by solutions of high ionic strength or alkaline pH, other proteins may in turn adhere to peripheral proteins.

- **Integral proteins** are positioned within the membrane from which they are not readily dislodged. The removal of integral proteins requires solubilization using detergents which damage the membrane.

  Integral proteins vary in their orientation, the number of times the phospholipid bilayer is spanned and the mode of attachment to the membrane (Figure 7.5):

- **The N-terminus and the bulk of the polypeptide chain is on the extracellular face** of the membrane. A single transmembrane region of hydrophobic amino acid residues interacts with the non-polar hydrocarbon chains of the membranous lipids. These hydrophobic regions are α-helical in nature and perpendicular to

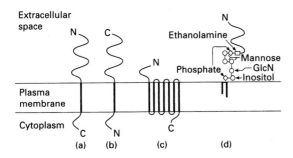

Figure 7.5 *Integral protein attachment to plasma membrane: (a) hydrophobic sequence close to the C-terminus; (b) hydrophobic sequence close to the N-terminus; (c) multiple-membrane spans; (d) glycosyl-phosphatidylinositol anchor*

the membrane surface. The C-terminus ends a short and hydrophilic cytoplasmic segment of the polypeptide chain (Figure 7.5a).

- **The C-terminus and the major proportion of the protein lie extracellularly** with a single hydrophobic transmembrane sequence close to the cytoplasmic N-terminus (Figure 7.5b).

- **Almost even distribution on both sides** of the membrane is a feature of some single-membrane spanning proteins.

- **Multiple-membrane spanning proteins** (Figure 7.5c) may contain up to 24 transmembrane segments.

- **Lipid-anchored proteins** are a separate group of glycoproteins in which the protein on the external face of the membrane is covalently attached to fatty acyl components of a membranous **glycosylphosphatidylinositol** (GPI) moiety (Figure 7.5d).

Proteins may span the membrane in such a manner as to create a **narrow channel** which may connect the cell cytoplasm to the outside milieu. These channels play an important role in the determination of the ionic status and thereby the activity of the cell.

The **single-membrane spanning proteins**, irrespective of orientation, may be subjected to limited proteolysis by proteases (also called **secretases**) or the action of phospholipases located in the membrane, a process referred to as **shedding**. Proteins released from the plasma membranes by these enzymes include some membrane receptors, e.g. tumour necrosis factor receptor (TNFR), some receptor ligands, e.g. transforming growth factor-α (TGF-α) and some **cell adhesion molecules,** e.g. L-selectin.

Many of the glycoproteins function as **cell-surface receptors,** i.e. as binding sites of unique molecular conformational shapes, each of which specifically binds a certain molecule of a complementary configuration called a ligand. When its ligand binds, the folding pattern of the polypeptide chains of the receptor changes to cause a conformational change in an associated membranous protein. In this way, a signal is transmitted across the membrane from its external face to the inside of the cell where an enzyme-mediated biological response is manifested. This process is called **signal transduction** (Chapter 8).

The plasma membrane also exhibits asymmetry with respect to some lipids. The outer monolayer of the plasma membrane of an erythrocyte, for example, contains only phosphatidylcholine and sphingomyelin (Chapter 6) whereas the inner monolayer contains phosphatidylethanolamine, phosphatidylserine and phosphatidylinositol. Glycolipids are located only in the outer monolayer. The monolayers exhibit large differences in enzymic activities.

Phosphoacylglycerols, sphingomyelins and cholesterol are incorporated into the lipid bilayer because of their amphipathic character. The bilayer formed from natural phospholipids is essentially a liquid in that it exhibits random motions consistent with the liquid state. Their hydrocarbon tails may move more freely about in the plane of the monolayer without losing their hydrophobicity which is responsible for their mutual attraction. Membranous proteins embedded within the membrane can also move laterally but are limited in the magnitude of such migrations by their interactions with other components located internal to the membrane. This property of molecular movement within the membrane is referred to as **membrane fluidity**.

Membrane fluidity is determined by the packaging of the hydrocarbon tails of the lipids within the membrane. The fluidity of biological membranes is influenced by the:

- **length** of the hydrocarbon chains;
- **degree of unsaturation** of the hydrocarbon chains;
- **cholesterol content** of the membrane.

Lipids with long saturated tails decrease membrane fluidity because their parallel tails may form extensive hydrophobic interactions. Shorter chain lengths increase membrane fluidity because of the limitations imposed upon interactions between adjacent chains. Unsaturation of a hydrocarbon tail introduces a *cis* double bond which causes a bend in the tail (Chapter 6). This lowers the numbers of hydrophobic interactions between adjacent tails and enhances membrane fluidity. Cholesterol molecules have a rigid planar non-polar ring structure which permits intercalation between the phospholipids near to their hydrophilic heads. The polar 3'-OH group of cholesterol molecules may interact with charged phospholipid groups. Cholesterol molecules may fit compactly with the kinked unsaturated hydrocarbon chains and promote hydrophobic interactions which reduce the fluidity of natural membranes.

Transport

Extracellular substances may gain access to the cell cytoplasm by a number of mechanisms dependent upon the chemistry of the molecule, the size of the molecule and the cell type. For **small molecules,** the available mechanisms are:

- **Passive diffusion.** This mechanism does not involve interaction with membranous proteins.

- **Facilitated diffusion.** Movement across the membrane is enhanced by specific integral membranous proteins called **carriers** or **transporters.**
- **Active transport** . This form of transport is also carrier-mediated but requires coupling to a source of energy, usually ATP.

These mechanisms may also apply to certain intracellular membranes, e.g in the mitochondrion and endoplasmic reticulum.

For **passive diffusion**, lipid solubility is the major criterion. The more non-polar a substance is, the greater its lipid solubility. Non-polar substances will pass through the plasma membrane readily by dissolving in the lipid regions of the membrane. Small lipid-soluble molecules, e.g. butyramide, may enter the cell by passive diffusion from a medium of high concentration to increase the low concentration within the cell. The migration of molecules in this case is simply dependent on their concentrations across the membrane.

Facilitated diffusion enables a variety of non-lipid soluble (lipophobic) small molecules, e.g. amino acids and monosaccharides, to pass through the plasma membrane. Carriers may transport more than one molecule simultaneously and may function in one or more direction(s). The relevant nomenclature, illustrated in Figure 7.6, is:

- a **uniport system** transports a single molecule in one direction;
- a **symport system** may carry two molecules simultaneously in the same direction;
- an **antiport system** transports two molecules in opposite directions by exchanging one molecule (or ion) for another molecule (or ion).

Carrier proteins demonstrate certain properties which are similar to enzymes:

- **they are permeant-specific,** e.g. glucose but not fructose may enter the erythrocyte by facilitated diffusion;
- **they are pH-dependent;**
- **they may be inhibited competitively** (Chapter 4) by compounds structurally similar to the permeant;
- **they exhibit saturation kinetics,** i.e. the rate of transport increases

> The **movement of glucose**, the major fuel molecule for most cells, between cells and the blood circulation is effected by facilitated diffusion employing a family of **tissue-specific glucose transporters** (GLUT). **GLUT 1, GLUT 3** and **GLUT 4** function in the cellular uptake of glucose. GLUT 1 is present in most cells but primarily in erythrocytes, placenta and brain. GLUT 3 is most abundant in the brain but is also found in heart, kidney and liver. GLUT 3 supplements the action of GLUT 1 during periods of high energy demand. GLUT 4 is present in insulin-target tissues, i.e. adipose tissue, cardiac and skeletal muscle.
>
> **GLUT 2** in liver, pancreatic β-cells and the small intestine senses low extracellular glucose levels and releases cellular glucose. GLUT 7 occurs in the ER of hepatocytes from where it transports glucose to the cytoplasm. GLUT 5 is now recognized as a fructose transporter and the *GLUT 6* gene is not expressed.
>
> In **brush border cells** of the small intestine and **kidney cells**, another mechanism operates. These cells may employ a **Na$^+$– glucose antiporter** which exchanges an intracellular Na$^+$ ion for extracellular glucose molecules.

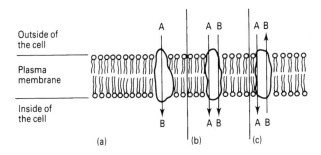

Figure 7.6 *Mechanisms for facilitated transport: (a) uniport mechanism; (b) symport mechanism; (c) antiport mechanism*

with increasing concentration of permeant until it becomes independent of concentration and remains constant (cf. V, Figure 4.2b).

Facilitated diffusion accelerates the rate at which the normal concentration equilibrium is established across the membrane but does not transport substances against a concentration gradient.

Active transport is the process which enables substances to enter the cell against a concentration gradient. The active transport carriers demonstrate the properties listed above for the carriers of facilitated diffusion. Although a source of energy is additionally required, the energy may not be used directly in the movement of the permeant in all active transport systems. Active transport is the mechanism by which cations are transported through specific narrow channels of the plasma membrane (Figure 7.4). K^+ ions are transported inwards whilst Na^+ ions travel outwards by the action of the $Na^+- K^+$-**exchanging ATPase** (also called the Na^+-K^+ pump). Ca^{2+}ions are pumped out of the cytosol by the Ca^{2+}-**transporting ATPase** at the expense of ATP.

Macromolecules and large particles penetrate the impermeable barrier of the plasma membrane by the process called **endocytosis**. In endocytosis, the matter to be absorbed is engulfed by an area of the plasma membrane which forms an enclosed vesicle. There are two possibilities for these particles:

- phagocytosis;
- receptor-mediated endocytosis.

In **phagocytosis**, large particles bind to the surface of the cell by non-specific interactions with receptors involving hydrophobicity and surface tension or through specific attachment to cell-surface receptors. Particle-receptor contact initiates a series of biochemical events which result in the envelopment of the particle by the plasma membrane to form a **phagosome**. The phagosome migrates inwards and fuses with a lysosome, the enzymes of which on activation degrade the ingested particle.

Receptor-mediated endocytosis is absolutely specific. The receptors may reside in specific areas of the plasma membrane called coated pits, e.g. low-density lipoprotein (LDL) receptors, or may be scattered over the membrane and, on ligand binding, migrate laterally to a specific area of the membrane, e.g. insulin receptors. The intracellular transport and processing of receptor–ligand systems in receptor-mediated endocytosis may be characterized into four general modes:

- recycling receptors which transport their ligand to lysosomes, e.g. LDL receptors;
- recycling receptors which do not transport their ligand to lysosomes, e.g. transferrin receptors;

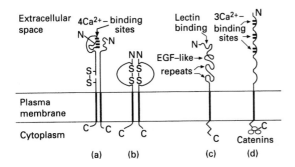

Figure 7.7 *Members of the family of cell-adhesion molecules: (a) integrin; (b) immunoglobin superfamily (CD8); (c) selectin (L-selectin); (d) cadherin*

- **non-recycling receptors** which transport their ligand to lysosomes, e.g. EGF (epidermal growth factor) receptors;
- **non-recycling receptors** which do not transport their ligand to lysosomes, e.g. IgA (immunoglobulin A) receptors.

Another endocytic intake mechanism is **pinocytosis**. Pinocytosis is a non-specific process in which minute droplets of extracellular fluid are engulfed by the plasma membrane. On detachment from the plasma membrane, pinocytic vesicles of less than 1 nm in diameter containing ions and small molecules migrate into the cytoplasm.

Cellular adhesion molecules

A **cellular adhesion molecule** is any cell-surface molecule which functions in increasing the affinity of a cell for either another cell or components of the extracellular matrix. Their adhesive properties may be inhibited by specific antibodies which prevent their association with their specific ligand(s). In addition to their effects on cellular affinities, adhesion molecules often play a role in cell signalling.

The majority of cellular adhesion molecules have been classified into four families (Figure 7.7):

- **The integrins** are a family of heterodimeric glycoproteins expressed on the surface of many cells.
- **The immunoglobulin superfamily** contains over 70 members which function in the control of cell function predominantly in the nervous and immune systems.
- **The selectins** are a family of three single polypeptide chains which function in the inflammatory response.
- **The cadherins** are a family of at least 11 different calcium-dependent molecules which generally mediate homotypic cell–cell adhesion. **Homotypic adhesion** occurs when the same molecule located on different cells functions as both the receptor and the ligand.

All **integrins** consist of two chains, α- and β-chains (Figure 7.7a).

There are at least 15 different α-chains and eight different β-chains. An individual α-chain may bind with different β-chains. The integrins are further subdivided on the basis of the β-chain, e.g. the β_2-integrins found on leukocytes each have a β_2-chain (also called CD18) but different α-chains such as α_L (CD11a), α_M (CD11b) and α_X (CD11c). The integrins bind to various extracellular matrix proteins, e.g. collagen, fibronectin and to members of the immunoglobulin superfamily, e.g. intercellular adhesion molecules ICAM-1 (CD54), ICAM-2 (CD102), ICAM-3 (CD50) and vascular intercellular adhesion molecule VCAM-1 (CD106). Most family members bind more than one ligand for which they exhibit different affinities. Both integrin chains participate in ligand binding. Both integrin chains are transmembranal and play important roles in connecting the extracellular matrix with components of the cytoskeleton. Through the integrins, the extracellular matrix may influence cellular behaviour.

Immunoglobulin superfamily members (Figure 7.7 b) are believed to be derived from a **common ancestral unit** which is composed of 70–110 amino acid residues organized into two parallel β-conformations stabilized by disulphide bonds as found in the immunoglobulin molecule. Although their primary structures are extremely varied, the tertiary structures displayed by family members are very similar. Immunoglobulin superfamily members function in organismal development especially of the nervous system and in the regulation of the immune system.

The **selectins** (Figure 7.7c) are single-chain glycoproteins. **E- and P-selectins** (CD62E and CD62P respectively) are located on endothelial cells whereas most leukocytes express L-selectin (CD62L). Each polypeptide chain contains three types of extracellular domains. Selectins contain a N-terminal calcium-dependent (C-type) carbohydrate-binding domain (lectin is the generic term for a carbohydrate-binding protein). Each selectin also contains a domain related to the repeat described in epidermal growth factor (EGF-like repeat), a variable number (two in L-, six in E- and nine in P-selectin) of a repeat found in some proteins which regulate the complement system, a transmembrane region and a short cytoplasmic sequence. The selectin molecules recognize numerous ligands and are responsible for the first adhesion event between leukocytes and the vascular endothelium which culminates in leukocyte migration into the tissues.

The **cadherins** (Figure 7.7d) were originally named after the cells on which they were identified. Therefore, **E-cadherin** was present on epithelial cells, **N-cadherin** on nerve cells and **P-cadherin** on placental cells. At least 12 different cadherins are known. Cadherins are single-pass glycoproteins, i.e. they pass directly through the plasma membrane. Their large extracellular domain usually contains five internal repeats, three of which may bind Ca^{2+} ions without which cell–cell adhesion does not occur and without which the cadherins are rapidly degraded by proteolytic enzymes.

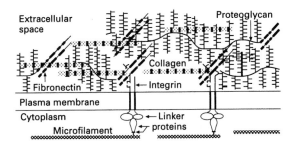

Figure 7.8 *Schematic structure of the extracellular matrix*

Their cytoplasmic sequences bind cytoplasmic proteins called **catenins**. The cadherins play important roles in development during which they direct different cell types to their required positions within tissues.

Extracellular matrix

The **extracellular matrix** is the relatively stable structural material which supports tissue cells and provides space for the diffusion of nutrients and oxygen to these cells through the tissue. The extracellular matrix comprises four major classes of macromolecules (Figure 7.8):

- **collagens** (Chapter 3) give strength or durability to the tissues;
- **proteoglycans** (Chapter 5)are essential for compressive resiliency of tissues;
- **elastin,** a fibrous protein, provides tear-resistant resiliency in elastic tissues, e.g. in arteries of the cardiovascular system and skin;
- **adhesion-promoting glycoproteins** provide cohesiveness in tissues.

The **adhesion-promoting glycoproteins** generally contain structural domains which provide binding sites for other molecules of the extracellular matrix, cell-surface receptors and sites for self-association or oligomerization through disulphide or non-covalent bonding. **Fibronectin** (Figure 7. 9) is a heterodimer, assembled from two similar but non-identical chains of ~ 2300 amino acid residues. The two subunits are linked near their C-termini by a pair of disulphide bonds. Each chain is a series of functional domains each of which permits a specific function, e.g. binding to collagen, heparin, fibrin and cells. Of the three fibrin binding sites, one is cryptic and only binds fibrin upon proteolytic release from the polypeptide chain. The cell-binding domain (75 kDa) contains the tripeptide **RGD motif** (Arg-Gly-Asp) to which an appropriate cell-surface receptor molecule (integrin $\alpha_5\beta_1$) may bind. In this way, fibroblasts may bind to fibronectin-coated surfaces and *in vivo* fibronectin is a major anchor for cells. On one chain only, an

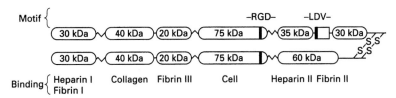

Figure 7.9   *The domain structure of fibronectin*

LDV motif (Leu-Asp-Val) provides a cell-type specific sequence to which activated T lymphocytes but not fibroblasts may bind.

Suggested further reading

Coux, O., Tanaka, K. and Goldberg, A.L. (1996). Structure and functions of the 20S and 26S proteasomes. *Annual Review of Biochemistry* **65**, 801–847.

Freemont, A.J. and Hoyland, J.A. (1996). Cell adhesion molecules. *Journal of Clinical Pathology and Molecular Pathology* **96**, M321–M330.

Halban, P.A. and Irminger, J.-C. (1994). Sorting and processing of secretory proteins. *Biochemical Journal* **299**, 1–18.

Haimo, L.T. (1997). Ordering microtubules. *Bioessays* **19**, 547–550.

Ruoslahti, E. (1996). RGD and other recognition sequences for integrins. *Annual Review of Cell and Developmental Biology* **12**, 697–715.

Warren, G. and Wickner, W. (1996). Organelle inheritance. *Cell* **84**, 395–400.

Goodsell, D.S. (1993). *The Machinery of Life*. New York: Springer.

Self-assessment questions

1. Identify the subcellular structures responsible for the following activities:
   (a) detoxification of H_2O_2; (b) ATP production in aerobic cells; (c) folding of newly synthesized proteins; (d) hydroxylation of procollagen chains; (e) storage of most of the cell's DNA.
2. With which membrane do you associate the following activities: (a) ATP production in hepatocytes; (b) Na^+–K^+ pump; (c) endocytosis; (d) facilitated diffusion of glucose by GLUT 1; (e) regulation of the export of ribosomal subunits; (f) synthesis of phospholipids?
3. In what way are the carriers of active transport similar to enzymes?
4. A member of which family of cellular adhesion molecules

assists in the responsiveness of cells to variations in the extracellular matrix?

5. Where in the mammalian cell would you find the following: (a) cisternae; (b) intermembrane space; (c) perinuclear space; (d) proteasomes; (e) cristae?

6. How does cholesterol influence plasma membrane fluidity?

7. Are multiple-membrane spanning proteins subject to shedding from the plasma membrane?

8. List the mechanisms by which macromolecules may gain entry to a cell.

9. Which of the following organelles are enclosed by a single membrane: (a) endoplasmic reticulum; (b) Golgi complex; (c) mitochondrion; (d) ribosome; (e) lysosome; (f) nucleus; (g) peroxisome?

10. How is autolysis by lysosomal enzymes prevented?

Key Concepts and Facts

Nucleus

- The nucleus stores most of the cell's DNA which is dispersed throughout the nucleoplasm as chromatin fibres.

- The nucleus is the site of DNA replication and RNA synthesis, the nucleolus being the site of rRNA synthesis.

- The nuclear envelope has pore complexes which regulate the import and export of large molecular complexes into and out of the nucleus.

Cytoplasm

- Membrane-bound organelles are suspended in the aqueous phase of the cytoplasm called the cytosol.

- The proteasome is a barrel-shaped structure in which intracellular proteins are degraded.

- Ribosomes, whether attached or not attached to the endoplasmic reticulum, synthesize proteins.

- The inner mitochondrial membranes hold the components for oxidative phosphorylation.

- The mitochondrial matrix houses most of the enzymes which function in aerobic oxidative pathways, some ribosomes, DNA and is a store for Ca^{2+} ions.

- The endoplasmic reticulum is the site of co- and post-translational modifications to newly synthesized proteins and a store for Ca^{2+} ions.

- The Golgi complex sorts proteins for secretion or delivery to intracellular locations.

Plasma Membrane

- The plasma membrane is a phospholipid bilayer which incorporates cholesterol and various proteins, e.g. receptors, ion channels, cell adhesion molecules and enzymes.

- The plasma membrane is an asymmetric and dynamic structure, supported by the cytoskeleton.

- Substances which enter or leave the cell may pass through the plasma membrane by a variety of mechanisms.

- Cellular adhesion molecules increase a cell's affinity for either another cell or the extracellular matrix.

Extracellular Matrix

- Collagens, proteoglycans, elastin and adhesion-promoting glycoproteins provide strength, resiliency and cohesiveness to tissues.

- The extracellular matrix may influence intracellular events through transmembrane molecular systems.

Answers to questions (Chapter 7)

1. (a) Peroxisome; (b) mitochondrion; (c) RER and *cis*-Golgi; (d) RER; (e) nucleus.
2. (a) Inner mitochondrial membrane; (b) plasma membrane; (c) plasma membrane; (d) plasma membrane; (e) nuclear envelope; (f) SER.
3. They are proteins, specific for permeant (substrate), pH-dependent, may be competitively inhibited and exhibit saturation kinetics.
4. Fibronectin receptor (integrin $\alpha_5\beta_1$).
5. (a) ER; (b) between the inner and outer mitochondrial membranes; (c) between the inner and outer nuclear membranes; (d) cytosol and nucleus; (e) inner mitochondrial membrane.
6. Its rigid planar non-polar ring structure intercalates between the phospholipids near to their hydrophilic charged heads which interact with the polar 3′-OH group of the cholesterol molecule. Cholesterol promotes hydrophobic interactions which reduce membrane fluidity.
7. No. This process only applies to single-membrane spanning proteins.
8. Phagocytosis and receptor-mediated endocytosis.
9. (e) and (g).
10. The enzymes are normally inactive until acidification of the organelle activates them by lowering the pH towards their optimum pH (pH 5.5).

Chapter 8
The principles of cellular metabolism

Learning objectives

After studying this chapter you should confidently be able to:

Apply the laws of thermodynamics to biochemical reactions.

Discuss the importance of free energy in biological systems.

Describe metabolic pathways as interconnected sequences of coupled enzyme-catalysed reactions.

Interrelate anabolism and catabolism.

Discuss intracellular strategies to regulate cellular metabolism.

Discuss extracellular control of metabolism in relation to hormonal influence on metabolic activity.

Discuss the generation and roles of second messengers in signal transduction.

Discuss the mechanisms of action of hydrophobic hormones.

Living cells require energy to survive, differentiate, function and reproduce. Mammalian cells acquire energy in chemical form from nutrient molecules. The chemical processes which occur within the cell are termed **cellular metabolism**. Cellular metabolism is organized into a network of **metabolic pathways**. A metabolic pathway may be defined as a sequence of **coupled enzyme-catalysed reactions**. Cellular metabolism is therefore the conversion of substrates into products through the activity of various enzymes. The normal function of metabolism is intimately associated with the:

- **release of energy** usually in the form of adenosine triphosphate (ATP);
- **biosynthesis** of macromolecules and important smaller molecules;
- **active transport** of molecules and ions across membranes;
- **movement of cells** or their component parts.

Cellular metabolism also provides much of the building materials for biosynthesis such as nucleotides, amino acids, monosaccharides and fatty acids for nucleic acid, protein, polysaccharide and lipid syntheses respectively. The demands for energy and building materials vary widely across different cell types and within the same cell under different conditions. Fluctuating needs demand mechanisms for adjustments to cellular metabolic activity. These variations within cells are managed so that the concentrations of key compounds are maintained within strict limits. Therefore, in healthy cells, the rate of biosynthesis of any compound compensates for the rate of its utilization. This balance is accomplished by the synthesis of enzymes required for the pathway to function or more immediately by the regulation of the activity of existent enzymes.

The laws which govern cellular energy transformations are also applicable to non-cellular processes. The discipline of physical science which considers energy changes is **thermodynamics** which was originally developed as a means to rationalize engineering processes. The principles of thermodynamics have subsequently been employed to underpin the release and utilization of energy in biological systems.

This chapter considers the source of energy for biological systems, equilibrium thermodynamics, coupled enzymic reactions, the role of ATP, metabolic pathways, and the intracellular and extracellular control of metabolism.

The carbon cycle

The **ultimate source of energy** used in biological systems is the thermonuclear fusion of hydrogen atoms to form helium which occurs at the surface of the **sun** according to the equation: $4H \rightarrow 1He + 2$ positrons + energy. (A positron is a particle which has the same mass as an electron but has a positive charge.) The energy is transported to earth as sunlight (light energy) which is converted into chemical energy by green plants and certain micro-organisms called **phototrophs** by the process of **photosynthesis**. The chemical energy is stored primarily in carbohydrates synthesized by the reduction of atmospheric carbon dioxide. Also, oxygen is produced from water as a by-product and released into the atmosphere. These products of photosynthesis are vital for aerobic organisms which do not contain the necessary molecular apparatus (light-harvesting complexes) for the above transformations of energy. Such organisms obtain their energy by utilizing molecular oxygen to oxidize energy-rich plant products. This process, called **respiration**, produces, amongst other products, carbon dioxide which is returned to the atmosphere to be subsequently utilized in photosynthesis. This cycle of events is called **the carbon cycle** (Figure 8.1).

During most of the inherent reactions of the cycle, energy is lost

Figure 8.1   *The carbon cycle*

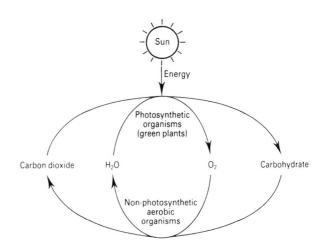

The **nitrogen cycle** comprises the circulation of nitrogen atoms from the atmosphere into the molecules of living organisms through ammonium ions (NH_4^+) and their return to the atmosphere by denitrifying bacteria. Ammonium ions may be incorporated into organic nitrogenous compounds such as amino acids and nucleotides through the formation of glutamate by **glutamate dehydrogenase**. Glutamate may be converted into glutamine by **glutamate–ammonia ligase**.

The formation of NH_4^+ may occur by two routes: **nitrogen fixation** and **nitrogen assimilation**. **Nitrogen-fixing bacteria** may live free in the soil but the most effective are of the genus **Rhizobium**, located in root nodules of leguminous plants, e.g. clover and soya bean, and of a few non-leguminous plants, e.g. alder. **Cyanobacteria** perform nitrogen fixation mainly in the oceans. These organisms all reduce N_2 to NH_4^+ by a **nitrogenase** in an energetically expensive reaction. **Nitrogen assimilation** involves soil nitrates, often the decay products from organic matter. Initially, **nitrate reductase** reduces nitrate (NO_3^-) to nitrite (NO_2^-) which is reduced to ammonia by **nitrite reductase**.

Ammonia may, however, be oxidized back to NO_3^- by **nitrifying bacteria**. **Nitrosomonas** converts NH_4^+ to NO_2^- and **Nitrobacter** converts NO_2^- to NO_3^-. Denitrifying bacteria release nitrogen back into the atmosphere from the nitrogen oxides.

and cannot be used profitably by the cells of the organism. Therefore, although chemical substances may recycle, energy flow is linear and irreversible.

Equilibrium thermodynamics

The study of the energetics of any system is described as thermodynamics, the principles of which are elucidated from the quantitative analysis of energy transformations in simpler physical and chemical systems. These principles have been applied in an attempt to explain energy flow in living organisms.

First law of thermodynamics

The first law of thermodynamics is related to the principle of **conservation of energy**. The law in essence states that, although energy can be converted from one form to another, it cannot be created or destroyed, so that whenever one form of energy is produced, there is a reduction of the same magnitude in another form of energy.

The system under consideration may gain or lose heat to its surroundings. Alternatively, the system may perform work on its surroundings or be modified by the work of its surroundings. **In a chemical reaction**, reactants A and B are converted to products C and D only when energy is obtainable from without the system, i.e.

$$A + B \underset{- \text{ energy}}{\overset{+ \text{ energy}}{\rightleftharpoons}} C + D$$

The quantity of energy absorbed in the forward reaction equals exactly the amount released during the reverse reaction. The **change in internal energy** of the system in both the forward and reverse reactions, and therefore the first law of thermodynamics, may be expressed as:

$$\Delta E = E_2 - E_1 = q - w$$

where ΔE = the change of the internal energy of the system, E_1 = the internal energy of the system initially, E_2 = the internal energy of the system at the end of a process, q = the heat flow and w = the work done.

At the molecular level, the internal energy of the system includes the **translational, rotational, vibrational** and **electronic energies** of the molecule. Electronic energies involve electron–electron, electron–nucleus and nucleus–nucleus interactions. Since thermodynamics is not concerned with reaction mechanisms but the difference in energy between reactants and products, interactions which do not change during the course of a chemical reaction are not considered. Although some categories of electronic energies, e.g. nucleus–nucleus interactions, do not change during a reaction, the overall magnitude of electronic energies involved in the reaction, e.g. through electron–electron interactions, make the major contribution to the internal energy of a chemical reaction.

Second law of thermodynamics

The second law of thermodynamics conveys the principle that all spontaneous reactions endeavour to achieve an equilibrium state. During the approach to equilibrium, energy is released so that the system under consideration becomes less ordered, i.e. more random. Consider a strong salt solution as a system separated by a semipermeable membrane from water (the surroundings). After some time, salt ions are lost from the system to its surroundings; the salt solution becomes dilute in the system and therefore the system is less ordered. Viable cells and organisms are never at equilibrium with their surroundings and are constantly at work to avoid the equilibrium state.

The second law does not consider internal energy in isolation but considers **enthalpy** (**H**) which may be regarded as 'internal energy plus'. In an ideal gas, enthalpy is the internal energy of the gas plus the changes in the pressure and volume of the system. In addition to internal energy, enthalpy takes into account the effects of the interactions between the molecules as a result of collisions, although a chemical reaction need not result. As biochemical reactions usually occur in solutions rather than in the gaseous state, volume changes are relatively small so that enthalpy and internal energy are often approximately equal.

Free energy

Biochemists consider enthalpy in relation to **entropy** (**S**), a measure

Thermodynamic principles are based on the concept of **a system** and **its surroundings**. The system may be a chemical reaction, a cell or an organism for which the surroundings are the reaction solvent, the extracellular fluid (or matrix) or the environment in which the organism survives respectively. Exchange of energy and/or matter may occur between the system and the surroundings depending on whether the system is **closed, isolated or open**. In a closed system, there is no exchange of matter or energy between the system and its surroundings. In an isolated system, only energy may be exchanged between the system and its surroundings. In an open system, both energy and matter may be exchanged between the system and its surroundings. Viable cells and organisms may exchange matter (e.g. gaseous exchange of carbon dioxide and oxygen) and energy (derived from metabolism in the form of heat) with their surroundings. Living cells and organisms are therefore examples of open systems.

The third law of thermodynamics states that the entropy of any crystalline substance at a temperature of absolute zero (0 K on the **Kelvin temperature scale**) is exactly zero. As the temperature descends towards 0 K, the entropy of a perfectly ordered substance approaches zero. A mathematical equation has been developed to relate entropy to the heat capacity of a substance which is pressure-dependent. The importance of absolute zero to considerations of entropy requires that the Kelvin temperature scale is employed in calculations related to thermodynamics.

It is generally considered that the **oxygenation of haemoglobin** (Chapter 3) is an **exothermic reaction** although within the animal kingdom some exceptions exist. In man, the ΔH for oxygenation is $-33.4 \, kJ \, mol^{-1}$ but in some arctic animals, ΔH is lower, e.g. in reindeer, ΔH is $-13.8 \, kJ \, mol^{-1}$. The lower ΔH permits the reindeer to survive in extremely cold temperatures since deoxygenation requires much less heat than in man, thus permitting an adequate delivery of oxygen to colder peripheral tissues.

of randomness. Entropy however cannot be measured directly. Enthalpy, the total heat energy of the system, consists of entropy and **free energy** (G). Entropy is associated with the randomness of molecular motions within the system and tends to increase as free energy is released during reactions. Free energy is available to perform useful work in the system until equilibrium is achieved. At any given temperature and pressure: $H = TS + G$, where T is the absolute temperature.

Since biochemists primarily use thermodynamics to consider the progress of a reaction, it is more pertinent to describe the effect of any change in free energy. Changes in free energy are accompanied by concomitant changes in enthalpy and entropy: $\Delta G = \Delta H - T\Delta S$, where Δ denotes change. A biochemical system:

- **At equilibrium** exhibits no change in its free-energy content, i.e. ΔG is zero, and entropy is maximal. Alteration may be effected only by the supply of free energy to the system. In this case, ΔG is positive and the entropy decreases. Reactions which consume free energy are **endergonic**. They consequently exhibit a positive enthalpy change and are thermodynamically unfavourable.

- **Not at equilibrium** may proceed spontaneously only by the liberation of free energy, i.e. ΔG is negative, and with a progressive increase in entropy. Reactions which liberate free energy and consequently undergo a negative enthalpy change are termed **exergonic**. Exergonic reactions are considered to be thermodynamically favourable. If the free energy contained within the reactant(s) is greater than that of the product(s), the reaction may proceed spontaneously since:

$$\Delta G = G_{(products)} - G_{(reactants)} = \textbf{negative value}.$$

To permit comparisons of free-energy changes during different reactions, evaluations must be made under agreed conditions, called the **standard thermodynamic conditions**, of a temperature of 298 K (25°C), a pressure of 1.0 atmosphere, with reactants and products at a concentration of 1.0 mol l^{-1}. For the general reaction, $A + B \rightarrow C + D$, the **actual** change in free energy (ΔG) is related to the **standard free-energy change** ($\Delta G°$) by the approximation:

$$\Delta G = \Delta G° + RT \ln \frac{[C][D]}{[A][B]}$$

where R = the gas constant = $8.3 \, J \, K^{-1} \, mol^{-1}$, T = temperature in K and ln = natural logarithm.

$\Delta G°$ may be determined when the system is at equilibrium since, under such conditions, $\Delta G° = 0$ and the above equation rearranges to:

$$\Delta G° = -RT \ln \frac{[C][D]}{[A][B]}$$

However, since the system is at equilibrium, the concentration

Table 8.1 *The numerical relationship between the equilibrium constant of biochemical reactions, standard free-energy change and the direction of a reaction at pH 7.0 and 25° C*

K'_{eq} value	$\Delta G'$ (kJ mol^{-1})*	Direction
10 000	−22.8 ⎫	
1000	−17.1 ⎪	
100	−11.4 ⎬	Forward reaction
10	−5.7 ⎭	
1	0	At equilibrium
0.1	+5.7 ⎫	
0.01	+11.4 ⎪	
0.001	+17.1 ⎬	Reverse reactions
0.0001	+22.8 ⎭	

* Calculated from $\Delta G^{\circ\prime} = RT \ln K'_{eq} = -2.3\, RT \log K'_{eq}$.

component is the equilibrium constant, $\boldsymbol{K}_{eq}$, so that: $\Delta G^{\circ} = -RT \ln K_{eq}$. Therefore at any temperature, ΔG° can be calculated from the equilibrium constant for that reaction. Also, since the $\ln K_{eq}$ component is dimensionless, the units of $R(\mathrm{J\,K^{-1}\,mol^{-1}})$ and $T(\mathrm{K})$ result in ΔG having the units of $\mathrm{J\,mol^{-1}}$. J denotes the unit of energy called the joule which has been adopted by the International System of Units (Le Système International, abbreviated to SI units).

Standard free-energy change (ΔG°) measurements demand that the initial concentrations of reactants and products are 1.0 mol l^{-1}. Many biochemical reactions liberate or consume protons. To comply with standard thermodynamic conditions, these reactions should proceed at pH 0 (Chapter 1). Since most biochemical reactions occur *in vivo* near pH 7.0, standard free-energy changes for biochemical reactions are measured at pH 7.0 and accordingly denoted as $\boldsymbol{\Delta G^{\circ\prime}}$. Table 8.1 relates $\Delta G^{\circ\prime}$ to the equilibrium constant and the direction of the reaction. Through the equation, $\Delta G^{\circ} = -RT \ln K'_{eq}$, a K'_{eq} greater than 1 gives a negative $\Delta G^{\circ\prime}$ and therefore the reaction will proceed in a forward direction.

Coupled reactions

A thermodynamically favourable reaction may be linked to an unfavourable reaction so that the free energy liberated may be employed to drive the energy-consuming reaction. Interconnected endergonic and exergonic reactions are termed **coupled reactions**. Two forms of coupling may occur:

- **Through a common intermediate.** Consider the following two reactions:

  $\mathrm{A \rightarrow B}; \Delta G^{\circ\prime} = -24\,\mathrm{kJ\,mol^{-1}}; K'_{eq} = 16\,645$ and

$$B \rightarrow C; \Delta G^{\circ\prime} = +15 \, \text{kJ mol}^{-1}; K'_{eq} = 0.0023$$

Under standard conditions, A can be spontaneously converted into B because $\Delta G^{\circ\prime}$ has a negative value and K'_{eq} is greater than 1. Since in the second reaction, $\Delta G^{\circ\prime}$ has a positive value and K'_{eq} is less than 1, B cannot form C. However, C may be produced by the coupling of the reactions since $A \rightarrow B \rightarrow C$ has an overall negative $\Delta G^{\circ\prime}$ and a K'_{eq} greater than 1, i.e.

$$A \rightarrow C; \Delta G^{\circ\prime} = -9 \, \text{kJ mol}^{-1}; K'_{eq} = 38.3.$$

Coupled reactions illustrate the principle that $\Delta G^{\circ\prime}$ values are **additive**. The logarithmic relationship between $\Delta G^{\circ\prime}$ and K'_{eq} results in $\Delta G^{\circ\prime}$ being a more convenient representation of the equilibrium constant.

- **Through the transfer of a chemical group**, e.g. **phosphoryl group**, **acyl group** or **hydrogen atoms** (hydride ions). Consider the following two reactions:

$$A \rightarrow B; \Delta G^{\circ\prime} = -\text{ve kJ mol}^{-1} \text{ and } Y \rightarrow Z; \Delta G^{\circ\prime} = +\text{ve kJ mol}^{-1}$$

but

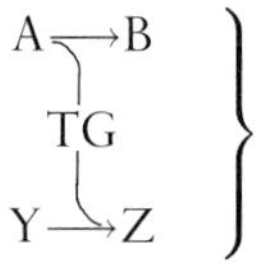

$$\left.\begin{array}{c} A \rightarrow B \\ TG \\ Y \rightarrow Z \end{array}\right\} \quad \Delta G^{\circ\prime} = -\text{ve kJ mol}^{-1}$$

The **transferable group** (TG) is chemically bonded to a carrier. The most important intracellular carriers are ADP (Figure 8.2) which is phosphorylated to ATP to transport a phosphoryl group, $NAD(P)^+$ (Figure 4.5a) which is reduced by hydride ions and coenzyme A (Figure 4.5d) which is acylated to carry an acyl group.

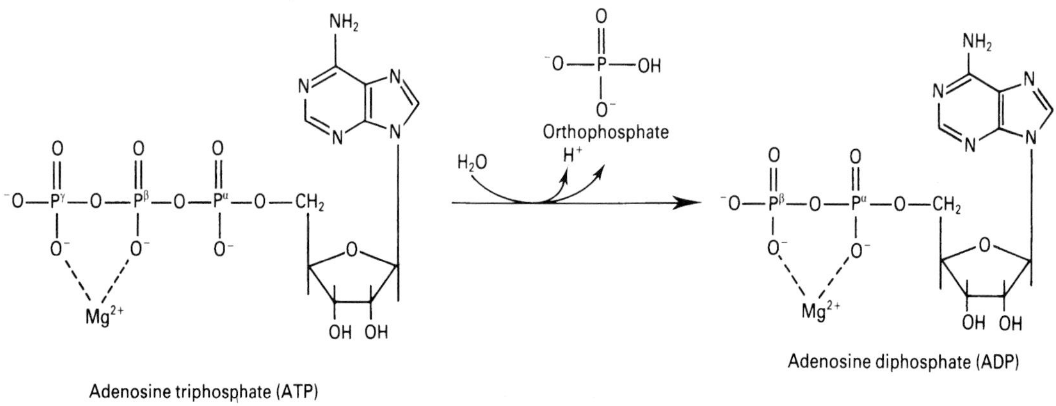

Figure 8.2   *Orthophosphate cleavage in the hydrolysis of ATP*

Table 8.2 *Standard free energy of hydrolysis of some phosphates*

Phosphate compound	$\Delta G^{\circ\prime}(kJ\ mol^{-1})$
Phospho*enol*pyruvate	−61.9
1,3-Bisphosphoglycerate	−49.4
Creatine phosphate	−43.1
Acetyle phosphate	−43.1
MgATP (to MgADP)	−30.5
MgADP (to AMP)	−30.5
Glucose 1-phosphate	−20.9
Fructose 6-phosphate	−15.9
Glucose 6-phosphate	−13.8

The role of ATP

The major link in cells between exergonic and endergonic reactions is ATP. Magnesium ions are found within the cell at relatively high concentrations so that ATP, ADP and AMP, because of their electronegativity, exist mainly as **magnesium complexes**. MgATP occupies an intermediate position on the list of standard free energy of hydrolysis, $\Delta G^{\circ\prime}$, of phosphate compounds (Table 8.2). This position enables the formation of ATP on the hydroiysis of a phosphoryl group from a phosphate compound with a higher $\Delta G^{\circ\prime}$ and permits the release of sufficient energy from ATP on its hydrolysis to drive the synthesis of a compound with a lower $\Delta G^{\circ\prime}$. This principle is illustrated during glycolysis where ATP provides the energy and the phosphoryl group for the production of glucose 6-phosphate and fructose 1, 6-bisphosphate but ATP is generated from 1,3-bisphosphoglycerate and phospho*enol*pyruvate (Chapter 9). By the removal of the negative signs, the data can be referred to as the **phosphate group transfer potential**, e.g. MgATP has a phosphate group transfer potential of 30.5 compared with 13.8 for glucose 6-phosphate. This means that the tendency for ATP to transfer a phosphoryl group is greater than that of glucose 6-phosphate.

The enhancement of phosphate group transfer potential in ATP has been accounted for in terms of:

- **Intra-molecular mutual repulsion.** At pH 7.0, the triphosphate moiety of ATP is almost fully deprotonated. The four electro-negative charges repel each other vigorously. When the γ-phosphoryl group is hydrolysed from ATP by orthophosphate cleavage (Figure 8.2), the electrostatic repulsion is reduced. The electrostatic repulsion is partially relieved by the binding of magnesium ions which results in the $\Delta G^{\circ\prime}$ value for MgATP being approximately 50% lower than that of free ATP.

- **Resonance stabilization.** Greater stability is conferred upon the hydrolysis products by their ability to oscillate rapidly between

The hydrolysis of ATP may proceed in an alternative manner to orthophosphate cleavage (Figure 8.2). **Pyrophosphate cleavage** produces pyrophosphate and AMP. This mechanism is important since a freely reversible coupled reaction may be converted into an essentially irreversible reaction by the subsequent removal of pyrophosphate by its hydrolysis catalysed by **inorganic pyrophosphatase**. Examples include the formation of UDP-glucose by UTP-glucose-1-phosphate uridylyltransferase in glycogen biosynthesis (Figure 9.6) and in the cytosolic activation of fatty acids by acyl-CoA synthase (Figure 12.1).

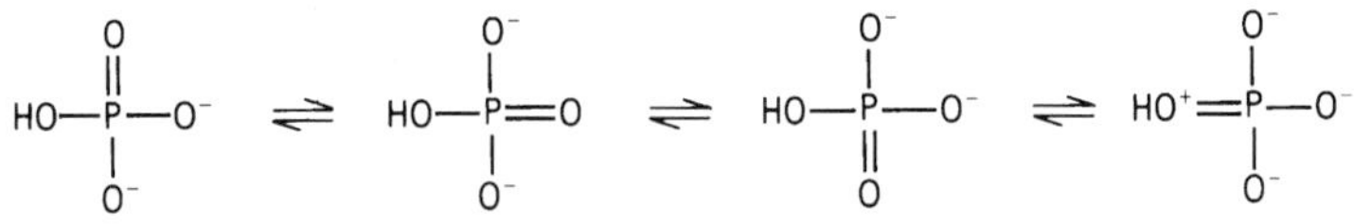

Figure 8.3 *The major resonance forms of orthophosphate*

ATP was discovered in 1929 and its ubiquitous role in cellular energetics has been long established. Although ATP has been viewed traditionally as functioning entirely within the cell, since 1985 it has been realized that ATP also has **extracellular functions** at micromolar concentrations.

ATP acts as a **cotransmitter** being released with **noradrenaline** from sympathetic nerves innervating blood vessels and is similarly involved in smooth muscle contraction. ATP is also released with **acetylcholine** from parasympathetic nerves and functions in the control of the urinary bladder. ATP has been shown to act as a neurotransmitter at neuroneuronal synapses in sympathetic ganglia and the brain.

On release from nerves, ATP interacts with subtypes of **P2 purinoceptors**, namely P2X$_1$, P2X$_2$ and P2X$_3$. P2X$_1$ and P2X$_2$ are ligand-gated cation channels of wide distribution in the human body but P2X$_3$ is of very limited distribution, being expressed at high levels in sensory C-fibre nerves entering the spinal cord. This location implicates ATP in the generation of **pain signals**. The highly restrictive localization of P2X$_3$ receptors suggests that suitable antagonists may be developed as pain-killing drugs.

different structures (Figure 8.3). This resonance enables the electrons in the products to orbit the atomic nucleus at a lower energy level than in ATP.

Other nucleoside 5′-triphosphates demonstrate a standard free energy of hydrolysis equivalent to that of ATP. Their intracellular concentrations are low which restricts their function to selected biosynthetic pathways, e.g. uridine triphosphate (UTP) in glycogen biosynthesis (Chapter 9). The enzyme, nucleoside-diphosphate kinase permits the phosphorylation of NDPs to NTPs at the expense of ATP and vice versa.

In mammalian cells, ATP may be synthesized by two mechanisms, each of which involves coupling:

- **Substrate-level phosphorylation,** which may be defined as the enzymic phosphorylation of ADP (or one other nucleoside 5′-diphosphate) employing energy derived from a coupled reaction involving a substrate with a large negative $\Delta G^{\circ\prime}$(Table 8.2). Such compounds are less stable than their free hydrolysis products.

- **Oxidative phosphorylation,** the process in which the transport of electrons from reduced coenzymes to molecular oxygen supplies the energy for ATP production (Chapter 11).

Metabolic pathways

A **metabolic pathway** is a sequence of coupled enzyme-catalysed reactions. Many metabolic pathways are linear sequences (Figure 8.4a) although some important pathways are cyclic. The enzymes of metabolic pathways are not generally organized intracellularly into defined rows but are available as random molecules in the aqueous milieu of a cellular compartment, e.g. cytosol, or as loosely or tightly bound membrane proteins. However, some enzymes are aggregated into **multi-enzyme complexes,** e.g. fatty acid synthase (Chapter 12). Substrates and products within a metabolic pathway are called **intermediates.** Certain intermediates may serve as substrates for more than one enzyme available within the same cellular compartment. This gives rise to **branch points** in metabolism (Figure 8.4b). Pertinent generation of products therefore requires the regulation of the activity of various metabolic pathways.

Capital letters = substrates/products
Small letters = enzymes

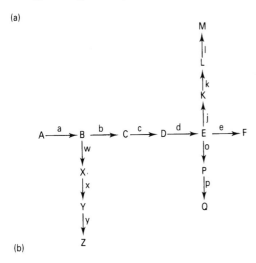

(a)

(b)

Figure 8.4 *Some principles of cellular metabolism: (a) a metabolic pathway; (b) branch points; (c) coupling of anabolism to catabolism*

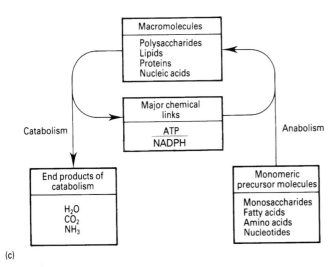

(c)

Anabolism and catabolism

Metabolic pathways conform to the principles of thermodynamics and may be classified as:

- **Anabolic pathways** (Greek, *ana* = up) which are concerned with **synthetic processes** and are overall **endergonic** sequences. Anabolism is a **reductive** process.

- **Catabolic pathways** (Greek, *kata* = down) which are concerned with **degradation** and are overall **exergonic** sequences. Catabolism is an **oxidative** process.

Figure 8.5 *Regulation of anabolism and catabolism: (a) exclusive pathways; (b) partially independent pathways; (c) a substrate cycle*

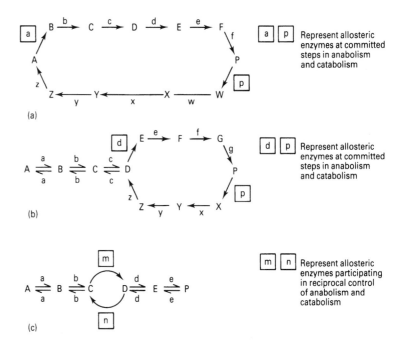

Catabolism may be considered as occurring in three stages:

- **Stage I** in which complex molecules, e.g. proteins, polysaccharides and non-steroidal lipids, are hydrolysed to amino acids, monosaccharides and fatty acids plus glycerol respectively.

- **Stage II** in which the products of stage I are further degraded mainly to acetyl-CoA.

- **Stage III** in which acetyl-CoA is oxidized to carbon dioxide and the coenzymes NAD^+ and FAD are reduced to NADH and $FADH_2$. These reduced coenzymes transfer their electrons across the respiratory chain of the inner mitochondrial membrane to drive oxidative phosphorylation.

Catabolism and anabolism are interconnected (Figure 8.4c) through the **major chemical links** of ATP and NADPH. NADPH provides energy in the form of **reducing power** necessary for certain biosyntheses. Catabolic and anabolic pathways are not always entirely exclusive. Frequently, these pathways share a number of common intermediates (Figure 8.5).

An important principle of cellular metabolism is that catabolic pathways are **convergent** whilst anabolic pathways are **divergent**. As many different macromolecules are degraded, the intermediates generated progressively enter into other pathways which terminate in a few end products. Conversely, anabolism utilizes a limited number of simple molecules which are processed through a number of major pathways from which, at many branch points, intermediates enter specific pathways leading to individual complex molecules. The intermediates of certain pathways are therefore present within the cell at high concentrations. These pathways constitute the **primary metabolism** of the cell. Pathways with relatively low concentrations of intermediates are referred to as **secondary metabolism**, e.g. pentose phosphate pathway (Chapter 9).

Compartmentalization

Anabolic and catabolic pathways may be segregated into different **cellular compartments**. In liver cells, the biosynthesis of fatty acids from acetyl-CoA occurs in the cytosol where the enzymes for both biosynthesis and the generation of NADPH are located. The degradation of fatty acids occurs within the mitochondria where the appropriate enzymes and the apparatus for oxidative phosphorylation are located (Chapter 7).

Compartmentalization of metabolic pathways necessitates the provision of mechanisms by which intermediates not soluble in lipids may move between compartments. The major mechanisms are:

- **Transport systems** in which integral membrane proteins called carriers specifically bind a molecule or ion and transport it across the membrane.
- **Shuttle systems** in which functional groups or atoms rather than actual molecules cross the membrane. The functional group is transferred to another substance which may then permeate the membrane, e.g. glycerone phosphate in the glycerol phosphate shuttle (Figure 9.5).

Creatine phosphate has a standard free energy of hydrolysis of -43.1 kJ mol^{-1} which is more negative than ATP. Vertebrate skeletal muscle employs creatine phosphate as a vehicle for the transport of energy from mitochondria to myofibrils. When the mitochondrial concentration of ATP is high, **creatine kinase** phosphorylates creatine at the expense of one ATP per creatine molecule. Creatine phosphate diffuses from the mitochondria to the myofibrils where the creatine kinase reaction operates in the thermodynamically favourable direction to generate ATP. During muscular exercise, a constant level of ATP is maintained whilst it is creatine phosphate that is consumed. Resting skeletal muscle has normally sufficient creatine phosphate to satisfy its energy requirements for several minutes but under conditions of maximum muscular activity, this period is reduced to a few seconds.

Regulation of metabolic pathways

The simultaneous operation of an anabolic and its opposing catabolic pathway would be unproductive and consume energy. At least a single difference between the synthetic and degradative pathways is required to facilitate selective regulation of the pathways. Sometimes this is achieved simply by the exploitation of different chemical mechanisms to reverse a reaction (Figure 8.5). **Control of metabolism** may be exerted from **within the cell**, i.e. intracellular control, or **from outside the cell**, i.e. extracellular control.

Intracellular control of metabolism

The regulation of metabolic pathways may be considered in terms of the characteristics of each constituent reaction. From the knowledge of actual intracellular concentrations of the substrate(s) and product(s) of a reaction, **the [product]/[substrate] ratio** may be calculated and compared with the established value of the equilibrium constant (K'_{eq}) of the reaction:

- A **near-equilibrium reaction** is one in which the [product]/[substrate] ratio is approximately equal to K'_{eq} and the resultant $\Delta G'$ is close to zero.

- A **non-equilibrium reaction** is one in which the [product]/[substrate] ratio varies appreciably from K'_{eq} and $\Delta G'$ is large.

A near-equilibrium reaction occurs if the catalytic activity of its enzyme is high relative to the activities of other enzymes in the pathway. Changes in the substrate concentration in a near-equilibrium reaction produce rapid concomitant alterations in product concentration. Near-equilibrium reactions may also be readily reversed by small additions of product. Their regulation tends to involve unsophisticated mechanisms such as alterations in substrate levels or variations in the concentrations of the appropriate form of a coenzyme.

A non-equilibrium reaction results when the activity of its enzyme is low compared with the activities of other enzymes in the pathway. This causes the concentration of its substrate to remain high whilst that of the product is greatly reduced due to removal by the successive enzyme. Increasing the activity of an enzyme catalysing a non-equilibrium reaction will convert larger quantities of its substrate to product and since the successive enzymes function at a higher rate, additional substrates are provided throughout the remainder of the pathway. Therefore, an increase in the activity of an enzyme which catalyses a non-equilibrium reaction may generate a significant change in **metabolic flux** or flow through that pathway whereas alterations in the activity of an enzyme catalysing a near-equilibrium reaction has less influence on the pathway flux. For this reason, non-equilibrium reactions tend to be subject to **allosteric regulation** (Chapter 4) which integrates the regulation of one pathway with that of other pathways.

Metabolic pathways often feature more than one non-equilibrium reaction. The first of these reactions controls the entry of a substrate into that pathway and thereby the generation of flux through the pathway. Subsequent non-equilibrium reactions cannot control the flux through the entire pathway but may regulate the operation of a section of the pathway and maintain levels of intermediates for diversion into branch pathways. Indeed, it is unlikely that any single enzyme is ever truly rate-limiting in a pathway. Quantitative analysis indicates that control of glycolysis (Chapter 9) is mainly distributed between hexokinase and 6-phosphofructokinase.

A variety of **intracellular strategies** are employed to effect control of the overall pathway and conserve cellular resources. These systems are focused on controlling the activities of existent enzymes and enzyme concentration:

- allosteric enzymes;
- substrate cycles;
- enzyme interconversion cycles;
- availability of substrates;
- energy status;
- enzyme levels.

The structure of **allosteric enzymes** (Chapter 4) is particularly suited to a role in the regulation of metabolic pathways. In general, pathways, whether exclusive or partially independent (Figure 8.5a, b) are regulated at the reaction which commits the flow of intermediates to the production of some necessary substance called the end product. The enzyme at the **flux-generating step** (non-equilibrium reaction) is usually an allosteric enzyme which can respond to cellular concentrations of a variety of modulators. In many cases, the concentration of end product determines the rate of metabolic flux through that pathway and thereby controls its own production. This form of control is called **feedback inhibition**. For example, in Figure 8.5a, as the end product P increases in concentration, it diffuses to the allosteric enzyme a causing a reduced synthesis of its product B which, in turn, lowers enzymic reaction rates in the remainder of the pathway. In Figure 8.5b, as the concentration of end product P increases, it inhibits allosteric enzyme d . Also, the first reaction after a branch point, e.g. enzymes b and w in Figure 8.4b, may be inhibited by specific end products. Sometimes, the first reaction in the overall pathway is inhibited by the end products from both branches. On occasion, allosteric enzymes are modulated by effectors which are not end products of pathways but are other metabolites that induce conformational changes in enzymes to enhance their activities.

Substrate cycles arise when the non-equilibrium step in both anabolic and catabolic pathways involves the same intermediates. In the absence of regulation, the two metabolites may be constantly re-formed (Figure 8.5c). Substrate cycles are the location of **reciprocal regulation** by different allosteric enzymes which catalyse the forward and reverse reactions.

Substrate cycles serve to determine the direction of and to amplify the variations in metabolic flux with respect to changes in the concentrations of allosteric effectors. For example, if the rate of flux from C → D (Figure 8.5c) is 3 'units' while the rate from D → C is 1 'unit', the net flux of the pathway will be 2 'units' in the direction of C → D. The pathway would then proceed to form P. If a single allosteric effector influences both enzymes m and n so that m is activated 10-fold and the activity of n is reduced 10-fold, the net flux of the pathway would be 29.9 'units' [(3 × 10) − (1 × 1/10)] in the direction of C → D. The change in the rate of flux is therefore amplified by reciprocal regulation of the substrate cycle. However, a variety of considerations, e.g. the

Phosphorylation is the most common **covalent modification** employed in the regulation of enzyme activity. Threonine, serine and tyrosine may be the target residues of various kinases, e.g. protein kinases and tyrosine kinases, because of the -OH groups in their side chains.

Other known covalent modifications include the **adenylylation** [the transfer of an adenylate (AMP) moiety from ATP] and the **uridylylation** [the transfer of a uridylate (UMP) moiety from UTP] of glutamate synthase in *Escherichia coli*. Adenylylation is reversed by deadenylylation whereas deuridylylation abolishes the impact of uridylylation.

activation or inhibition of only one of the enzymes by an effector or the collective consequence of numerous effectors, influence the relationship between substrate cycles and changes in metabolic flux.

Enzyme interconversion cycles are employed to 'fine-tune' metabolic flux. The enzymes involved may exist in two forms, the predominating form being determined by the simultaneous activities of additional enzymes which catalyse the interconversions. The conversion of one form to the other involves covalent modification of the enzyme, frequently by the addition or removal of phosphate groups. Since at physiological pH the phosphate group carries two negative charges, **phosphorylation** results in the introduction of a charged group which induces new bonding arrangements within the protein. The conformational change may be reversed by **dephosphorylation**. Protein phosphorylation is therefore controlled by the interplay of kinases and phosphatases. The phosphorylation and dephosphorylation reactions are non-equilibrium reactions which are regulated by allosteric effectors.

An important example of an enzyme interconversion cycle is the reciprocal control of glycogen metabolism involving glycogen synthase and glycogen phosphorylase (Chapter 9). The activities of both enzymes are regulated in concert by phosphorylation and dephosphorylation reactions so that when the synthetic pathway is in operation, the degradative pathway is reciprocally reduced. In mammals, glycogen synthesis is promoted (Figure 8.6) by an **active glycogen synthase** (called synthase *a*) and a less active glycogen phosphorylase *b*. Both are dephosphorylated forms. Glycogen synthase *a* is converted progressively into a **less active synthase *b*** by the protein kinase A-catalysed phosphorylation of specific seryl residues. Glycogen phosphorylase *b* is phosphorylated at a specific seryl residue (residue 14) on each of two identical subunits. Upon phosphorylation by phosphorylase kinase, two dimers may form a more active tetrameric structure. The phosphorylation of the synthase and phosphorylase is not long lasting since the enzymes are rapidly dephosphorylated by specific phosphatases (glycogen-synthase phosphatase and glycogen-phosphorylase phosphatase respectively) and return to conformations favouring the synthetic pathway.

The catalytic powers of the **less active forms** of the synthase and phosphorylase may be enhanced without the attainment of the catalytic capability of the fully active *a* forms. Glycogen synthase *b*, but not synthase *a*, may be allosterically modulated by glucose 6-phosphate which serves as its positive effector. Similarly, phosphorylase *b* may be activated by its positive effector, AMP.

The **availability of substrates** influences metabolic flux. The control may operate at various cellular levels:

• **The plasma membrane** may prevent entry to nutrients. Hormones may be required to effect the uptake of certain nutrients, e.g. insulin promotes the entry of glucose into target cells (Chapter 7).

- **Intracellular membranes.** By controlling the rate of entry of a metabolite into a particular compartment, the metabolic flux through that pathway may be controlled by limiting the concentration of a substrate, e.g. the rate of entry of acyl-CoA into the mitochondrial matrix modulates the rate of β-oxidation of fatty acids (Chapter 12).

- **Metabolic activity of other pathways.** Low substrate concentrations influence enzymic activity (Figure 4.2b). The tricarboxylic acid cycle may be inhibited through the utilization of acetyl-CoA and oxaloacetate in other pathways (Chapter 10).

The **energy status** of the cell is another regulatory parameter which influences the cell's metabolic activity. Anabolic pathways may be regulated by the availability of energy to drive endergonic reactions. Similarly, catabolic pathways operate in response to demands for energy by anabolic processes. Since ADP phosphorylation couples energy into biosynthetic pathways, adenine nucleotide levels may indicate the energy available for essential functions and biosynthesis. One indicator of energy status is the **adenylate energy charge** which interrelates the adenine nucleotide levels to the availability of chemical energy. Adenylate energy charge is defined by the equation:

$$\text{Adenylate energy charge} = \frac{[\text{ATP}] + 0.5[\text{ADP}]}{[\text{ATP}] + [\text{ADP}] + [\text{AMP}]}$$

Corynebacterium diphtheriae **toxin** is responsible for the disease **diphtheria**. The toxin inhibits eukaryotic protein synthesis by catalysing the **ADP-ribosylation** (the transfer of an ADP-ribosyl moiety from NAD^+) of an elongation factor (eEF-2). This covalent modification prevents the participation of eEF-2 in the translocation step during the elongation of the growing polypeptide chain (Chapter 13).

Vibrio cholerae **toxin** is responsible for the symptoms of **cholera** which include electrolyte loss and dehydration. This toxin catalyses the **ADP-ribosylation** of the α-subunit of G_s subunits of G-proteins inhibiting their GTPase activity. The resultant high [cAMP] results in the continuous secretion of Cl^-, HCO_3^- and H_2O into the lumen of the gut, producing diarrhoea and water loss.

Bordetella pertussis **toxin** is responsible for **whooping cough**. This toxin catalyses the ADP-ribosylation of the α-subunit of G_i subunits of G-proteins, inhibiting the displacement of GDP by GTP which blocks the inhibition of adenylate cyclase by G_i.

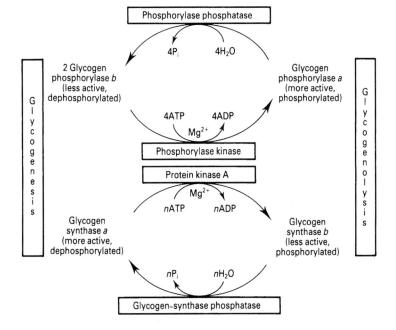

Figure 8.6 *Reciprocal regulation of glycogen metabolism by phosphorylation/dephosphorylation reactions*

The 0.5 in the denominator takes into account the possible interconversion of 2 ADP into 1 ATP + 1 AMP by the enzyme **adenylate kinase**. In theory, the adenylate energy charge may range from 0 (when only AMP is present) to 1 (when only ATP is present). In viable cells, the adenylate energy charge is held within narrow limits around 0.9. The maintenance of this value requires the continual balancing of the ATP, ADP and AMP concentrations which explains why these adenine nucleotides feature as major allosteric effectors.

Intracellular concentrations of **NAD$^+$ and NADPH** also play an important role in the determination of the metabolic flux through certain pathways. Low adenylate energy charge values indicate the requirement for energy whilst low [NAD$^+$]/[NADH] ratios imply that energy demands may be satisfied through oxidative phosphorylation. Low [NADP$^+$]/[NADPH] ratios suggest that reducing power is readily available. In the mitochondrial matrix, [NAD$^+$]/[NADH] ratios are more important because mitochondrial adenine nucleotide concentrations exhibit little variation because of the export of ATP to the cytosol (Chapter 11).

The intracellular **concentration of enzymes** may be used in the regulation of cellular metabolism. The level of a single enzyme may differ widely in different cells. A high substrate concentration may bring about the synthesis of new enzyme molecules, a phenomenon known as **enzyme induction**. Enzyme induction primarily occurs in the liver and involves the initiation of the transcription of the specific gene encoding the required enzyme followed by the translation of the mRNA to generate additional enzyme molecules.

The presence of the end product of a pathway may stop the synthesis of an enzyme required for its production, an event called **enzyme repression**. In the presence of a **repressor** (end product) molecule, synthesis of a pertinent enzyme may be inhibited by blocking gene transcription. The result is a progressive decline in the concentration of enzyme through normal degradative processes involving cytoplasmic proteasomes (Chapter 7). Induction and repression mechanisms may be considered as important coarse controls over metabolism.

Extracellular control of metabolism

Intracellular metabolic activity may be modulated in response to extracellular conditions by hormones. Hormones are substances which act as chemical messengers between cells in different locations to alter the activity of the recipient cell. Three classes of hormones have been identified:

- **Polypeptide hormones**, e.g insulin and glucagon.
- **Tyrosine-derived hormones** of which there are two distinct groups, the **catecholamines** and the **thyroid hormones**. The

catecholamine hormones, i.e. **adrenaline and noradrenaline**, are produced by and secreted from the adrenal medulla. The thyroid hormones, i.e. **thyroxine and 3, 5, 3′-triiodo-L-thyronine**, are elaborated by and secreted from the thyroid gland.

- **Steroid hormones,** e.g oestradiol and progesterone.

Hydrophilic hormones are water soluble but lipid insoluble and therefore cannot cross the plasma membrane of cells. **Polypeptide and catecholamine hormones** therefore do not enter their target cells but interact with cell-surface receptors (Chapter 7). The occupancy of the receptor initiates a series of reactions from which a specific intracellular response ultimately ensues. A polypeptide or catecholamine hormone transmits its message to the cell and is termed the **first messenger**. Any mediator produced in response to the first messenger is the **second messenger** which is responsible for a series of intracellular events culminating in biological action.

Cell-surface receptors

There are three general classes of cell-surface receptors:

- ligand-gated ion-channel-linked receptors;
- catalytic receptors;
- G-protein-coupled receptors.

Ligand-gated ion-channel-linked receptors are transmembrane proteins or multisubunit protein complexes with an extracellular receptor domain directly linked to a transmembrane channel-forming domain. They are found in nerve and muscle cells in which the binding of a neurotransmitter, e.g. acetylcholine, causes within milliseconds the opening of ion-specific channels to permit an influx of ions through the open channel.

Catalytic receptors are single transmembrane proteins or transmembrane protein complexes in which an extracellular hormone-binding domain is **directly linked** to a cytoplasmic domain possessing a **protein-tyrosine kinase activity**. These catalytic receptors are further classified according to structural features. Extracellular signals utilizing this mechanism include the receptors of some polypeptide hormones, e.g. insulin (protein complex, Class II receptor), and some growth factors, e.g. epidermal growth factor (EGF, single protein, Class I receptor) and platelet-derived growth factor (PDGF, single protein, Class III receptor). Growth factors are polypeptides or glycoproteins involved in the regulation of cell proliferation. They are required for the long-term growth and metabolism of most mammalian cells. When insulin occupies its receptor, the intrinsic tyrosine kinase activity phosphorylates tyrosyl residues in target proteins. The effect of this activity is

The term **hormone** (Greek *horman* = to excite) was introduced by Ernest Starling in 1905 to describe **'the internal secretions'** of the body. Earlier, in 1855, the physiologist, Claude Bernard had distinguished between two types of secretions: sweat and tears which he called the 'external secretions' and secretions which entered the blood circulation, i.e. 'the internal secretions'.

Hormones have wider effects than the control of cellular metabolism. In the whole human organism, hormones may regulate physiological phenomena such as heart rate (increased by adrenaline), blood pressure (increased by adrenaline and antidiuretic hormone, ADH), kidney function (water reabsorption is promoted by ADH), movements of the gut (motilin increases the contraction of small intestine, adrenaline contracts sphincters), acid secretion in the stomach (stimulated by gastrin) and lactation (promoted by prolactin).

Hormone binding to its cellular receptor is estimated by the use of a **Scatchard plot** in which $[L_{bound}]/[L_{free}]$ is plotted as a function of $[L_{bound}]$, where L = ligand (hormone) and [] = concentration. Hormone binding is measured by mixing the receptor, either present in whole cells, in membrane fragments, in cytosol, in nuclear preparations or as purified molecules, with radiolabelled hormone. The free hormone is separated from the hormone–receptor complex (L_{bound}) by rapid filtration. The levels of radioactivity in each fraction are measured by **liquid scintillation counting**.

The graph may demonstrate a straight line, the slope of which equals $-1/K_d$ where K_d = the dissociation constant. The intercept on the x-axis (L_{bound}) represents **B**, the maximal binding capacity, from which the concentration of binding sites may be calculated. Curved plots may be obtained which suggest cooperativity, either positive or negative, between binding sites.

terminated by the removal of the phosphate groups by a tyrosine phosphatase.

G-protein-coupled receptors are receptors which are **indirectly coupled** to an effector mechanism through a G-protein (G = Guanine nucleotide-binding regulatory protein). G-proteins are **heterotrimeric proteins**, i.e. they contain three dissimilar subunits called **α, β** and **γ**. These subunits are polymorphic in that some 20 different α-chains, five β-chains and 10 γ-chains have been reported. G-proteins are located attached to the inside of the plasma membrane through **lipidic feet** created by the myristoylation or palmitoylation (Chapter 6) of the G_{α} subunit and the farnesylation or geranylgeranylation (Chapter 12) of the G_{γ} subunit. From this site, G-proteins can interact with both receptor and effector components of the signalling system. Four families of G-proteins have been reported: the G_s **family** which activates adenylate cyclase to increase the level of intracellular cAMP, the G_i **family** which inhibits adenylate cyclase, the G_q **family** which activates specific isoenzymes of phospholipase C and the G_{12} **family**, the targets of which are poorly defined but include cell growth regulatory pathways.

Signal transduction

Two important mechanisms of signal transduction involving secondary messengers have been identified:

- the **cyclic AMP** (cAMP, adenosine 3′,5′-cyclic monophosphate) **system**;
- the **phosphoinositide** (PI) **system**.

The cyclic AMP system

In the cyclic AMP system, the interaction between an **appropriate stimulatory receptor** in the plasma membrane and its complementary hormone triggers the activation of adenylate cyclase via G-proteins (Figure 8.7). All these receptors are members of the **seven-helical transmembrane receptor family**. These receptors have an extracellular N-terminus which contains the hormone-binding domain, seven α-helical sequences of 20–25 hydrophobic residues between which form three interhelical extracellular loops and three interhelical intracellular loops, and a cytoplasmic tail to which a particular G-protein binds.

The **contact** between a stimulatory STR and a GDP-bound G_s-protein heterotrimer drives the release of GDP from the $G_{s\alpha}$ subunit. Cytoplasmic GTP and GDP levels are relatively high. Therefore, GTP replaces GDP in the $G_{s\alpha}$ subunit to initiate a conformational change in the $G_{s\alpha}$ subunit which decreases the affinity of $G_{s\alpha}$ for both the STR and the $G_{s\beta\gamma}$ subunit complex. This results in the dissociation of the complex into $G_{s\alpha}$ (GTP-

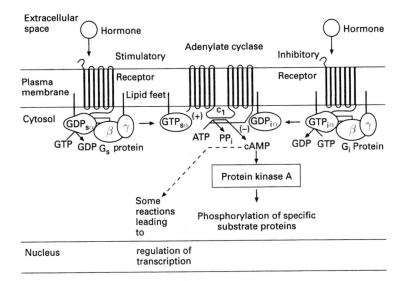

Figure 8.7 *The cyclic AMP system of extracellular signal transduction: the regulation of adenylate cyclase by G_s and G_i proteins*

bound), $G_{s\beta\gamma}$ components and the receptor. The receptor has a decreased affinity for the hormone which is thereby released. The $G_{s\alpha}$ (GTP-bound) diffuses laterally along the plasma membrane and interacts with a specific effector enzyme, **adenylate cyclase** to bring about the production of the secondary messenger, **cyclic AMP**. (In some systems, $G_{\beta\gamma}$ complex may activate its own effector molecule.) Cyclic AMP may activate **protein kinase A** (cAMP-dependent protein kinase) which phosphorylates specific target proteins. In addition, cyclic AMP may interact with DNA-binding proteins to form complexes which ultimately control the transcription of genes.

Mammalian adenylate cyclase exists in nine isoforms which are activated by $G_{s\alpha}$ but variable in their responses to $G_{i\alpha}$ subunits. Adenylate cyclases consist of a repeated motif of six hydrophobic transmembrane regions (12 in total) with both the *N*- and *C*-termini being cytoplasmic. Two well conserved cytoplasmic domains called C_1 and C_2 confer the catalytic activity. Activation of the effector enzyme is transient since G_α contains an intrinsic GTPase activity. The bound GTP is therefore hydrolysed to GDP and the concomitant conformational change permits the return of the system to the heterotrimeric resting state by the reassociation of the G_α and $G_{\beta\gamma}$ subunits. The production of cyclic AMP reverts to resting levels.

The binding of a hormone to an **appropriate inhibitory receptor** in the plasma membrane results in the guanine nucleotide exchange and dissociation of $G_{i\alpha}$(GTP) from $G_{i\beta\gamma}$. Inhibition may occur through two mechanisms:

- **by the binding of $G_{i\alpha}$(GTP) to adenylate cyclase to directly inhibit the enzyme;**
- **by the interaction of $G_{i\beta\gamma}$ with $G_{s\alpha}$(GTP) complexes which prevents the association of $G_{s\alpha}$(GTP) with adenylate cyclase.**

Therefore the same hormone may create stimulatory effects by binding to one of its receptors but may cause inhibition by binding to another type of receptor.

The cyclic AMP system and the hormonal regulation of glycogen metabolism

The role of the **cyclic AMP system** can be exemplified by consideration of the **hormonal regulation of glycogen metabolism.** The activity of glycogen synthase and phosphorylase are controlled by two hormones, adrenaline and the pancreatic polypeptide hormone, glucagon. **Adrenaline** stimulates glycogenolysis in both muscle and liver by increasing the amount of the more active phosphorylase *a* relative to that of phosphorylase *b* whilst reciprocally reducing the ratio of glycogen synthase *a* to glycogen synthase *b* (Figure 8.6). The main site of **glucagon** activity is the liver where it plays a major role in the release of glucose for the maintenance of blood glucose levels.

Adrenaline, for example, is released from the **adrenal medulla** in response to the activity of the sympathetic nervous system. Adrenergic plasma-membrane receptors are classified into $\alpha_1, \alpha_2, \beta_1$ or β_2 with respect to their response to adrenaline. The binding of adrenaline to α_1 receptors has no effect on adenylate cyclase activity whereas binding to α_2 receptors is inhibitory and binding to β_1 or β_2 receptors is stimulatory. The β_1 and β_2 receptors interact only with the G_s complex whereas α_2 receptors bind only to G_i proteins. In glycogen degradation, adrenaline exerts its influence by interaction with β-adrenergic receptors which results in activation of adenylate cyclase (Figure 8.8).

The resultant cyclic AMP interacts with protein kinase A which is a tetrameric structure, composed of two regulatory (R) and two catalytic (C) subunits. The binding of four molecules of cyclic AMP to sites on the regulatory subunits results in the dissociation of the enzyme. This activation releases the active monomeric form of the protein kinase and an inactive R_2–cyclic AMP_4 complex. There are two substrates for the protein kinase in this system:

- **phosphorylase kinase** which is activated by the phosphorylation of a specific serine residue and which phosphorylates its substrate, glycogen phosphorylase *b*;
- **glycogen synthase** *a* which is rendered less active by phosphorylation.

Glycogen synthesis is therefore inhibited whilst glycogen phosphorylase becomes more active thereby stimulating the degradative pathway.

When the production, and thereby the blood concentration, of adrenaline declines, adrenaline diffuses from the β-receptors. Adenylate cyclase is no longer activated, cyclic AMP production

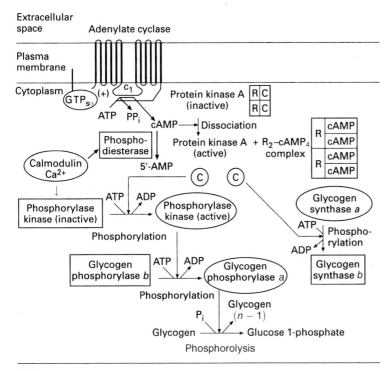

Figure 8.8 *The amplification cascade in the regulation of glycogen metabolism in skeletal muscle cells by adrenaline*

ceases and the cytosolic concentrations of cyclic AMP are returned to basal levels by the action of **3′,5′-cyclic nucleotide phosphodiesterase** which may catalyse the hydrolytic cleavage of cyclic AMP and some other cyclic nucleotides. Protein kinase A reassociates into its inactive form and the inhibition of **phosphorylase phosphatase** (Figure 8.6) is terminated, signalling the stimulation of the synthetic pathway.

The system is called an **amplification cascade** since the binding of one molecule of adrenaline may cause the formation of numerous molecules of cyclic AMP which may dissociate protein kinase A molecules. This then sequentially promotes the activation of more molecules of phosphorylase kinase and the inhibition of glycogen synthase to effect the reduction of synthesis and the stimulation of the degradation of glycogen.

The cascade is also subjected to regulation by calcium ions (Ca^{2+}) through **calmodulin**. Most of the intracellular effects of Ca^{2+} ions involve a member of the family of calcium-binding proteins. Calmodulin, a single polypeptide chain of 148 amino acid residues, has the widest distribution of these proteins being present in most cells. It may bind up to four calcium ions per molecule to negatively charged amino acid R groups contained within four domains. On binding one or more Ca^{2+} ions, calmodulin undergoes conformational change to form different Ca^{2+}–calmodulin complexes with different compactness and activities. Through influence on the activity of **3′,5′-cyclic nucleotide phosphodiesterase**, activated calmodulin regulates intracellular cyclic AMP levels.

Calmodulin is also involved in the regulation of phosphorylase kinase which has the subunit structure $(\alpha, \beta, \gamma, \delta)_4$. The δ-subunit is calmodulin which remains bound to the enzyme even if Ca^{2+} ions are absent. Through binding to this subunit, Ca^{2+} ions may control the activity of this enzyme. Phosphorylase kinase may therefore be regulated by both protein kinase A and Ca^{2+} ions. The cytosolic concentrations of Ca^{2+} ions may increase in response to **inositol trisphosphate**, another secondary messenger, which is generated in the phosphoinositide system.

The phosphoinositide system

The **phosphoinositide system** transduces the extracellular signal delivered by numerous agents including **bradykinin, histamine, vasopressin** and **adrenaline**. In this case, adrenaline binds to **α_1-adrenergic receptors** (Figure 8.9). The binding of these substances to their specific cell-surface receptors triggers the dissociation of the $\mathbf{G_{q\alpha\beta\gamma}}$ heterotrimeric protein. The released $G_{q\alpha}$ subunit activates an isoform of **phospholipase C** attached to the plasma membrane. Phosphatidylinositol-specific phospholipase C exists as at least eight isoenzymes (denoted as $PLC_{\beta1-4,\gamma1,\gamma2,\beta1,\delta2}$). $PLC_{\beta,\gamma,\delta}$ are Ca^{2+}-dependent. $PLC_{\beta1-3}$ are stimulated by G_q proteins whereas PLC_γ is activated through a receptor protein-tyrosine kinase. The function of PLC_δ is less well defined. PLC_β hydrolyses membraneous **phosphatidylinositol-4, 5-bisphosphate** (PIP_2) into:

- **1,2-diacylglycerol** (DAG);
- **inositol 1,4,5-trisphosphate** (IP_3).

PIP_2 is present in very small quantities but may be synthesized from, and degraded to, **phosphatidylinositol 4-phosphate** (**PIP**) which, in turn, may be produced from **phosphatidylinositol** (**PI**) by specific phosphorylation as part of an enzymically regulated network of various PIP, PIP_2 and PIP_3 molecules, e.g. phosphatidylinositol 3-phosphate, which exists. These three substances are maintained at appropriate intramembraneous concentrations by the action of specific kinases and phosphatases which constitute two substrate cycles. The substrate (PIP_2) for the production of second messengers is provided by delicate adjustments in the activities of the kinases and phosphatases which preserve the equilibrium between the phosphoinositides.

Diacylglycerol (DAG) is lipophilic and remains in the plasma membrane where it promotes the binding of an isoform of **protein kinase C** (**PKC**) to the plasma membrane. PKCs were originally defined as protein serine or threonine kinases, the activity of which is dependent upon Ca^{2+} ions and phospholipids. At least 11 different isoforms of PKC are known and have been classified into:

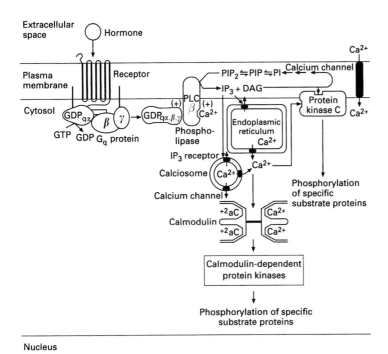

Figure 8.9   *The phosphoinositide system of extracellular signal transduction*

- conventional protein kinase C isoforms denoted as $PKC_{-\alpha,\beta I,\beta II,\gamma}$;
- novel protein kinase C isoforms denoted as $PKC_{-\delta,\varepsilon,\zeta,\eta,\iota,\theta,\mu}$ (human).

The occurrence of the PKC isoforms differs in different tissues.

At low concentrations of Ca^{2+} ions and in the absence of DAG, PKCs are inactive, soluble cytosolic proteins. The binding of DAG causes a conformational change through which the affinity of PKCs for Ca^{2+} ions and DAG is enhanced. On binding to the plasma membrane, the isoenzyme becomes activated. PKCs catalyse the phosphorylation of seryl and threonyl residues of a broad spectrum of cellular proteins. Alternatively, DAG may serve as a substrate for enzymes including the Ca^{2+}-dependent **phospholipase A_2**, which removes from the *sn*-2 position **arachidonate**, the precursor of some eicosanoids (Chapter 6).

Inositol trisphosphate (IP_3) is water soluble and diffuses from the membrane and across the cytosol to bind to specific receptors on parts of the endoplasmic reticulum (ER) closely associated with the plasma membrane and calciosomes (Chapter 7) to open Ca^{2+} ion channels and release Ca^{2+} from these intracellular stores. The draining of the ER stores induces a conformational change in the IP_3 receptor complex which causes the opening of the plasma membrane Ca^{2+} ion channels. It is believed that **inositol 1,3,4,5-tetraphosphate** also plays a role in effecting calcium influx from the extracellular environment. The principal receptor protein for Ca^{2+} ions is calmodulin. Calcium–calmodulin complexes are capable of

Steroid and thyroid hormones are transported in the blood circulation by specific binding glycoproteins, e.g. **sex hormone-binding globulin** and **thyroxine-binding globulin**. However, when bound to their binding glycoproteins, they are devoid of biological activity. It is only the unbound hormone which is available to the tissues to influence cellular function via intracellular receptors. For this reason, clinical biochemists may measure the free hormone and/or binding glycoprotein plasma levels for the diagnosis of patients with suspected gonadal or thyroid disorders.

activating another family of protein kinases, **calmodulin-dependent protein kinases**, and thereby control the phosphorylation of certain proteins. The transmission of the signal is terminated by the dephosphorylation of IP_3 by the hydrolytic action of **inositol trisphosphatase** to produce **inositol-1,4-bisphosphate**. Ca^{2+} ions may be returned to their intracellular stores by the action of a Ca^{2+}-transporting ATPase at the expense of ATP.

Steroid and thyroid hormones

Steroid and thyroid hormones, being hydrophobic and lipid soluble, enter their target cells to exert their effect through changes in the cellular pattern of protein synthesis. Regulation by these hormones occurs at the level of transcription of responsive genes. Whereas polypeptide and tyrosine-derived hormones effect rapid change (within seconds or minutes) through the activation or inhibition of pre-existing enzymes, steroid and thyroid hormone action involves longer time-scales (days or weeks).

The activity of these hormones is limited to eukaryotic cells containing receptor molecules. Steroid and thyroid hormones may enter a non-target cell by diffusion but, in the absence of appropriate receptor molecules, depart from the cell. In target tissues, steroid and thyroid hormones interact with receptor proteins located as follows:

- **glucocorticoid receptors** are predominantly found in the cytoplasm complexed with **heat-shock proteins** [heat-shock protiens (hsps) of 90 kDa and 70 kDa are induced by insults to cells such as temperature stress];

- **oestradiol and progesterone receptors** are predominantly found in the nucleus complexed with hsp 90 and hsp 70;

- **thyroid hormone receptors** are always bound to DNA.

Intracellular hormone receptors exist at levels of only about 100–10 000 molecules per cell and have a very high affinity for their ligand. The receptors display a modular structure, the major regions being:

- the *N*-terminal region, essential for the activation of transcription;

- a central highly conserved domain, essential for DNA binding for which it has two Zn^{2+}-containing motifs comprising a conserved sequence of cysteine residues;

- the *C*-terminal region which contains the ligand-binding domain and participates in hormone binding, homo- and hetero-dimerization, formation of heat-shock protein complexes and transcriptional activation.

Glucocorticoids bind to receptor–heat-shock protein complexes predominantly in the cytoplasm (Figure 8.10a). Hormone binding induces changes in receptor conformation with the result that the heat-shock proteins dissociate from the complex. The occupied receptors dimerize and bind to a specific DNA site called a **hormone-response element (HRE)** whose **consensus sequence** (the sequences determined in different DNAs exhibit only limited variations) is an inverted repeat separated by three nucleotides. Glucocorticoid and progesterone receptors bind to the same sequence, i.e.

AGAACAnnnTGTTCT

TCTTGTnnnACAAGA

The receptor dimers then interact with transcription factors, other DNA-binding proteins and cofactors to effect transcription of the target gene into mRNA which serves as a template for the ribosomal synthesis of protein.

Oestradiol binds to receptor–hsp complexes loosely associated with the nucleus (Figure 8.10b). Following hsp dissociation and receptor dimerization, the receptor dimers bind to a HRE, the consensus sequence of which is

AGGTCAnnnTGACCT

TCCAGTnnnACTGGA

Transcription and protein synthesis follow.

Thyroid hormone receptors differ from steroid hormone receptors in that they are bound to their HREs in the absence of hormone

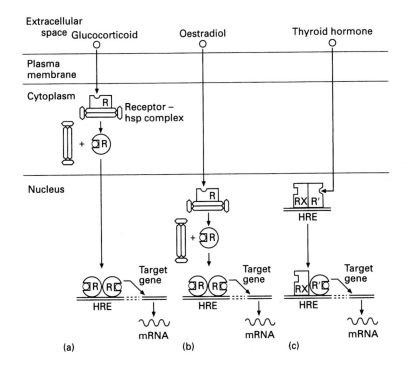

Figure 8.10 *The activation of transcription by steroid and thyroid hormones: (a) glucocorticoids; (b) oestradiol; (c) triiodothyronine*

Hypothyroidism results from the underactivity of the thyroid gland. About 10% of middle-aged women suffer from some degree of the condition. The symptoms are due to an insufficiency of thyroid hormone production which results in lethargy, weight gain, constipation, cold intolerance and a deepening of the voice which becomes hoarse. Diagnosis of hypothyroidism involves the measurement of components of the **hypothalamic-pituitary-thyroid axis**. The plasma levels of triiodothyronine (T_3) and thyroxine (T_4) decline whilst the level of thyroid-stimulating hormone (TSH), the pituitary hormone which stimulates T_3 and T_4 production in the thyroid, is elevated. TSH in turn is released in response to thyrotropin-releasing hormone (TRH) of hypothalamic origin.

The most common cause of hypothyroidism is **Hashimoto's thyroiditis**, an **autoimmune disease** which results in the progressive destruction of the thyroid gland. Recent evidence suggests that, in Hashimoto's disease, thyroid cells die not because of a direct antibody-mediated cytotoxic activity of the immune system but as a result of the activation of **apoptosis**, the self-destruction mechanism which causes cells to commit suicide (Chapter 7).

(Figure 8.10c). Thyroid hormone receptors belong to the family of **retinoid X receptors**. The receptor dimer is a heterodimer with a retinoid receptor (RX), the complex repressing transcription of the target gene. The binding of hormone changes the conformation of the receptor to activate transcription. Protein synthesis follows.

Suggested further reading

Böhm, S.K., Grady, E.F. and Bunnett, N.W. (1997). Regulatory mechanisms that modulate signalling by G-protein-coupled receptors. *Biochemical Journal* **322**, 1–18.

Fields, T.A. and Casey, P.J. (1997). Signalling functions and biochemical properties of pertussis toxin-resistant G-proteins. *Biochemical Journal* **321**, 561–571.

Mendes, P. (1997). Biochemistry by numbers: simulation of biochemical pathways with Gepasi 3. *Trends in Biochemical Sciences* **22**, 361–363.

Weigel, N.L. (1996). Steroid hormone receptors and their regulation by phosphorylation. *Biochemical Journal* **319**, 657–667.

Zhang, G., Liu, Y., Ruoho, A.E. and Hurley, J.H. (1997). Structure of the adenylyl cyclase catalytic core. *Nature* **386**, 247–253.

Fell, D. (1997). *Understanding the Control of Metabolism.* Colchester: Portland.

Gokcen, N.A. and Reddy, R.G. (1996). *Thermodynamics*, 2nd edn., New York: Plenum.

Self-assessment questions

1. In an experiment, when $0.02 \, mol\,l^{-1}$ glucose 1-phosphate was incubated at 25°C in pH 7.0 buffer in the presence of phosphoglucomutase, the final equilibrium mixture contained $0.001 \, mol\,l^{-1}$ glucose 1-phosphate and $0.019 \, mol\,l^{-1}$ glucose 6-phosphate. Calculate the standard free-energy change, given that $R = 8.3 \, J\,K^{-1}\,mol^{-1}$.
2. A cell contains ATP at $2.7 \, mmol\,l^{-1}$, ADP at $0.18 \, mmol\,l^{-1}$ and P_i at $45 \, mmol\,l^{-1}$ at 37°C. Calculate the actual free energy of ATP hydrolysis given that $\Delta G^{\circ\prime}$ for $ATP + H_2O \leftrightarrow ADP + P_i = -30.5 \, kJ\,mol^{-1}$ and $R = 8.3 \, J\,K^{-1}\,mol^{-1}$.
3. Distinguish between the modes of action of a steroid and a thyroid hormone.
4. Draw out the cyclic AMP system as it applies to the hormonal regulation of glycogen metabolism, and the phosphoinositide system of extracellular signal transduction.
5. Distinguish between the terms 'substrate cycle' and 'enzyme conversion cycle'.
6. List four differences between anabolic and catabolic pathways.

7. What advantages does compartmentalization bestow on cellular metabolism?
8. Explain how adrenaline can act as a stimulatory or inhibitory signal and utilize different signal transduction pathways.
9. Which enzymes remove second messengers in the cyclic AMP and phosphoinositide systems of signal transduction?
10. What constitutes the internal energy of a molecular system?

Key Concepts and Facts

The Carbon Cycle
- Living cells require energy to survive, differentiate, function and reproduce.

- The ultimate source of energy in biological systems is the sun.

Equilibrium Thermodynamics
- The principles of thermodynamics have been applied to explain energy flow in living organisms.

- All spontaneous reactions endeavour to achieve an equilibrium state.

- Free energy performs useful work in biological systems and changes in free energy are accompanied by alterations in the enthalpy and entropy of the system.

Coupled Reactions
- An exergonic reaction may be employed to drive an energy-consuming reaction.

- Coupling may involve a common intermediate or a transferable chemical group.

- ATP and NADPH are major links between exergonic and endergonic reactions.

Metabolic Pathways
- A metabolic pathway is a sequence of coupled enzymic reactions.

- Metabolic pathways may be classified as anabolic and catabolic pathways.

Regulation of Metabolism
- Regulation of metabolic pathways may be exerted from within or outside cells.

- Metabolic flux may be regulated at non-equilibrium reactions.

- Intracellular regulatory strategies include allosteric enzymes, substrate cycles, enzyme interconversion cycles, energy status, substrate and enzyme concentrations.

- The cyclic AMP and phosphoinositide systems are major mechanisms of signal transduction.

- Hydrophobic hormones enter their target cells and interact with intracellular receptor molecules.

- Steroid and thyroid hormones effect metabolic regulation at the level of transcription of responsive genes.

Answers to questions (Chapter 8)

1. $-7.28 \text{ kJ mol}^{-1}$:

$$\Delta G' = \Delta G^{\circ\prime} + RT \ln K'_{\text{eq}}$$

$\therefore$ at equilibrium

$$\Delta G' = 0 \quad \therefore \quad \Delta G^{\circ\prime} = RT \ln K'_{\text{eq}}$$

But

$$K'_{\text{eq}} = [\text{G-6-P}]/[\text{G-1-P}] = 0.019/0.001 = 19$$

$$\therefore \quad \Delta G^{\circ\prime} = RT \ln K'_{\text{eq}}$$

$$\therefore \quad \Delta G^{\circ\prime} = -[(8.3 \times 298)] \ln 19 \text{ J K}^{-1} \text{ mol}^{-1} \text{ K}$$

$$= -(2473.4)(2.944) \text{ J mol}^{-1} = -7282 \text{ J mol}^{-1}$$

$$\therefore \quad \Delta G^{\circ\prime} = -7.28 \text{ kJ mol}^{-1}$$

2. $-45.45 \text{ kJ mol}^{-1}$:

$$\Delta G' = \Delta G^{\circ\prime} + RT \ln \frac{[\text{ADP}][\text{P}_{\text{i}}]}{[\text{ATP}]}$$

$$= -30.5 + [(8.3 \times 310)/1000]$$

$$\times \ln [0.00018][0.045]/[0.0027] \text{ kJ mol}^{-1} \text{ J K}^{-1} \text{ mol}^{-1} \text{ K mol mol mol}^{-1}$$

(Note: R in J but $\Delta G^{\circ\prime}$ in kJ $\therefore$ divide by 1000)

$$= -30.5 + [(2.573) \ln 8.1 \times 10^{-6}/2.7 \times 10^{-3}] \text{ kJ mol}^{-1}$$

$$= -30.5 + [(2.573) \ln 3 \times 10^{-3}] \text{ kJ mol}^{-1}$$

$$= -30.5 + [(2.573) \times -5.81] \text{ kJ mol}^{-1}$$

$$= -30.5 + [(-14.95] \text{ kJ mol}^{-1} = -45.45 \text{ kJ mol}^{-1}$$

3. Both hormones are lipid soluble and interact with intracellular receptors. In the absence of hormone, steroid hormone receptors are in inactive soluble complexes with hsps whereas thyroid hormone receptors are always attached to the HRE as heterodimers with retinoid receptors. On dissociation from hsps, activated steroid receptors dimerize and subsequently bind to the corresponding HRE. Refer to Figure 8.10.

4. For cyclic AMP join Figure 8.7 (stimulatory aspects) to Figure 8.8. Refer to Figure 8.9.

5. Substrate cycles arise where different enzymes catalyse the forward and reverse directions of a reaction. Without adequate regulation, usually reciprocal regulation, the metabolites would not proceed through the metabolic pathway but re-form each other, wasting energy. Enzyme conversion cycles effect regulation by allowing enzymes to be enzymatically converted between more active and less active forms by the addition

and removal of phosphate groups (due to their influence on protein structure). Usually two or more enzymes are involved.

6. Anabolic pathway features are listed first with catabolism in parentheses: reductive (oxidative); synthetic (degradative), uses ATP (generates ATP), divergent (convergent).

7. Separation of pathways which may use identical or similar intermediates. Exchange between compartments affords opportunities for regulation.

8. Adrenaline may bind to different adrenergic receptors linked to different G-proteins. Through their α-subunits, G_s proteins are stimulatory whereas G_i proteins are inhibitory for adenylate cyclase. G_q proteins are stimulatory for PLC in the phosphoinositide system.

9. Phosphodiesterase and inositol trisphosphatase respectively. DAG may serve as a substrate for a number of enzymes.

10. Translational, rotational, vibrational and electronic energies of the molecule.

Chapter 9
Carbohydrate metabolism

Learning objectives

After studying this chapter you should confidently be able to:

Interrelate the principal pathways of carbohydrate metabolism, namely glycolysis, glycogen synthesis and degradation, gluconeogenesis and the pentose phosphate pathway.

Identify the major tissue and subcellular locations for each pathway.

Discuss the important biological roles of each pathway.

Describe the reactions of these pathways with discussion of the major features of key enzymes.

Discuss alternative fates for intermediates and coenzymes within the metabolic network.

Relate thermodynamic principles to carbohydrate metabolism.

Calculate the energy release or utilization of each pathway in terms of numbers of ATP molecules.

Discuss the flux of carbohydrate metabolism.

Discuss the role of nucleotides and metabolic intermediates in the regulation of carbohydrate metabolism.

Carbohydrates produced during photosynthesis (Chapter 8) are utilized as a source of energy and as precursors for the synthesis of many structural and metabolic components. These requirements are satisfied in mammalian and human cells primarily by D-**glucose**, obtained from the diet or the storage compound, **glycogen** (Chapter 5). This glucose is degraded by a metabolic pathway called **glycolysis**.

In cells functioning aerobically, pyruvate, the considered end-product of glycolysis, is transported from the cytoplasm into the mitochondria where, in the presence of oxygen, further metabolism yields additional energy. In the absence of oxygen, cells do not utilize this organelle but convert glycolytic intermediates into a

The **secret of studying metabolic pathways** is to refer to the illustration of the pathway of interest. In this publication, pathways are shown in their entirety in one figure whenever possible. Locate the **initial substrate(s)** (usually on the top/ left of the figure). Scan the **intermediates** and note their **sequence** in the pathway. Identify the **functional group** of each intermediate and the nature of its change as the next intermediate is formed. **Classify** the changes, e.g. as a phosphorylation, dehydrogenation, intramolecular rearrangement, to identify the type of enzyme involved, e.g kinase, dehydrogenase, mutase. Phosphorylations must have a source of phosphate, e.g ATP. Dehydrogenases must have an electron acceptor, e.g. NAD^+. Learn to spot the situations in which a particular reaction may occur, e.g. when a CHOH (secondary alcohol) group appears in the formula, will it be dehydrogenated to a C=O (carbonyl group)? The names of specific intermediates and enzymes may be worked out systematically as well as the cofactor requirements. You will realize that metabolic pathways operate by reactions, the nature of which occur repetitively throughout metabolism. Finally, if knowledge of structural formulae is required, ensure that you know that of the initial substrate and proceed through the pathway focusing your attention on the functional groups.

variety of end products, e.g. skeletal muscle cells convert pyruvate to lactate.

A key glycolytic intermediate is **glucose 6-phosphate** which may serve as a substrate for more than one cytosolic enzyme (Chapter 8). Glucose 6-phosphate is the branch point for glycogen synthesis (**glycogenesis**) and the **pentose phosphate pathway**. It may be formed by two routes on the degradation of glycogen (**glycogen-olysis**). **Gluconeogenesis** is the sequence of reactions by which glucose or glycogen is synthesized from a wide variety of non-carbohydrate precursors, e.g. lactate and some amino acids. The interrelationships of these pathways are shown in Figure 9.1.

This chapter considers the metabolic roles, the tissue and subcellular locations, the energetics, the regulation and other key features of glycolysis, glycogenesis, glycogenolysis, gluconeogenesis and the pentose phosphate pathway.

Glycolysis

Glycolysis (Greek *glykos* = sweet and *lysis* = a loosening) is the major pathway by which glucose is degraded to pyruvate in animals, plants and many micro-organisms under both aerobic and anaerobic conditions. Carbohydrate is the only fuel which can be used to generate ATP under anaerobic conditions because glycolysis does not require oxygen. For this reason, glycolysis has a vital role in the energetics of many anaerobic organisms.

The glycolytic pathway (Figure 9.2) is located in the cytosol of all mammalian and human cells. The pathway can be divided into three phases:

- the **priming stage** in which energy is put into the system in the form of two molecules of ATP;
- the **splitting stage** in which a six-carbon molecule is cleaved into two three-carbon molecules;
- the **energy-conservation stage** in which molecules with large negative standard free energy of hydrolysis are used to produce ATP.

The priming stage

This stage is from **glucose to fructose 1,6-bisphosphate** and consists of three enzymic reactions. The first reaction involves the phosphorylation of glucose. The main group of enzymes which catalyse phosphorylation reactions are called **kinases**. Kinases bind the $MgATP^{2-}$ complex more readily than free ATP^{4-} (Chapter 7). Phosphorylation by **hexokinase** ensures that the glucose molecules are retained within the cytosol since charged molecules do not cross cellular membranes in the absence of specialized transport mechanisms (Chapter 8). Hexokinase occurs in a wide variety of

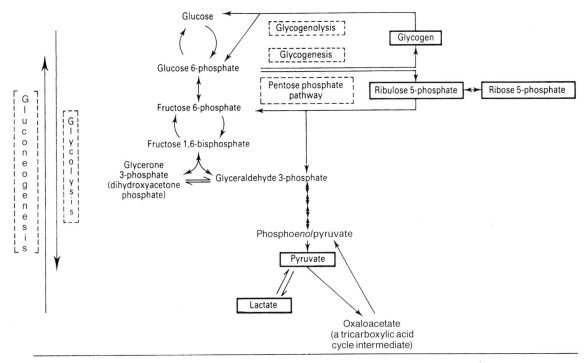

Figure 9.1   *Summary of carbohydrate metabolism*

animals, plants and micro-organisms. It is an example of the induced-fit model of substrate binding (Chapter 4) in which glucose induces significant alterations in the tertiary structure of the enzyme. The positional changes of the amino acid within the protein molecule create a more non-polar environment which is conducive to the transfer of the terminal phosphoryl group of ATP to the substrate.

The readily reversible isomerization of glucose 6-phosphate, an aldose, into its corresponding ketose involves a change of anomeric carbon atom (Chapter 5). The magnesium-ion-requiring **glucose-6-phosphate isomerase** exhibits absolute specificity and establishes the equilibrium at the ratio of 7:3 in favour of glucose 6-phosphate. Progression through the pathway proceeds by the utilization of fructose-6-phosphate as substrate in the following reaction. The second phosphorylation reaction, in which fructose 6-phosphate is phosphorylated at the expense of ATP, is catalysed by allosteric isoenzymes of **6-phosphofructokinase** which is regulated by a variety of effectors.

The splitting stage

In this stage, **fructose-bisphosphate aldolase** cleaves fructose 1,6-bisphosphate into **glycerone phosphate** (also called dihydroxyace-

Figure 9.2   *The glycolytic pathway*

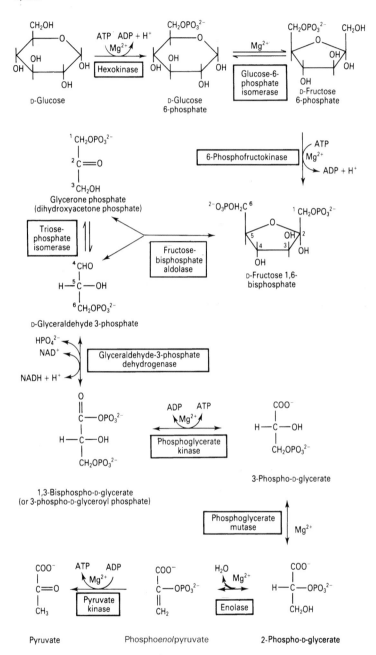

tone phosphate) **and glyceraldehyde 3-phosphate.** The name of the enzyme is derived from the chemical nature of the reverse reaction, an aldol condensation. The equilibrium remains vastly in favour of the substrate ($K'_{eq} = 10^{-4}$M) but the reaction proceeds by the mechanism of removal of products further along the reaction sequence. Another isomerization enables the utilization of the glycerone phosphate (ketose) in the pathway by its conversion into glyceraldehyde 3-phosphate.

The energy-conservation stage

In this stage, **glyceraldehyde 3-phosphate is sequentially metabolized to pyruvate.**

The conversion of glyceraldehyde 3-phosphate into **1,3-bisphosphoglycerate** by **glyceraldehyde-3-phosphate dehydrogenase** without the involvement of ATP reveals the secret of glycolysis as an energy-releasing pathway (Figure 9.3). The aldehydic group of the substrate reacts with the side chain of a cysteinyl residue in the active site of the enzyme to form a **thiohemiacetal** intermediate. Enzyme-bound NAD^+ accepts a hydride ion and a proton (H^+) is released from the OH group to produce a **thioester**. The enzyme-bound NADH in turn reduces coenzymic NAD^+. These two steps effect the oxidation of the aldehyde group of the substrate. **Phosphorolysis**, the cleavage of a bond by the introduction of an orthophosphate group, yields a mixed anhydride (**1,3-bisphosphoglycerate**) which has a large negative standard free energy of hydrolysis (Chapter 8).

The destruction of the phosphoanhydride bond of 1,3-bisphosphoglycerate during the following reaction releases sufficient free energy to enable ATP synthesis although the reaction is freely reversible. This reaction, catalysed by **phosphoglycerate kinase**, is termed a **substrate-level phosphorylation** (Chapter 8) and produces **3-phosphoglycerate**. **Phosphoglycerate mutase** catalyses the transfer of a phosphoryl group from the C-3 position of **3-phosphoglycerate** to the C-2 position to produce **2-phosphoglycerate**. In general, intra-molecular rearrangements of chemical groups are performed by enzymes called mutases. The reaction is freely reversible and proceeds in mammalian tissues through the utilization of an obligatory intermediate, 2,3-bisphosphoglycerate. In erythrocytes, however, 2,3-bisphosphoglycerate has the additional important role as an allosteric effector in the binding of oxygen by haemoglobin.

2-Phosphoglycerate is converted into **phospho*enol*pyruvate** by the elimination of the elements of water from its C-2 (H) and C-3 (OH) atoms. The reaction is catalysed by **phosphopyruvate hydratase** which is more commonly called **enolase**. Phospho*enol*pyruvate is an intermediate which demonstrates a large negative standard free energy of hydrolysis. In the final reaction of glycolysis, allosteric isoenzymes of **pyruvate kinase** catalyse the second substrate-level phosphorylation of ADP; the metabolic product is **pyruvate**. Unlike phosphoglycerate kinase, the pyruvate kinase reaction is not reversible under intracellular conditions.

NAD$^+$ and glycolysis

The operation of the glycolytic pathway is dependent upon the

---

The name of the enzyme **hexokinase** (EC. 2.7.1.1) implies that the enzyme can catalyse the phosphorylation of a number of six-carbon monosaccharides, i.e. D-glucose, D-mannose, D-fructose and D-glucosamine. Different isoenzymes of hexokinase are located in different mammalian body tissues. Each of the isoenzymes exhibits different kinetic properties. Human and mammalian liver cells (hepatocytes) contain exclusively **hexokinase Type IV** (also called glucokinase) which differs from the skeletal muscle isoenzymes. The catalytic action of Type IV is restricted to D-glucose and D-mannose and has a K_m of $\sim 10\,mM$ for glucose. This isoenzyme therefore requires much higher glucose levels for maximum activity (the K_m of the other isoenzymes is $\sim 0.1\,mM$).

In some micro-organisms and invertebrates, there is a different **glucokinase** (EC 2.7.1.2) which is a group of enzymes highly specific for glucose. In these organisms, glucokinase catalyses the initial reaction of glycolysis.

The K_m value for hexokinase Type IV is a useful feature in the control of high blood glucose levels. The K_m of Type IV is higher than the normal concentration of glucose in the blood of man (range: 4–5.5 mM). When the blood glucose levels rise after a carbohydrate-rich meal, the excess blood glucose is transported into the liver cells in which it is converted to glucose 6-phosphate by the appropriate isoform. The Type IV isoenzyme may be induced and its concentration in the liver is controlled by the pancreatic hormone insulin.

In the commonest endocrine disorder, **diabetes mellitus**, patients produce insufficient insulin and consequently have low levels of hexokinase Type IV. Their livers produce little glycogen.

These patients may be damaged by the levels of glucose remaining high in their blood. The complications of prolonged diabetes mellitus may be severe, including thickening of basement membranes leading to amputations, renal failure, blindness and premature coronary heart disease.

availability of NAD in the oxidized state which participates as the electron acceptor in the oxidation catalysed by **glyceraldehyde-3-phosphate dehydrogenase**. As is the case with coenzymes, NAD^+ is in limited supply. The reduced NADH must be converted back into NAD^+. Different types of cells achieve the regeneration of NAD^+ by the employment of different metabolic reactions in which a convenient molecule is utilized as an acceptor of NADH-derived electrons. The fate of NADH (Figure 9.4) depends on the existent intracellular conditions:

- Under anaerobic conditions, highly active skeletal muscle cells and homolactic bacteria employ pyruvate, conveniently available as the end product of glycolysis, as a hydride ion (two electrons) acceptor to yield **lactate**. This reaction is catalysed by **lactate dehydrogenase**.

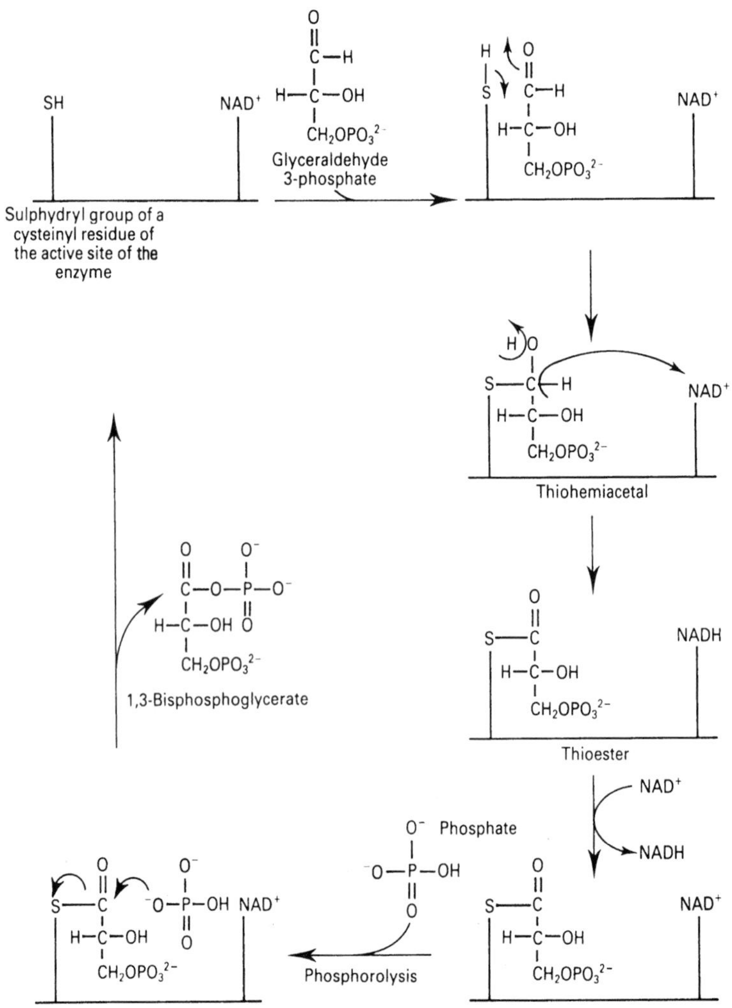

Figure 9.3 *Mechanism of action of glyceraldehyde-3-phosphate dehydrogenase. Only one of four identical subunits is shown; the reaction mechanism proceeds simultaneously in each subunit. The arrows indicate the migration of electrons to effect new bonding arrangements*

- Under **anaerobic conditions, yeast cells** also employ pyruvate which is initially decarboxylated into **acetaldehyde**. This reaction involves the coenzyme **thiamin diphosphate**, a derivative of the vitamin thiamin (vitamin B_1). The acetaldehyde is then reduced to ethanol by **alcohol dehydrogenase**. These anaerobic processes, called **fermentations**, are of major importance, e.g. in the baking industry as a source of CO_2 to raise dough and in the brewing industry to produce alcohol. Other adaptations are found in micro-organisms and invertebrates.

- Under **aerobic conditions**, a greater energy yield may be derived from the electrons contained within the NADH molecule by their participation in the process of oxidative phosphorylation (Chapter 11). Access to the electron-transport assemblies within the inner mitochondrial membrane necessitates the penetration of the membrane by NADH. The inner mitochondrial membrane is, however, impermeable to NADH molecules. This obstacle is circumvented by the use of shuttle systems (Chapter 8).

Shuttle systems for NADH

Shuttle systems do not transport the NADH molecules across the membrane but transfer the electrons as components of another substance which can traverse the membrane. Two tissue-dependent systems exist for this purpose:

Some poisons act by the inhibition of **glyceraldehyde-3-phosphate dehydrogenase**. Arsenate (AsO_4^{3-}) resembles phosphate (PO_4^{3-}) in shape. Thus, arsenate may bind to the active site of the enzyme and may participate in the 'phosphorolysis' of the thioester intermediate. The product, **1-arseno-3-phosphoglycerate**, spontaneously hydrolyses to yield 3-phosphoglycerate which proceeds through the remainder of glycolysis. However, the formation of 1,3-bisphospho-glycerate is lost and consequently the formation of an ATP. This process is termed uncoupling since the link between oxidation and phosphorylation is destroyed.

The enzyme may be inactivated by sulphydryl group reagents such as iodoacetate, 2-mercaptoethanol and mercury compounds (e.g. *p*-chloromercuribenzoate) which interfere with the critical role of the side chain of cysteine.

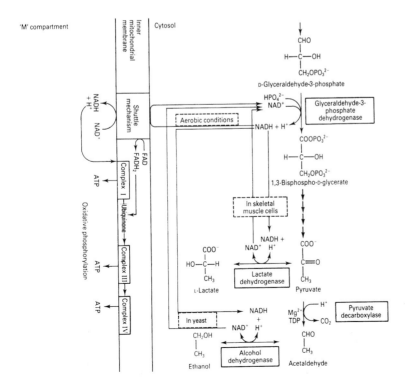

Figure 9.4 *Some fates of NADH produced in the glyceraldehyde-3-phosphate dehydrogenase reaction under anaerobic and aerobic conditions*

Fructose, produced mainly from the hydrolysis of dietary sugar, may enter the pool of glycolytic intermediates by different pathways in different tissues. In liver cells, fructose is phosphorylated at C-1 by **fructokinase**. The resultant **fructose 1-phosphate** is cleaved by **fructose-1-phosphate aldolase** into glyceraldehyde plus glycerone phosphate. Glyceraldehyde may be converted to glyceraldehyde 3-phosphate by **triokinase** (also called triose kinase) at the expense of a second ATP. In kidney and muscle cells, fructose 6-phosphate is produced directly by hexokinase.

Mannose is phosphorylated by hexokinase and the resultant mannose 6-phosphate is isomerized by **mannose-6-phosphate isomerase** to fructose 6-phosphate.

- the **glycerol phosphate shuttle** predominates in cells of mammalian skeletal muscle and brain;
- the **malate–aspartate shuttle** is important in liver, kidney and cardiac muscle cells.

The **glycerol phosphate shuttle** (Figure 9.5) utilizes the glycolytic pathway intermediate glycerone phosphate as an acceptor of electrons from NADH. The reversible reaction is catalysed by the cytosolic form of **glycerol-3-phosphate dehydrogenase**. The product, *sn*-**glycerol 3-phosphate**, can diffuse into the membrane and the reducing equivalents thus carried are transferred not to mitochondrial NAD^+ but to FAD (Figure 4.5b) bound as a prosthetic group to a different enzyme, mitochondrial glycerol-3-phosphate dehydrogenase. The oxidation of glycerol 3-phosphate produces glycerone phosphate which diffuses back into the cytosol. The FAD-linked enzyme is an integral membrane protein suitably positioned on the outside of the inner membrane to effect the transfer of the electrons to ubiquinone of the respiratory chain (Chapter 11). Glycerol-3-phosphate molecules therefore do not enter the mitochondrial matrix. The employment of FAD creates a free-energy differential which drives the transport of the electrons into the membrane and renders the shuttle mechanism irreversible.

In the **malate–aspartate shuttle**, the acceptor of reducing equivalents from NADH is oxaloacetate which is reduced to L-**malate** by cytosolic **malate dehydrogenase**. The inner mitochondrial membrane has an antiport transport system for malate which is carried into the 'M' compartment by a conformational change in the carrier protein in exchange for **2-oxoglutarate**. Malate is oxidized to **oxaloacetate** with concomitant NADH production. Oxaloacetate cannot permeate the inner membrane but is converted to 2-oxoglutarate by the action of mitochondrial **aspartate transaminase** at the expense of glutamate (Chapter 13). The 2-oxoglutarate may be exchanged for cytosolic malate. The action of cytosolic aspartate transaminase on 2-oxoglutarate provides the oxaloacetate for the regeneration of NAD^+. Both isoenzymes of malate dehydrogenase are NAD-linked so that the shuttle in essence transfers electrons from the cytosolic pool of NADH to the mitochondrial pool of NAD^+.

The use of different mitochondrial coenzymes as electron acceptors has implications for the energetics of aerobic carbohydrate metabolism. Electrons from NADH enter the respiratory chain at Complex I and provide ~ 2.5 ATP whereas $FADH_2$ transfers its electrons to ubiquinone and provides ~ 1.5 ATP.

The energetics of glycolysis

Glycolysis, like all pathways of carbohydrate metabolism, is exergonic overall (Chapter 7). As calculated from thermodynamic

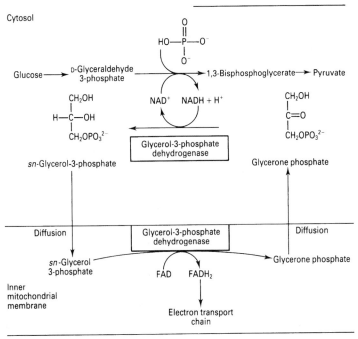

Cytosol

Glucose →

Figure 9.5 *The glycerol phosphate shuttle*

Galactose enters glycolysis by a more complex route. A hereditary disease called **galactosaemia** results from an inability to utilize this pathway. Various forms of galactosaemia exist: all are due to genetic defects in the enzymes of this pathway. Galactosaemia may result in cataracts and neurological disorders.

A major source of galactose is milk which contains **lactose**. **Lactase** in the brush border epithelial cells of the small intestine hydrolyses the disaccharide to galactose and glucose. **Genetic lactase deficiency** results in **lactose intolerance**, the major symptoms of which include abdominal cramps, bloating and diarrhoea. This common world-wide metabolic disorder is the result of an inability to digest lactose and may be relieved by abstinence from milk. Alternatively, lactose-containing yoghurt enhances lactose tolerance of these patients. Various species of *Lactobacillus* used in yoghurt production contain lactase activity.

data, the degradation of glucose to two lactate molecules proceeds with the release of free energy according to the equation:

$$\text{Glucose} \rightarrow 2 \text{ lactate} + 2\text{H}^+; \Delta G^{o\prime} = -196.6 \text{ kJ mol}^{-1}$$

In mammalian skeletal muscle cells, the degradation occurs according to the following equation:

$$\text{Glucose} + 2\,\text{ADP} + 2 \text{ phosphate} \longrightarrow$$
$$2 \text{ lactate} + 2\text{H}^+ + 2\,\text{ATP} + 2\,\text{H}_2\text{O}; \Delta G^{o\prime} = -135.6 \text{ kJ mol}^{-1}$$

Thus, during glycolysis, part of the energy released is conserved by the substrate-level phosphorylation reactions which synthesize ATP. The greater proportion of energy is dissipated as heat.

Table 9.1 indicates the standard free-energy changes for individual reactions of glycolysis. Over half of the reactions are endergonic, i.e. $\Delta G^{o\prime} = +\text{ve}$. However, when the actual free-energy changes, ΔG, are calculated employing available data on intracellular concentrations of metabolites, only three reactions, i.e. the triose-phosphate isomerase, phosphoglycerate kinase and phosphoglycerate mutase reactions, are energy requiring, but by such small amounts that their energetic deficiencies can be accommodated by the mechanism of coupling reactions (Chapter 8). Accurate assessments of ΔG necessitate that the reaction achieves a steady state. However, metabolic flow through pathways implies that none of the intermediate reactions is at equilibrium so that ΔG values must also be considered to be of limited value although useful as a basis for understanding fundamental principles.

The net yield of ATP from the anaerobic catabolism of glucose can be calculated as shown in Table 9.2. Glycolysis yields two molecules of ATP per molecule of glucose consumed.

Glycogen

Glycogen, the major storage polysaccharide found in animal and human tissues, is a polymer of glucose in which glucose residues are linked by α-(1 → 4) glycosidic linkages with branching by α-(1 → 6) glycosidic linkages (Figure 5.6a and c). Although glycogen synthesis may occur in nearly all animal tissues, the major tissues of storage are skeletal muscles and liver. Glycogen is stored as granules which also incorporate the enzymes for its synthesis and intracellular degradation.

An important consideration in the storage of glucose as a polymer is that large quantities of small molecules lead to high osmotic pressures (Chapter 1) within the cells. Since osmotic pressure is concentration dependent, polymerization reduces the concentration of free glucose molecules and thereby retains glucosyl residues in a form which does not risk membrane lysis.

Liver and muscle glycogen

In man, glycogen may account for up to 10% and 2% of the wet weight of the liver and skeletal muscle respectively. Since the total

Table 9.1   *The standard and actual free-energy changes during the reactions of glycolysis*

Enzyme	Free energy change (kJ mol^{-1})	
	Standard, $\Delta G^{o\prime}$	Actual, ΔG
Hexokinase	−16.7	−33.4
Glucose-6-phosphate isomerase	+ 1.7	− 2.5
6-Phosphofructokinase	−14.2	−22.2
Fructose-bisphosphate aldolase	+23.8	− 1.3
Triose-phosphate isomerase	+ 7.5	+ 2.5
Glyceraldehyde-3-phosphate dehydrogenase	+ 6.3	− 1.7
Phosphoglycerate kinase	−18.8	+ 1.3
Phosphoglycerate mutase	+ 4.6	+ 0.8
Enolase	+ 1.7	− 3.3
Pyruvate kinase	−31.4	−16.7

Table 9.2   *The role of ATP in glycolysis*

Stage	Enzymic reaction	ATP change per molecule of glucose	
		Utilization	Production
Stage 1: priming	Hexokinase	1	–
	6-Phosphofructokinase	1	–
Stage 2: splitting	–	–	–
Stage 3: energy conservation	Phosphoglycerate kinase	–	$1 \times 2^*$
	Pyruvate kinase	–	$1 \times 2^*$
Totals		2	4
Net yield of ATP $= 4 - 2 = 2$ molecules			

*Stages 1 and 2 degrade each glucose molecule into two molecules of glyceraldehyde 3-phosphate so that stage 3 occurs twice per glucose molecule

quantity of skeletal muscle exceeds that of liver about 10-fold, approximately twice as much glycogen is stored in muscle.

The roles of liver and skeletal muscle glycogen, however, differ:

- **Liver glycogen** functions as a reservoir of glucose which is released to maintain the concentration of glucose in the blood circulation from which other tissues, e.g. brain, draw their supply of glucose. Liver glycogen levels increase following a meal and progressively decrease to maintain an almost constant blood glucose level.

- **Muscle glycogen** serves as a reservoir of glucose mainly for use within the same tissue. Glucose metabolism provides ATP which is necessary during mechanical work. Muscle glycogen levels vary less markedly with food intake than those of liver and its mobilization is triggered by increased muscular activity.

Glycogenesis

Glycogen synthesis commences from glucose 6-phosphate (Figure 9.6) which may be produced from glucose transported from the bloodstream (Chapter 7) as in skeletal muscle or by gluconeogenesis from C_3 compounds, e.g. lactate, as in liver. An intra-molecular transfer of the phosphate from the C-6 position to the C-1 position is performed by phosphoglucomutase.

The next reaction is unique to the synthetic pathway and involves the formation of **uridine diphosphate glucose** (UDP-glucose) which serves as the carrier of the glucosyl residue which participates in the elongation of an existent molecule of glycogen, called the primer molecule. The enzyme, **UTP-glucose-1-phosphate uridylyltransfer-ase** utilizes both UTP and glucose 1-phosphate in a readily reversible reaction. Synthesis is promoted by the irreversible hydro-lysis of pyrophosphate by **inorganic pyrophosphatase**. The removal

Ethanol is a drug which gives pleasure to some individuals and is responsible for the misery of others. In the UK, the maximum blood alcohol level at which driving is legally permitted (1997) is $0.8 \, g \, l^{-1}$ (17.6 mM). Ethanol may be metabolized in the liver to acetaldehyde by two main pathways depending on the blood concentration. At ethanol levels of approximately 1–5 mM, **alcohol dehydrogenase** is active. At higher concentrations, the principal pathway involves a **cytochrome P_{450} system** in liver microsomes. The acetaldehyde is converted to acetyl-CoA for entry into the tricarboxylic acid cycle (Chapter 10).

Some unfortunate persons may drink **ethylene glycol** and **methanol** (both available in antifreeze solutions for vehicle cooling systems). Alcohol dehydrogenase converts these substances to toxic **oxalic acid** and **formic acid** respectively. Administration of ethanol may protect these cases from poisoning. Indeed, ethylene glycol has been employed commercially as a flavour enhancer in wine!

of the pyrophosphate commits the uridylyltransferase reaction to the direction of glycogen synthesis (Chapter 8).

Glycogen synthesis involves both **chain elongation and branching**:

- **Chain elongation** is performed by **glycogen synthase** which transfers the glucosyl moiety of UDP-glucose to the non-reducing end (Chapter 5) of a glycogen primer containing at least four glucosyl residues. Glycogen synthase is highly specific: it will only produce a new α-(1 → 4) glycosidic bond. The released UDP may be phosphorylated to UTP (at the expense of ATP) which may participate in the formation of another UDP-glucose. Glycogen synthase may repeatedly add glucosyl groups to the primer molecule.

- **Branching** through α-(1 → 6) glycosidic bonds occurs by the action of another enzyme, **glycogen branching enzyme**, which transfers terminal hexa- or septasaccharide units from growing chains of at least 11 residues to the hydroxyl group of glucose residues in internal positions. Branch points are not created closer than every fourth residue. Since similar chemical linkages are involved, the free-energy change is very small.

Branching increases the number of non-reducing ends which may be simultaneously elongated by glycogen synthase or degraded.

Glycogenolysis

Glycogen degradation involves both **chain shortening and debranching**:

- **Chain shortening** proceeds by the action of the **glycogen phosphorylase** (Figure 9.6) which cleaves the α-(1 → 4) glycosidic linkage between the terminal glucose residue of a branch and its neighbour by phosphorolysis. The products of the reaction are glucose 1-phosphate which retains the α-configuration and a glycogen molecule which is one glucosyl residue smaller. Glycogen phosphorylase may sequentially remove residues from the non-reducing ends of glycogen chains until it approaches a branching point. Like glycogen synthase, glycogen phosphorylase cannot negotiate α-(1 → 6) glycosidic bonds and its activity ceases at the fourth residue from such a linkage.

- **Debranching** proceeds by an enzyme system called the **glycogen debranching system**, involving two enzymic activities. **4-α-Glucanotransferase** transfers a trisaccharide unit to the end of another chain, and **amylo-1,6-glucosidase** removes the solitary glucose remaining at the end of the branch.

The non-phosphorylated glucose accounts for about 10% of the cleavage products since branches occur approximately every eight

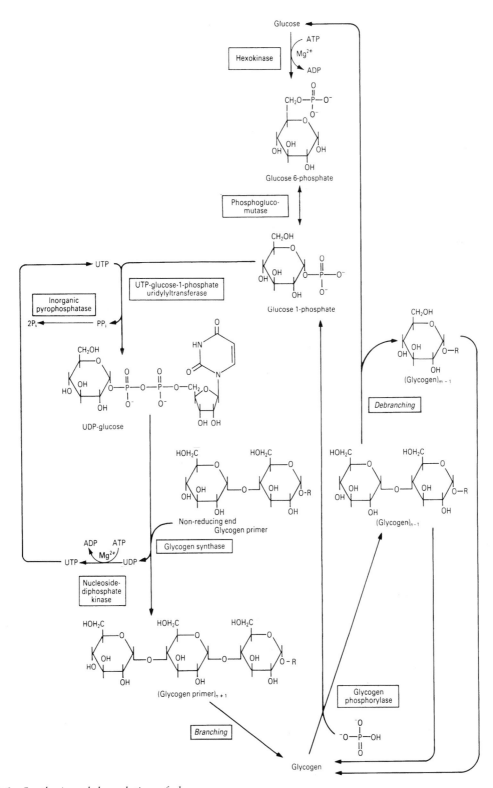

Figure 9.6 *Synthesis and degradation of glycogen*

to 12 glucose residues. Glycogen phosphorylase then resumes its activity.

The fate of glucose 6-phosphate and glucose depends on the nature of the tissue:

- **In skeletal muscle cells,** glucose may be phosphorylated into glucose-6-phosphate by hexokinase. Glucose-6-phosphate from either route may be utilized in energy release through glycolysis.
- **Liver cells** utilize glucose 6-phosphatase to remove the phosphate from glucose 6-phosphate. Non-phosphorylated glucose from liver glycogen can traverse the plasma membrane and be transported via the blood circulation to other tissues.

Glucose-6-phosphatase is absent from skeletal muscle and brain and so glucose is retained by these tissues as glucose 6-phosphate which cannot permeate the plasma membrane.

The energetics of glycogenesis and glycogenolysis

Glycogen is a highly efficient way of storing glucose. Only one equivalent of ATP (i.e. UTP) is utilized in the elongation of a glycogen chain by one glucose residue. Phosphorolysis cleaves glycogen to glucose-1-phosphate which is readily converted into glucose-6-phosphate. Each glucose released by the debranching enzyme may be phosphorylated into glucose 6-phosphate at the expense of one ATP. Under anaerobic conditions, each glucose-6-phosphate will yield three molecules of ATP.

Gluconeogenesis

The daily glucose requirement for the human body is about 160 g. Body fluids contain ~20 g of glucose, and glycogen may provide ~180–200 g. of free glucose. If dietary glucose is not available, glucose must be generated from other sources. Gluconeogenesis is the process by which glucose is synthesized from non-carbohydrate precursor molecules.

The role of gluconeogenesis

As glycogen stores are utilized, gluconeogenesis promotes the continuance of the supply of glucose to the blood circulation. This is of paramount importance since certain tissues, including the brain, erythrocytes and renal medulla, utilize glucose as their primary source of energy although their gluconeogenic capacity is almost negligible. The brain accounts for approximately 75% of all the glucose degraded in the body. These cells depend upon the liver (the major site of gluconeogenesis) and the kidney (renal cortex) to support their glucose catabolism during periods of glycogen depletion.

There are a number of conditions collectively known as **glycogen-storage diseases**. They are classified as **Types I–VIII** and are often referred to by the name of the physician who first described them.

Type I (von Gierke's disease) is caused by a defective glucose-6-phosphatase or a genetic mutation in a glucose 6-phosphate transporter (Chapter 7) in the endoplasmic reticulum. Liver and kidneys are affected with massive enlargement of the liver due to increased amounts of glycogen in this organ.

Other forms involve defects in lysosomal 4-α-glucano-transferase (Type II), amylo-1,6-glucosidase (Type III), branching enzyme (Type IV), glycogen phosphorylase (Types V and VI), the glycolytic enzyme 6-phosphofructokinase (Type VII) and the regulatory enzyme phosphorylase kinase (Type VIII).

Sources of gluconeogenic precursors

The principal precursors are:

- lactate;
- alanine;
- glycerol.

Lactate is produced during periods of strenuous muscular activity, e.g. sprinting, when rapid provision of ATP by glycolysis in highly active muscle is necessitated. Gluconeogenesis aids the restoration of glycogen levels in skeletal muscle. This lactate, together with some pyruvate, diffuses through the permeable plasma membrane into the blood circulation. These substances are sequestered by the liver and, in the cytosol of hepatocytes, the lactate is oxidised to pyruvate which is converted by the gluconeogenic pathway into glucose. The resultant glucose may diffuse into the blood circulation and be absorbed by skeletal muscle cells to replenish their depleted glycogen stores. This sequence of events, called the **Cori cycle** (Figure 9.7), operates between tissues in which glucose is not completely oxidized and the liver.

Alanine is available from dietary proteins. However, during a fast or starvation, a major contribution is made by alanine which is released along with other amino acids from skeletal muscle. Since labile proteins rich in alanine are not present in muscle, the released alanine appears to result from the activity of alanine transaminase which produces alanine from cytosolic pyruvate. This is the basis of the **pyruvate–alanine cycle** which also operates between skeletal muscle and the liver. This cycle functions only when peripheral tissues reoxidize glycolytic NADH through the oxidative phosphorylation pathway. In the presence of oxygen, pyruvate is not utilized in lactate production and is available for the transaminase reaction.

Glycerol is yielded by the enzymic hydrolysis of triacylglycerols (Chapter 12). Glycerol may enter gluconeogenesis or glycolysis through the common intermediate, glycerone phosphate. The other hydrolytic product, fatty acids, may undergo β-oxidation (Chapter 12) to acetyl-CoA which cannot significantly contribute to gluconeogenesis. However, fatty acids which are branched or have an odd number of carbon atoms also yield some propionyl-CoA which may be metabolized to succinyl-CoA, a tricarboxylic acid intermediate (Chapter 11). Additional production of tricarboxylic acid intermediates, e.g. from glutamine (Chapter 13), makes the cycle available as a source of gluconeogenic precursors which may enter the pathway through the reversal of anaplerotic pathways (Chapter 10).

The bypass reactions of gluconeogenesis

The synthesis of glucose from pyruvate is not simply a reversal of glycolysis despite the participation of all glycolytic intermediates

Figure 9.7 *The Cori cycle*

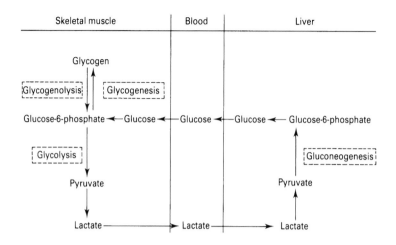

(Figure 9.8). Seven reactions which are freely reversible are shared by both pathways. Three glycolytic reactions are essentially irreversible in the cell because of their standard free energies of hydrolysis:

- hexokinase, $\Delta G^{o\prime} = -16.7\,\text{kJ mol}^{-1}$;
- 6-phosphofructokinase, $\Delta G^{o\prime} = -14.2\,\text{kJ mol}^{-1}$;
- pyruvate kinase, $\Delta G^{o\prime} = -31.4\,\text{kJ mol}^{-1}$.

In gluconeogenesis, more favourable alternative reactions, termed the bypass reactions, are exploited.

Lactate and **alanine** enter as pyruvate following the activities of lactate dehydrogenase (Figure 9.4) and alanine transaminase (Chapter 13) respectively. In **the first bypass reaction**, the objective of which is to overcome the unfavourable energetics of a reversal of the pyruvate kinase reaction, seems a tortuous route (Figure 9.8). The reaction sequence relies on two important enzymes: **pyruvate carboxylase** and **phospho***enol***pyruvate carboxykinase**. Since pyruvate carboxylase is located exclusively in the mitochondrion, pyruvate must cross the inner mitochondrial membrane (Chapter 10). Oxaloacetate produced by pyruvate carboxylase cannot traverse the inner membrane and is reduced by malate dehydrogenase to L-malate. This step is the reversal of the tricarboxylic acid cycle reaction. Malate may, of course, be formed by the sequential action of the cycle enzymes following increased levels of cycle intermediate pools, e.g. 2-oxoglutarate and succinyl-CoA. Malate may be translocated out of the mitochondrion in exchange for phosphate by the **malate–phosphate antiport system**. Oxaloacetate is reformed from the malate by the cytosolic isoenzyme of malate dehydrogenase. Oxaloacetate is the substrate for phospho***enol***pyruvate carboxykinase which produces phospho***enol***pyruvate: the enzyme specifically requires GTP to act as phosphate group

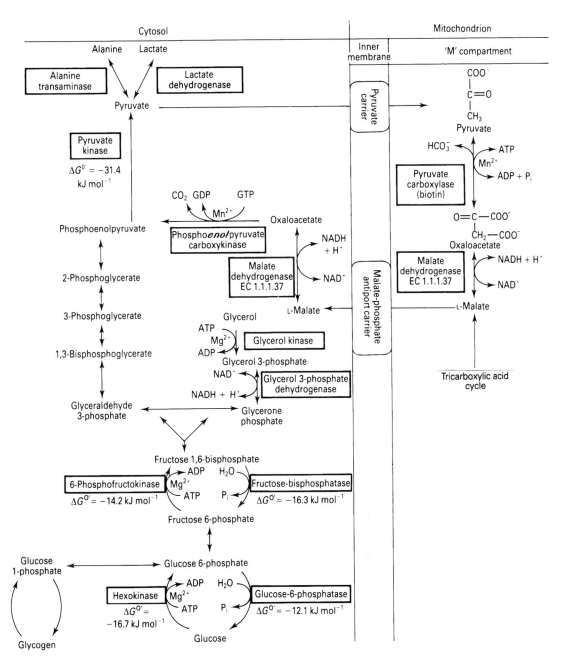

Figure 9.8 *Pathway for gluconeogenesis from lactate, alanine and glycerol*

donor. GTP may be formed from ATP through the action of
nucleoside-diphosphate kinase.

From phospho*enol*pyruvate, the gluconeogenic pathway proceeds through the reversal of glycolytic reactions as far as the
formation of fructose 1,6-bisphosphate. ATP must be supplied for
the phosphoglycerate kinase reaction whilst NADH and phosphate
are necessary for the glyceraldehyde-3-phosphate dehydrogenase

Carboxylation reactions utilize carbon dioxide either in gaseous form or derived from the solubilized form of bicarbonate. A number of important carboxylations use HCO_3^- and ATP, including pyruvate carboxylase, acetyl-CoA carboxylase (Chapter 12), propionyl-CoA carboxylase (Chapter 12) and **methylcrotonyl-CoA carboxylase** (in leucine degradation). These enzymes all utilize **biotin** (Figure 4.5) as a prosthetic group which is covalently bound through the ε-amino group of a lysyl residue of the protein.

Bicarbonate is readily available from body fluids (adult human normal range in serum is 21–28 mM) but is a weak electrophile. Bicarbonate is therefore converted to CO_2 in an ATP-dependent reaction in which its cleaved phosphate group forms a carbonyl-phosphate mixed anhydride intermediate. Phosphate is then released from this intermediate and the CO_2 formed at the active site adds to biotin which, by movement of the flexible lysyl side chain, is translocated to another subsite in the active site for transfer to the substrate.

Some important carboxylations, however, do not use biotin. **Ribulose-1,5-bisphosphate carboxylase** in photosynthetic organisms fixes gaseous CO_2 during the formation of two molecules of 3-phosphoglycerate ($2 \times C_3$) from ribulose 1,5-bisphosphate (C_5).

reaction. When lactate is the source of cytosolic pyruvate, as in the liver, this NADH is generated by the lactate dehydrogenase reaction. However, if pyruvate arises from other sources, e.g. alanine, the NADH is made available through the cytosolic malate dehydrogenase reaction of the first bypass.

Glycerol released from triacylglycerol storage undergoes phosphorylation in gluconeogenic tissues to form *sn*-glycerol 3-phosphate which is then reduced to glycerone phosphate and subjected to the activity of fructose-bisphosphate aldolase. **The second bypass reaction** involves **fructose-bisphosphatase**. This enzymic reaction circumvents the irreversible glycolytic reaction catalysed by 6-phosphofructokinase. Fructose-bisphosphatase irreversibly cleaves a phosphate group from the C-1 position of fructose 1,6-bisphosphate to yield fructose 6-phosphate. Fructose 6-phosphate is converted into glucose 6-phosphate by isomerization. Glucose 6-phosphate may be processed to glycogen and thereby employed to replenish depleted glycogen stores. Alternatively, **the third bypass reaction** involves **glucose-6-phosphatase**. This reaction operates when glucose is required to maintain blood glucose levels. This enzyme, present in the liver but absent from muscle, permits glucose to be released from the liver to the blood circulation.

The energetics of gluconeogenesis

The multistep route of the first bypass reaction requires only 0.84 kJ mol^{-1} under standard conditions. On consideration of actual intracellular conditions, the reaction is exergonic (ΔG is approximately -25 kJ mol^{-1}). Dephosphorylation reactions catalysed by fructose-bisphosphatase and glucose-6-phosphatase provide exergonic reactions which reverse exergonic glycolytic reactions by a different mechanism. However, it should be noted that ATP participates in the phosphorylation reaction whereas the hydrolytic cleavage of the phosphate group releases energy in the opposite reaction (Figure 9.8).

Gluconeogenesis from pyruvate is an energy-requiring process. The pyruvate kinase bypass utilizes ATP in the pyruvate carboxylase step and GTP (equivalent to ATP) in the PEP carboxykinase step. Reversal of the phosphoglycerate kinase and glyceraldehyde-3-phosphate dehydrogenase reactions consumes ATP and NADH respectively. To attain glyceraldehyde 3-phosphate from pyruvate requires three ATP. Two glyceraldehyde 3-phosphate are needed to produce one glucose. The synthesis of glucose from pyruvate therefore requires six ATP. Glycolysis only yields two ATP. Gluconeogenesis must therefore be considered as energetically expensive, a feature of fundamental importance in the starving individual.

The pentose phosphate pathway

The pentose phosphate pathway is also known as the hexose monophosphate shunt and the phosphogluconate pathway because of the variety of intermediates formed under different conditions. The pathway, which occurs in a wide variety of organisms including animals, plants and micro-organisms, is classifiable as secondary metabolism (Chapter 8) due to the relatively small quantity of glucose catabolized by this route.

The importance of the pentose phosphate pathway

In mammalian tissues, the pathway is particularly important as it yields:

- reduced nicotinamide adenine dinucleotide phosphate (NADPH);
- pentose sugars.

A major requirement for **NADPH** is in the biosynthesis of saturated **fatty acids** and **steroids**. Appreciable quantities of fatty acids are synthesized in adipose (fat) tissue, liver and mammary glands. Steroid biosynthesis is particularly active in adrenal cortex, testes and ovaries. Since reducing power in the form of NADPH is utilized in these pathways, the pentose phosphate pathway is highly active in these tissues. The pathway occurs in the cell cytosol where the syntheses of fatty acids and steroids occur. Tissues which are less active in NADPH-dependent reductive biosyntheses generally exhibit markedly less pathway activity, e.g. skeletal muscle.

The reducing power of NADPH plays other important roles:

- **In certain biological hydroxylation reactions.** A series of over 100 **cytochrome P$_{450}$ enzymes**, located predominantly in the endoplasmic reticulum and also in the mitochondrion, catalyse these hydroxylations. In contrast to cytochrome a_3 of the respiratory chain which can also reduce oxygen and react with carbon monoxide, reduced cytochrome P$_{450}$ enzymes when complexed with CO exhibit maximum absorption of light at 450 nm, hence their name. The activity of cytochrome P$_{450}$ enzymes is called **monoxygenase activity** since one atom of molecular O_2 is employed in the formation of a hydroxyl group, the other being reduced by NADPH$+$H$^+$ to water (Figure 9.9). Cytochrome P$_{450}$ enzymes participate in a variety of reactions involving numerous different substrates, e.g. the biosynthesis of steroid hormones (Chapter 12) and the hydroxylation of drugs and other foreign substances (**xenobiotics**) largely by the liver during **detoxification** processes.
- **In erythrocytes.** Red blood cells require NADPH to protect indirectly against both the oxidation of sulphydryl groups of haemoglobin with concomitant impairment of its performance in

After strenuous physical exertion such as playing squash or hill-walking, it is customary to celebrate with the consumption of a few beers. This practice, however, has metabolic consequences. **Ethanol** is an inhibitor of gluconeogenesis and can cause hypoglycemia, a low blood glucose level. This is because **alcohol dehydrogenase** converts NAD$^+$ to NADH. This reduces the [NAD$^+$]/[NADH] ratio in the liver cytosol with two results: lactate dehydrogenase produces lactate instead of pyruvate, and, in the first bypass reaction, cytosolic oxaloacetate tends not to be produced from malate. Both effects inhibit gluconeogenesis. Biochemically speaking, it would be preferable to celebrate with a cup of sugary tea!

The major biological roles of **NADH** and **NADPH** are rather different although the coenzymes differ structurally only by a phosphate group (Figure 4.5). Reduced NAD is of importance in catabolism especially in the generation of ATP through oxidative phosphorylation (Chapter 11) whilst the primary metabolic function of reduced NADP is as **reducing power** in certain biosyntheses. Reducing power is required, for example, to convert double bonds to single bonds.

Figure 9.9 *Role of NADPH in hydroxylation reactions catalysed by cytochrome P$_{450}$ enzymes*

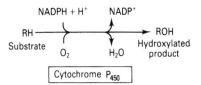

oxygen transport and cell lysis due to the oxidation of unsaturated lipids of the cell membrane.

- **In neutrophilic polymorphonuclear leukocytes** which provide the first line of defence against bacterial infection. These white blood cells use NADPH to produce microbicidal **reactive oxygen radicals.**

Pentose sugars are required for the synthesis of nucleotides:

- **Ribose 5-phosphate** is utilized in the synthesis of purine and pyrimidine deoxyribo- and ribonucleotides. Since neonatal and foetal thymuses and bone marrow are highly active in nucleic acid synthesis, these tissues have an active pentose phosphate pathway to furnish ribose-5-phosphate.

- **Ribonucleotides** are also needed for the synthesis of some major coenzymes such as NAD(P)$^+$, coenzyme A and FAD (Figure 4.5).

The pentose phosphate pathway can be sectioned into two phases: the oxidative phase and the non-oxidative phase.

The oxidative phase of the pentose phosphate pathway

This stage is from **glucose-6-phosphate to ribose 5-phosphate** and consists of four enzymic reactions. The first reaction of the oxidative phase (Figure 9.10) involves the oxidation of glucose 6-phosphate by the NADP$^+$specific enzyme, **glucose-6-phosphate dehydrogenase**, with the concomitant reduction of NADP$^+$ to produce **6-phosphoglucono-1,5-lactone**. This lactone, although unstable and liable to revert to the open-chain form (Chapter 5), is rapidly hydrolysed by a specific **lactonase** to yield **6-phosphogluconate** which undergoes **oxidative decarboxylation**. NADP$^+$ again participates as electron acceptor. Both the removal of firstly electrons and secondly the carboxylate group are catalysed by the same enzyme, **phosphogluconate dehydrogenase (decarboxylating)**. The product, **ribulose 5-phosphate** (ketose), is isomerized into the corresponding aldose phosphate. **Ribose 5-phosphate** may also be generated by **phosphopentomutase** from **ribose 1-phosphate**, the product of nucleic acid and nucleotide degradation.

In some tissues, the pathway is terminated at ribose 5-phosphate which is utilized in nucleotide biosynthesis. During the oxidative

NADPH oxidase is an enzyme which is located on the outside of the plasma membrane of neutrophils. During neutrophil activation, a **phagosome** is formed from the plasma membrane with the result that the enzyme is located in the inside of the phagosome membrane. Activation of the cell also increases its oxygen consumption by 10- to 15-fold. Since neutrophils have very few mitochondria and the oxygen increase is cyanide-insensitive, this oxygen cannot be necessary to satisfy an increase in oxidative phosphorylation. Instead, NADPH oxidase utilizes the molecular O$_2$ as a cosubstrate to produce the **superoxide anion** (·O$_2^-$, which contains one electron more in its outer electronic orbital than oxygen). The electron is donated by NADPH. Through a series of reactions, superoxide is used to generate **hydroxyl radicals** (·OH), **hydrogen peroxide** (H$_2$O$_2$), **hypochlorite** (ClO$^-$) and **singlet oxygen** (^{1}O$_2$, which contains one electron fewer than molecular O$_2$). Each of these **reactive oxygen intermediates** is toxic to different bacteria.

phase of the pathway, the processing of one molecule of D-glucose generates one D-ribose 5-phosphate, one CO_2 and two NADPH.

The non-oxidative phase of the pentose phosphate pathway

This phase is from **ribulose 5-phosphate to glycolytic intermediates.** It will be considered as it occurs within adipose tissue, a tissue which is more active in the synthesis of fats than nucleotides and therefore has a predominant NADPH requirement. In such a tissue, the ribose 5-phosphate enters a series of **sugar interconversion reactions** which connect the pentose phosphate pathway with glycolysis and gluconeogenesis. These interconversion reactions constitute the non-oxidative phase of the pathway (Figure 9.11) and since oxidation is not involved, NADPH is not produced.

Two enzymes, which function in the transfer of carbon units, catalyse the important reactions:

- **transketolase**, which contains **thiamin diphosphate** (Figure 10.3a) as its prosthetic group, transfers two-carbon units;

- **transaldolase** transfers three-carbon units.

The transfer occurs from a ketose donor to an aldose acceptor. The interconversion sequence requires the oxidative phase to operate three times, i.e. three molecules of glucose 6-phosphate yield three molecules of ribulose 5-phosphate.

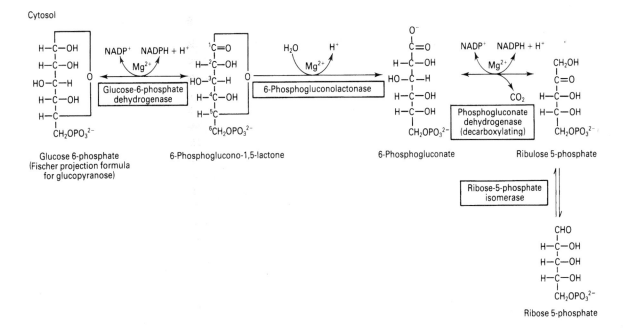

Figure 9.10 *The oxidative phase of the pentose phosphate pathway*

The most common form of **glucose-6-phosphate dehydrogenase deficiency** is found in Afro-Americans. Deficiency of this enzyme may protect the individual against a form of **malaria**. The causative protozoa, *Plasmodium falciparum*, requires reduced glutathione without which its growth is impaired. Glutathione is maintained in the reduced state by NADPH, produced by the pentose phosphate pathway.

Some **drugs** cause **haemolytic anaemia** in some recipients due to their deficiency in glucose-6-phosphate dehydrogenase or by lowering the intracellular concentration of NADPH by acting as an electron acceptor. Lysis of erythrocytes occurs because of insufficient levels of reduced glutathione which is necessary to maintain the integrity of their plasma membranes. Drugs reported as responsible for haemolytic anaemia in deficient patients include **some antimalarials**, e.g. primaquine and chloroquine, **analgesics** (pain-killers), e.g. acetylsalicylic acid (aspirin), and **antibacterials**, e.g. most sulphonamides and chloramphenicol.

The first of the interconversions features **xylulose 5-phosphate** and **ribose 5-phosphate**. Because transketolase has the specific requirement that the hydroxyl group at C-3 must be in the xylulose configuration, xylulose 5-phosphate is produced from ribulose-5-phosphate by epimerization involving the enzyme **ribulose-phosphate 3-epimerase**. Epimers are sugars which differ only in the configuration of the hydroxyl group on one specific chiral carbon atom (Chapter 5), in this case C-3, and hence the name of the enzyme. The C-1 and C-2 atoms of xylulose 5-phosphate are transferred to ribose-5-phosphate to synthesize **sedoheptulose 7-phosphate**. The C-1, C-2 and C-3 atoms of sedoheptulose 7-phosphate are transferred as a three-carbon unit, under the influence of transaldolase, to convert glyceraldehyde 3-phosphate (the other product of the transketolase reaction) into fructose 6-phosphate. The remainder of the carbon chain of sedoheptulose 7-phosphate forms **erythrose 4-phosphate**.

A second transketolase reaction converts the erythrose 4-phosphate into another molecule of fructose 6-phosphate. Because of the specificity of the enzyme, a second xylulose 5-phosphate contributes two carbon atoms to yield the ketose phosphate and glyceraldehyde-3-phosphate. Thus, three molecules of ribulose 5-phosphate are required for the entire interconversion from the pentose to glycolytic intermediates which are two molecules of fructose 6-phosphate and one molecule of glyceraldehyde 3-phosphate. The fructose 6-phosphate molecules enter the cytosolic pool of fructose 6-phosphate and may be utilized in energy release through the glycolytic pathway. Alternatively, they may be isomerized into glucose 6-phosphate and reprocessed through the oxidative phase of this pathway.

It may appear that glyceraldehyde 3-phosphate may only participate in glycolytic degradation. However, if the oxidative phase of the pathway operates another three times, two molecules of glyceraldehyde 3-phosphate would be produced, one of which could be converted by triose-phosphate isomerase to glycerone phosphate. Glucose 6-phosphate could be synthesized through gluconeogenic reactions (Figure 9.8). The pentose phosphate pathway may therefore operate as a cycle which in effect processes one molecule of glucose-6-phosphate to six CO_2 with an appreciable yield of reduced NADP (Table 9.3).

The energetics of the pentose phosphate pathway

The energetics of the pathway differs depending upon which cellular requirement applies. Diversion of glucose 6-phosphate into the pentose phosphate pathway in adipose tissue reduces the direct ATP yield during its oxidation to pyruvate since three glucose 6-phosphate molecules generate only eight molecules of ATP.

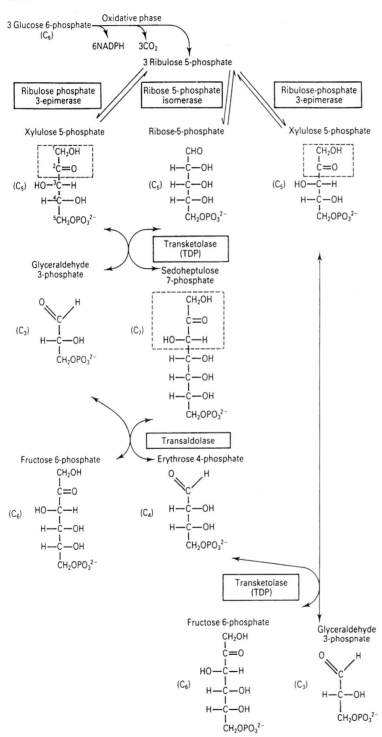

Figure 9.11 *The non-oxidative phase
of the pentose phosphate pathway in
adipose tissue*

Table 9.3   *The operation of the pentose phosphate pathway as a cycle*

Stage number	Reaction sequence	Equation
Stage 1	Oxidative phase	6 Glucose 6-P_i + 12 $NADP^+$ + 6 $H_2O \longrightarrow$ 6 ribulose 5-P_i + 6 CO_2 +12 NADPH + 12 H^+
Stage 2	Non-oxidative phase	6 Ribulose 5-$P_i \longrightarrow$ 4 fructose 6-P_i + 2 glyceraldehyde 3-P_i
Stage 3	Gluconeogenesis	2 Glyceraldehyde 3-P_i + 1 $H_2O \longrightarrow$ 1 glucose 6-P_i + 1 P_i
Stage 4	Isomerization	4 Fructose 6-$P_i \longrightarrow$ 4 glucose 6-P_i
	Sum of stages	6 Glucose 6-P_i + 12 $NADP^+$ + 7 $H_2O \longrightarrow$ 5 glucose 6-P_i + 6 CO_2 + 12 NADPH + 12 H^+ + 1 P_i
	Net reaction	1 Glucose 6-P_i + 12 $NADP^+$ + 7 $H_2O \longrightarrow$ 6 CO_2 + 12 NADPH + 12 H^+ + 1 P_i

The regulation of carbohydrate metabolism

Various enzymic reactions contribute collectively to the control of the metabolic flux through carbohydrate metabolism. The regulation of **glycogen metabolism** primarily involves:

- **glycogen synthase;**
- **glycogen phosphorylase.**

The principal aspects of reciprocal regulation by interconversions between active and less active forms of both enzymes have been discussed in Chapter 8.

Glycolysis is regulated by two reactions:

- **hexokinase;**
- **6-phosphofructokinase.**

These reactions are bypassed in gluconeogenesis by alternative reactions.

Hexokinase activity promotes the intracellular retention of glucose and thereby controls its rate of entry into carbohydrate metabolism whereas glucose-6-phosphatase activity permits the release of glucose from hepatic tissue. This substrate cycle (Chapter 8) is therefore functional in the regulation of blood glucose concentrations. The isoenzymes of hexokinase (already discussed) play a role in the regulation of glucose metabolism according to available glucose concentrations. The reaction product, glucose 6-phosphate, inhibits only Types I, II and III isoenzymes to prevent depletion of intracellular inorganic phosphate required for other cellular reactions.

Glycolytic **6-phosphofructokinase** together with **fructose-bisphosphatase** catalyse the reactions of another substrate cycle in mammalian gluconeogenic tissues. 6-Phosphofructokinase functions under the influence of a number of positive and negative effectors (Table 9. 4) depending on the tissue under consideration. Intracellular concentrations of ATP and ADP contribute to the intracellular energy status and the control of the activity of an enzyme. A high **adenylate energy charge** (Chapter 8) results in ATP binding to a regulatory site with concomitant reduction in product formation. A low charge implies an energy requirement, therefore the operation of the glycolytic pathway is desirable and 6-phosphofructokinase becomes more active. High levels of NADH, citrate and long-chain fatty acids imply that the energy needs of the cell may be satisfied by the utilization of oxidative phosphorylation for which most of the reduced coenzymes are supplied through the tricarboxylic acid cycle and the β-oxidation pathway respectively. Fructose-bisphosphatase is inhibited by AMP and fructose 2,6-bisphosphate. AMP therefore serves to amplify the net flux through the glycolytic pathway.

Gluconeogenesis is allosterically controlled at the first and second bypass reactions:

- **pyruvate carboxylase** is influenced by positive effectors, acetyl-CoA and ATP, and the negative effector, ADP;
- **fructose-bisphosphatase** regulation is described above.

There are, however, additional complications to consider. Enzymes, e.g. 6-phosphofructokinase, fructose-bisphosphate aldolase and glyceraldehyde-3-phosphate dehydrogenase, may bind to the cytoskeleton and cellular membranes. Particle-bound enzymes *in vitro* differ in enzyme kinetics from soluble-phase enzymes. 6-Phosphofructokinase relinquishes its conformational flexibility which is accompanied by a switch from allosteric to Michaelis–Menten kinetics (Chapter 4). Unlike soluble-phase 6-phosphofructokinase, the membrane-bound enzyme is not inhibited by ATP and the plot of its velocity versus fructose 6-phosphate is non-sigmoidal. Moreover, under various physiological conditions, the degree of binding of glycolytic enzymes and their isoenzymic forms to the aforementioned structures may markedly differ. In addition, such binding interactions effectively compartmentalize the glycolytic enzymes within the cytoplasm. This means that, because of compartmentalization, the actual available concentrations of effectors in mammalian cells are unknown.

The rate of the **pentose phosphate pathway** is primarily controlled at the first reaction of the oxidative phase. The major

A number of scenarios are possible for the **pentose phosphate pathway**. If the cell requires **both ribose 5-phosphate** and **NADPH**, only the oxidative phase functions. If the cell requires **more NADPH than ribose 5-phosphate**, the cycle described in the text may apply.

In cells in which the availability of **ribose 5-phosphate for nucleotide synthesis** predominates, this demand may be satisfied through the reversal of the sugar interconversion reactions. In other words, glycolysis may be employed to generate fructose-6-phosphate and glyceraldehyde 3-phosphate from which transketolase and transaldolase produce ribose 5-phosphate. By this route, five molecules of glucose 6-phosphate may yield six molecules of ribose 5-phosphate at the expense of five ATP employed in the 6-phosphofructokinase reaction.

If the cell requires **both NADPH and ATP but not ribose 5-phosphate**, the products fructose 6-phosphate and glyceraldehyde 3-phosphate, may be oxidized to pyruvate which may yield additional ATP molecules via the tricarboxylic acid cycle and oxidative phosphorylation (Chapters 10 and 11).

Since NADPH and NADH are interconvertible through the action of **NAD(P)$^+$ transhydrogenase**, the pentose phosphate pathway under aerobic conditions may contribute electrons for energy production.

Table 9.4   *Principal allosteric effectors of 6-phosphofructokinase*

Positive effectors	Negative effectors
Fructose 1.6-bisphosphate	ATP
Fructose 2.6-bisphosphate	NADH
ADP	Citrate
AMP	Long-chain fatty acids
Phosphate	H$^+$
K$^+$	Ca^{2+}

The **6-phosphofructokinase/ fructose-bisphosphatase cycle** is subject to extracellular influences.

Investigations into the mechanism of action of the peptide hormone **glucagon** on liver gluconeogenesis led to the discovery in 1980 of **fructose 2,6-bisphosphate** which is present at low intracellular levels (nanomoles per gram wet weight of tissue). Fructose 2,6-bisphosphate is a major effector of both enzymes. In liver, fructose 2,6-bisphosphate activates 6-phosphofructokinase and inhibits fructose-bisphosphatase to amplify the glycolytic flux. The presence of fructose 2,6-bisphosphate in all mammalian cells suggests that its main role is to control 6-phosphofructokinase and thereby glycolysis. Fructose 2,6-bisphosphate is synthesized by **6-phosphofructo-2-kinase** from fructose 6-phosphate and ATP and degraded by **fructose-2,6-bisphosphatase** to fructose 6-phosphate and ortho-phosphate. Both reactions constitute a substrate cycle in which 6-phosphofructo-2-kinase is activated by orthophosphate but inhibited by citrate, phospho*eno*lpyruvate and *sn*-glycerol 3-phosphate while fructose 2,6-bis-phosphatase is stimulated by *sn*-glycerol-3-phosphate and nucleoside triphosphates and inhibited by fructose 6-phosphate. Both 6-phospho-fructo-2-kinase and fructose 2,6-bisphosphatase are subjected to further control by the phosphorylation/ dephosphorylation reactions of their interrelated enzyme interconversion cycles (Chapter 8).

regulatory factor governing glucose-6-phosphate dehydrogenase activity is the cytosolic ratio of $[NADP^+]/[NADPH]$. When the ratio lies markedly in favour of NADPH, the reduced coenzyme competes with $NADP^+$ for its binding site on the enzyme and inhibits the essentially irreversible reaction. Higher $NADP^+$ concentrations enhance the metabolism of glucose 6-phosphate through the pathway. In addition, ATP acts as a competitive inhibitor of the enzyme. The non-oxidative phase of the pathway is regulated through the availability of intermediates.

Suggested further reading

Agius, L., Peak, M. and van Schaftingen, E. (1995). The regulatory protein of glucokinase binds to the hepatocyte matrix, but, unlike glucokinase, does not translocate during substrate stimulation. *Biochemical Journal* **309**, 711–713.

Bernstein, B.E., Michels, P.A.M. and Hol, W.G.J. (1997) Synergistic effects of substrate-induced conformational changes in phosphoglycerate kinase activation. *Nature* **385**, 275–278.

Cadefau, J., Bollen, M. and Stalmans, W. (1997). Glucose-induced glycogenesis in the liver involves glucose-6-phosphate-dependent dephosphorylation of glycogen synthase. *Biochemical Journal* **322**, 745–750.

Pilkis, S.J., Claus, T.H., Kurland, I.J. and Lange, A.J. (1995) 6-Phosphofructo-2-kinase/fructose-2,6-bisphosphatase: A metabolic signaling enzyme. *Annual Review of Biochemistry* **64**, 799–836.

Srere, P. (1994). Complexities of metabolic regulation. *Trends in Biochemical Sciences* **19**, 519–520.

Wood, T. (1985). *The Pentose Phosphate Pathway*. New York: Academic Press.

Self-assessment questions

1. Assuming anaerobic conditions, calculate the number of ATP molecules produced during the catabolism of each monosaccharide residue released by the action of glycogen phosphorylase.

2. Which of the following enzyme systems, sucrose phosphorylase (sucrose + P_i ⇌ fructose + glucose-1-phosphate) or invertase (sucrose + H_2O ⇌ fructose + glucose), offers an energetic advantage in the preparation of sucrose for entry into glycolysis?

3. What is the effect of the intracellular production of AMP on carbohydrate metabolism?

4. In the phosphorolysis of muscle glycogen by glycogen phosphorylase, shortened glycogen and glucose 1-phosphate are produced. The equilibrium constant for the reaction is 3.45. Assuming that K'_{eq} is independent of the concentrations of both glycogen and shortened glycogen and that the intracellular phosphate concentration is 1 mM, calculate the maximum concentration of glucose 1-phosphate obtainable.

5. Show that the diversion of three glucose 6-phosphate molecules into the pentose phosphate pathway generates only eight molecules of ATP.

6. If glucose, labelled with radioactivity (^{14}C) at the anomeric carbon atom (C-1), is used as a substrate for the glycolytic pathway, which carbon atom of glyceraldehyde 3-phosphate would you expect to be labelled?

7. Identify in which human tissues the following pathways predominate: (a) gluconeogenesis; (b) pentose phosphate pathway; (c) glycogen synthesis.

8. You have available various samples of glucose radioactively labelled at only one carbon atom. You wish to assess the relative importance of the pentose phosphate pathway to glycolysis in the degradation of glucose in a cell under study *in vitro*. You are allowed to chose two samples. Which labelled carbon atoms do you select and why?

9. In what way does fructose-2,6-bisphosphatase influence gluconeogenesis?

10. What structural feature in one of its substrates does transketolase require?

Carbohydrate metabolism is also controlled from outside the cell by hormonal action. The pancreatic hormones **insulin** and **glucagon** promote an increase in intracellular glucose concentration by enhancing uptake and glycogenolysis respectively. **Adrenaline** (also called epinephrine), produced by the **adrenal medulla**, also promotes glycogenolysis. Glucagon, which is released when blood glucose levels fall, is active only in liver and adipose tissue whereas adrenaline acts on liver and muscle cells. They function through the regulation of the extended enzyme interconversion cycle governing the reciprocal control of glycogen synthase and glycogen phosphorylase (Chapter 8).

Insulin secretion is a response to elevated blood glucose levels. It acts rapidly to reduce high levels by stimulating glycogenesis and inhibiting glycogenolysis in liver and skeletal muscle cells. Insulin also increases glucose metabolism by the induction of hexokinase Type IV, phosphofructokinase and pyruvate kinase. Insulin also inhibits the enzymes responsible for the regulation of gluconeogenesis.

Cortisol is a corticosteroid hormone produced by the **adrenal cortex**. Cortisol promotes protein degradation (and decreased protein synthesis) in skeletal muscle. In the liver, it stimulates gluconeogenesis primarily from amino acids and glycogenesis.

Key Concepts and Facts

Glycolysis
- Glyceraldehyde-3-phosphate dehydrogenase switches glycolysis from an energy-utilizing to energy-releasing pathway.

- A net yield of 2 ATP per glucose as a glycolytic substrate is realized under anaerobic conditions.

- NAD^+ is regenerated from NADH by a variety of routes.

- Tissue-specific shuttle mechanisms are involved in the supply of cytosolic NADH to the respiratory chain.

Glycogen Metabolism
- Glycogen in liver and skeletal muscle is mainly used for different purposes.

- Glycogen synthesis proceeds by the addition of single glucose units to an existing molecule.

- Glycogen synthase cannot synthesize branches, a function which is performed by the glycogen branching enzyme.

- Glycogen degradation proceeds by phosphorolysis and debranching.

- Glycogen storage has important benefits to the cell and is energetically efficient.

Gluconeogenesis
- Gluconeogenesis operates to maintain blood glucose levels in the absence of carbohydrates.

- The major precursors are lactate, alanine and glycerol.

- Gluconeogenesis contains three bypass reactions to avoid reversal of exergonic glycolytic reactions.

Pentose Phosphate Pathway
- The products of major importance are NADPH and pentose sugars.

- The pathway is divided into an oxidative and a non-oxidative phase.

Regulation
- Different pathways function in different cells according to the product requirements of that cell.

- Metabolic pathways are regulated by a variety of methods, e.g allosteric activators and inhibitors, adenine nucleotide ratios, end-product inhibition and enzyme interconversion cycles.

Answers to questions (Chapter 9)

1. Three ATP. Glycogen phosphorylase produces glucose 1-phosphate which is rearranged to glucose 6-phosphate. Glucose 6-phosphate to lactate will produce three ATP; two from each of the reactions catalysed by phosphoglycerate kinase and pyruvate kinase but one ATP is utilized by phosphofructokinase action.

2. Sucrose phosphorylase. Glucose 1-phosphate can be readily converted by phosphoglucomutase into the glycolytic intermediate, glucose-6-phosphate. Glucose requires phosphorylation by hexokinase utilizing ATP.

3. AMP increases the activity of 6-phosphofructokinase and reduces the activity of fructose-bisphosphatase and therefore promotes glycolysis and inhibits gluconeogenesis. Do not confuse AMP with cyclic AMP (cAMP) involved in the hormonal regulation of glycogen metabolism.

4. $775\,\mu M$: If $[P_i]$ is reduced by y M at equilibrium, then $[G\ 1\text{-}P] = y$ M and the remaining $[P_i] = (10^{-3} - y)$ M then $K'_{eq} = [G\ 1\text{-}P]/[P_i]$ and $3.45 = y/(10^{-3} - y)$, $3.45\ (10^{-3} - y) = y$, $3.45 \times 10^{-3} = 4.45y$ and $y = 0.775 \times 10^{-3}$ M or $775\,\mu M$.

5. Refer to Figure 9.11. Three glucose-6-phosphate produces two fructose 6-phosphate and one glyceraldehyde-3-phosphate. Each fructose 6-phosphate utilizes one ATP in the phosphofructokinase reaction and produces four (2×2) ATP in the substrate-level phosphorylation reactions. Thus, the yield from fructose 6-phosphate is six and glyceraldehyde 3-phosphate produces two ATP, giving a total of eight ATP.

6. C-3. The label at C-1 will appear in the $CH_2OPO_3^{2-}$ of glycerone phosphate which after isomerization will become the C-3 of glyceraldehyde 3-phosphate. (Refer to Figure 9.2.)

7. (a) Liver, renal cortex; (b) liver, adipose tissue, mammary gland, adrenal cortex, testes, ovaries; (c) liver, skeletal muscle.

8. ^{14}C-1 and ^{14}C-6 of glucose. The sample with ^{14}C-1 will release $^{14}CO_2$ in the pentose phosphate pathway. C-6 of glucose is not released, allowing assessment of the relative rates of the two pathways.

9. Fructose 2,6-bisphosphate activates 6-phosphofructokinase but inhibits fructose-bisphosphatase. Fructose-2,6-bisphosphatase hydrolyses fructose 2,6-bisphosphate and thereby promotes gluconeogenesis.

10. Transketolase requires that the hydroxyl group at C-3 be in the xylulose configuration. (Refer to Figure 9.11.)

Chapter 10
The tricarboxylic acid cycle

Learning objectives

After studying this chapter you should confidently be able to:

Describe the catabolic and anabolic roles of the tricarboxylic acid (TCA) cycle.

Describe the translocation of pyruvate from the cytosol into the mitochondrial matrix.

Describe the mechanism of the reaction by which the major substrate of the TCA cycle is formed.

Discuss the important features of all the reactions comprising the TCA cycle.

Discuss the role of nucleotides and metabolic intermediates in the regulation of the TCA cycle.

Small quantities of ATP are yielded when carbohydrate substrates are degraded to pyruvate via glycolysis (Chapter 9). Under anaerobic conditions, pyruvate is frequently converted into another substance to effect the regeneration of NAD^+. Much of the energy contained within the initial monosaccharide structure is retained in the end product of the fermentation. Under **aerobic** conditions, however, a higher ATP yield can be achieved by the complete degradation of substrate to carbon dioxide and water. In eukaryotes, this degradation occurs within the mitochondrial matrix through the reactions of:

- **the tricarboxylic acid cycle** in which the carbon atoms of the acetyl group of acetyl-CoA derived from pyruvate are oxidized to CO_2;
- **oxidative phosphorylation** in which coenzymes reduced during cycle reactions are oxidized indirectly by molecular oxygen and are thus regenerated with a further yield of ATP and the formation of water (Chapter 11).

The overall process is called **respiration** to differentiate from fermentation which occurs in the absence of oxygen.

This chapter considers the metabolic roles, reactions and the energetics of the tricarboxylic acid cycle, the generation of its major

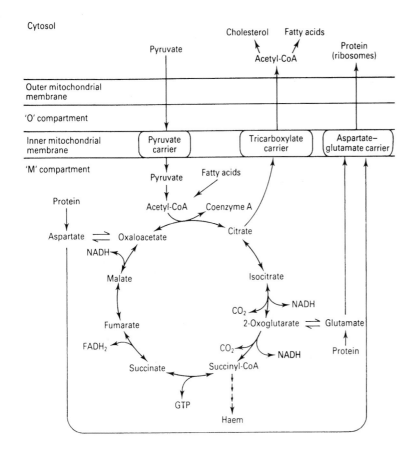

Figure 10.1 *Role of the tricorboxylic acid cycle in catabolism and anabolism*

substrate, the maintenance of metabolite levels and the subcellular locations of these metabolic events.

Roles of the tricarboxylic acid cycle in metabolism

Acetyl-CoA is not exclusively produced from pyruvate within the mitochondrion but is also the oxidation product of the catabolism of fatty acids (Chapter 12) and some amino acids (Chapter 13). Although the degradation of other amino acids yields tricarboxylic acid (TCA) cycle intermediates, the major substrate of the cycle is acetyl-CoA derived primarily from the breakdown of carbohydrate and fatty acids.

The TCA cycle is a central metabolic pathway involved in both catabolic and anabolic processes (Figure 10.1). The major catabolic function of the cycle involves the conversion of the carbon atoms of acetyl-CoA to CO_2 and the generation of reduced hydrogen carriers.

A number of **biosynthetic pathways** use TCA cycle intermediates:

When **yeast cultures** metabolizing glucose under anaerobic conditions were exposed to air, the rate of glucose utilization declined about seven-fold. This observation made by **Louis Pasteur**, and known as the **Pasteur effect**, is due to the indirect inhibition of glycolysis by oxygen. Much later experiments by others involving the technique of **freeze-clamping**, in which tissue is rapidly solidified between metal plates cooled to $-196°C$ by liquid nitrogen, have shown that the levels of glucose, glucose 6-phosphate and fructose 6-phosphate increase whilst those of fructose 1,6-bisphosphate and subsequent glycolytic intermediates decline. The Pasteur effect is mainly the result of the allosteric inhibition of 6-phosphofructokinase by the tricarboxylic acid cycle intermediate citrate and ATP generated by oxidative phosphorylation.

- Oxaloacetate and 2-oxoglutarate may be converted into **aspartate** and **glutamate** respectively by **transaminase reactions** (Chapter 13) and thereby be employed as sources of these amino acids for protein synthesis.

- **2-Oxoglutarate** may serve as an important source of **glutamate** through the action of **glutamate dehydrogenase** (Chapter 13). Since protein synthesis is a cytoplasmic event, these amino acids must be transported across the inner mitochondrial membrane by a specific carrier. (During protein degradation, the same reactions in reverse permit the entry of these amino acids into the TCA cycle.)

- **Citrate** may serve as a source of acetyl-CoA for the biosynthesis of fatty acids and cholesterol which occur in the cytosol (Chapter 12). Citrate may be translocated out of the mitochondrion whereas acetyl-CoA cannot leave the matrix.

- **Succinyl-CoA** may serve as a starting material in animals and micro-organisms for the synthesis of protoporphyrin IX which forms the basis of **haem**, the oxygen-binding component of haemoglobin and the electron-binding component of the cytochromes of the electron-transport system.

- **Oxaloacetate** and **malate** may serve as gluconeogenic precursors (Chapter 9).

Entry of pyruvate into the mitochondrion

Aerobic utilization of pyruvate in eukaryotes necessitates its entry into the mitochondrial matrix where the reactions of the tricarboxylic acid cycle are considered to occur. In actuality, some of the enzymes are bound or may bind to the inner membrane. The translocation is achieved by a **pyruvate carrier.** This carrier is either a pyruvate–hydroxyl ion antiport system which exchanges the pyruvate for a hydroxyl ion or a symport system by which pyruvate enters the 'M' compartment together with a proton. In both situations, the pH balance is maintained across the membrane.

The oxidative decarboxylation of pyruvate

Upon entry into the mitochondrial matrix, pyruvate may be converted into acetyl-CoA by the action of a multi-enzyme complex called the **pyruvate dehydrogenase complex.** The overall non-equilibrium reaction (Figure 10.2a) is exergonic to an extent which appears capable of supporting the substrate-level phosphorylation of ADP. However, ATP synthesis does not occur. The large negative $\Delta G^{o\prime}$ renders the reaction essentially irreversible under physiological conditions so that acetyl-CoA from fatty acid oxidation cannot be employed to produce carbohydrate via this route.

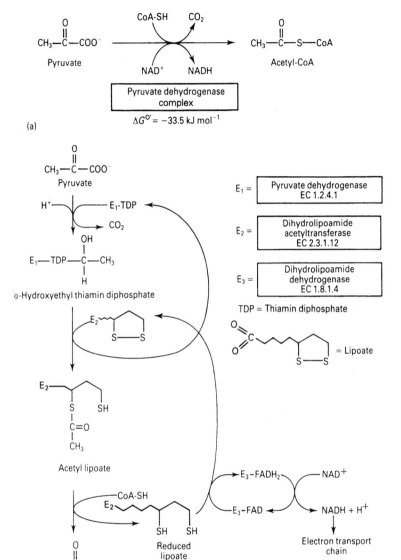

Figure 10.2 *Oxidative decarboxylation of pyruvate: (a) overall reaction; (b) mechanism of action of the pyruvate dehydrogenase complex*

The mammalian pyruvate dehydrogenase complex exists as a complex (approximate molecular weight 9 000 000) of three enzymes plus regulatory enzymes:

- **pyruvate dehydrogenase,** of which there are some 20–30 molecules;

- **dihydrolipoamide acetyltransferase,** of which there are 60 molecules;

Figure 10.3 *Structure of two coenzymes involved in the pyruvate dehydrogenase complex:(a) thiamin diphosphate (TDP); (b) lipoate*

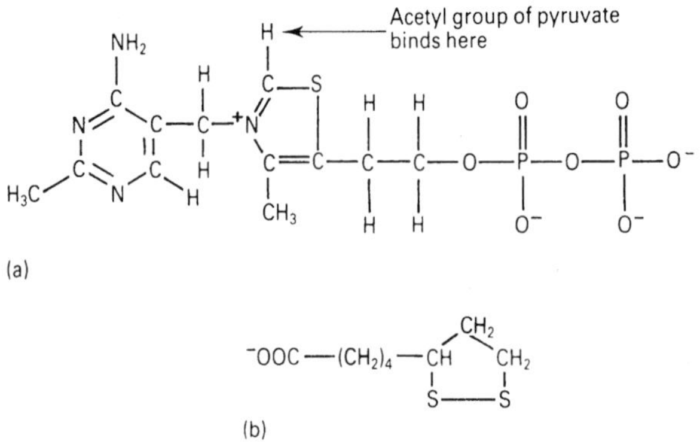

Thiamin (vitamin B_1) is a cofactor of numerous enzymic reactions. With regards to the tricarboxylic acid cycle, **thiamin diphosphate (TDP)** is the prosthetic group of pyruvate dehydrogenase and oxoglutarate dehydrogenase where it performs the transfer of a two-carbon unit. Thiamin is found in many foodstuffs so that the recommended daily requirement of 1 mg is normally achieved without difficulty.

Thiamin deficiency manifests itself as **beriberi** in the malnourished poor of Asia. Rice forms the staple diet and part of the problem lies in its preparation. Rice has a low content of thiamin which is located in the husk. Milling to produce polished rice severely reduces the amount of thiamin available for nutrition. Changes in the preparation of rice, e.g. undermilling or part cooking, and the consumption of thiamin-rich peas and beans may prevent the disease.

The initial symptoms of beriberi are heaviness and stiffness of the legs which progress to weakness and numbness, due to damage of the peripheral nervous system. Oedema may extend throughout the body with consequences for the cardiovascular system, i.e. increased blood pressure and eventual heart failure.

- **dihydrolipoamide dehydrogenase**, of which there are some 20–30 molecules;
- **Mg^{2+}-dependent pyruvate dehydrogenase kinase**, which phosphorylates three specific serine residues of pyruvate dehydrogenase;
- **Ca^{2+}-activated pyruvate dehydrogenase phosphatase**, which removes these phosphate groups.

(The numbers of molecules quoted for these enzymes may vary depending upon the actual source. The microbial complex contains fewer molecules of each enzyme.)

The mammalian and microbial systems employ five different coenzymes, some as prosthetic groups. They are thiamine diphosphate (TDP; Figure 10.3a), **lipoate** (Figure 10.3b), NAD^+ (Figure 4.5a), coenzyme A (Figure 4.5d) and FAD (Figure 4.5b).

Pyruvate (Figure 10.2b) is initially decarboxylated by the enzyme, pyruvate dehydrogenase, the prosthetic group of which is TDP. To the **thiazole ring** of TDP is bound a hydroxyethyl group which pyruvate dehydrogenase utilizes in the reduction and acetylation of a lipoate prosthetic group of dihydrolipoamide acetyltransferase. The pyruvate dehydrogenase may then repeat the process with another pyruvate molecule. Next, coenzyme A accepts the acetyl group to yield reduced lipoate and acetyl-CoA. The latter may enter the TCA cycle. The remaining two stages in the mechanism relate to the oxidation of the reduced lipoate involving the FAD prosthetic group of another enzyme, dihydrolipoamide dehydrogenase, which is regenerated to its oxidized state at the expense of free NAD^+. The reduced NAD may be utilized in oxidative phosphorylation.

The multi-enzyme complex retains the product of one reaction and transfers it to the active site of another enzyme by the movement of a flexible group, namely lipoate bound covalently to an ε-amino group of a lysyl residue of dihydrolipoamide acetyltransferase. This improves catalytic efficiency by increasing the chances of contact with the next active site and by providing immunity from other reactions. Regulation of the series of reactions is simplified since only one of the participating enzymes, pyruvate dehydrogenase, is subject to control.

The reactions of the tricarboxylic acid cycle

The TCA cycle is a series of reactions involving initially the anions of tricarboxylic acids and subsequently those of **dicarboxylic acids**. The operation of the cycle may be subdivided for convenience into:

- the condensation reaction;
- the intramolecular rearrangement reaction;
- the oxidative decarboxylation reactions;
- the substrate-level phosphorylation reaction;
- the dicarboxylic acid reactions.

In **the condensation reaction**, the acetyl groups of **acetyl-CoA** enter the TCA cycle (Figure 10.4) by condensation with **oxaloacetate** to form the tricarboxylate **citrate**. The reaction, catalysed by **citrate synthase**, occurs in two stages: the formation of **citryl-CoA** (Figure 10.5a), an enzyme-bound intermediate, followed by the hydrolysis of citryl-CoA to produce **citrate** and release **coenzyme A**. The cleavage of the thioester bond of citryl-CoA accounts for the high negative $\Delta G^{o\prime}$ value and the irreversibility of the reaction. Intracellular levels of acetyl-CoA and oxaloacetate, together with the concentrations of some cycle intermediates, modulate the activity of citrate synthase and are important influences on flux through the cycle.

In **the intramolecular rearrangement reaction, citrate**, because the position of its hydroxyl group prevents its direct oxidation, is converted into another tricarboxylate, **isocitrate**, by the enzyme **aconitate hydratase**. This enzyme contains an iron–sulphur centre (Chapter 11) which functions stereospecifically both in removal of the elements of water to produce an enzyme-bound intermediate called *cis*-**aconitate** and in the replacement of the proton and hydroxyl ion to form **isocitrate** (Figure 10.5b). The reaction proceeds because of coupling to citrate production.

The switch from the participation of tricarboxylate to dicarboxylate anions in the TCA cycle occurs by the next reaction, one of **the oxidative decarboxylation reactions**. The first of these two reactions is catalysed by allosteric **isocitrate dehydrogenase** and occurs in two stages. In the initial stage, isocitrate is oxidized to the corresponding keto acid (Figure 10.5c), the enzyme-bound intermediate **oxalosuccinate**. This involves the reduction of NAD^+ and the release of a proton. Oxalosuccinate is then decarboxylated to **2-oxoglutarate**, a reaction which employs the proton previously released.

During the first turn of the cycle, the C–C covalent bond of the introduced acetyl group remains intact and is retained within the structure of **oxaloacetate**, the final TCA product (Figure 10.4). During subsequent turns of the cycle, this bond is cleaved by

Thiamin deficiency in the west is found mainly among chronic alcoholics who may suffer from neurological disorders such as dementia. Prompt treatment with thiamin may reverse the dementia, but if left untreated, thiamin deficiency may result in permanent neurological damage.

A **diagnosis** of thiamin deficiency is confirmed by the assay of transketolase in erythrocytes. Transketolase is a TDP-dependent enzyme of the non-oxidative phase of the pentose phosphate pathway (Chapter 9). Its activity is measured in the presence and absence of added TDP; a TDP-induced increase of 30% in enzyme activity intimates thiamin deficiency.

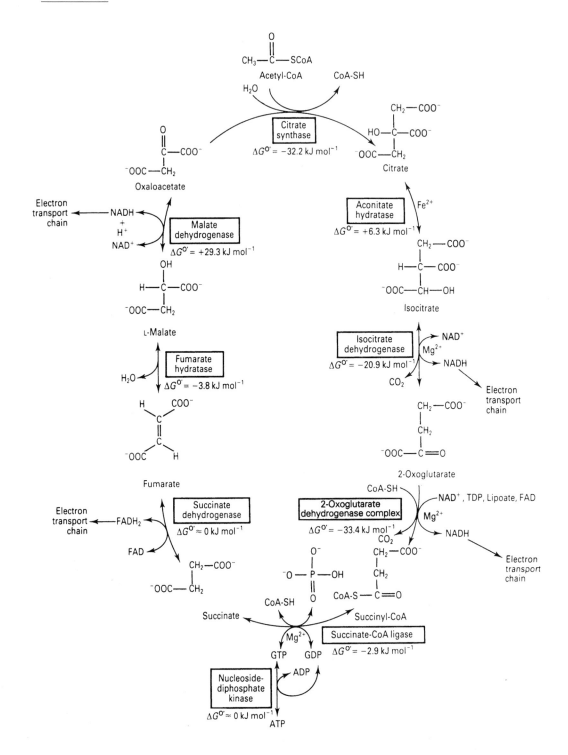

Figure 10.4 *The tricarboxylic acid cycle*

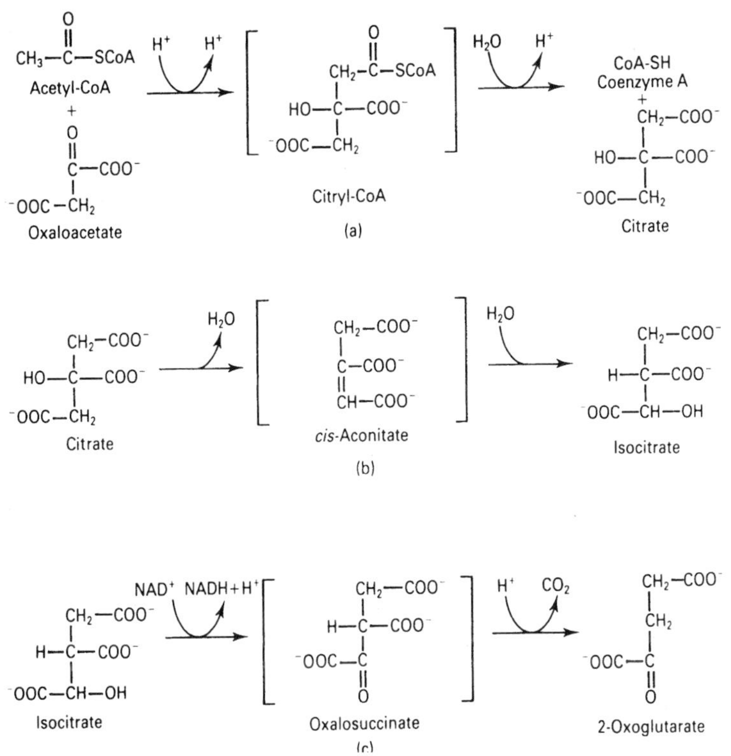

Figure 10.5 *Intermediates of TCA cycle reactions: (a) citrate synthase reaction; (b) aconitate hydratase reaction; (c) isocitrate dehydrogenase reaction*

isocitrate dehydrogenase with the loss of one carboxylate group as CO_2. There are **two different enzymes** called isocitrate dehydrogenase (NAD^+), EC 1.1.1.41 which is NAD-inked and EC 1.1.1.42 which is NADP-linked. Isocitrate dehydrogenase ($NADP^+$) is the only form present in most micro-organisms.

In the second oxidative decarboxylation, 2-oxoglutarate forms **succinyl-CoA** by the action of the **2-oxoglutarate dehydrogenase complex**. The reaction proceeds by a mechanism identical to that employed by the pyruvate dehydrogenase complex. The 2-oxoglutarate dehydrogenase complex is also a complex of three enzymes and has identical cofactor requirements. The reaction mechanism is as shown in Figure 10.2 when E_1 = oxoglutarate dehydrogenase (EC 1.2.4.2), E_2 = dihydrolipoamide succinyltransferase (EC 2.3.1.61), E_3 = dihydrolipoamide dehydrogenase (EC 1.8.1.4) and formulae are modified as appropriate.

In **the substrate-level phosphorylation reaction**, hydrolysis of the thioester bond of succinyl-CoA to form **succinate** releases a quantity of free energy in excess of that required for ATP synthesis. The cleavage of the bond is therefore coupled to an energy-conservation reaction. The excess amount of free energy is so small that the reaction is reversible. The name of the enzyme, **succinate-CoA ligase**, reflects the involvement of a nucleotide in the reaction (Chapter 4). In mammalian systems, GDP is phosphorylated and

The tricarboxylic acid cycle is inhibited by **fluoroacetate**, a well-known rodent poison. Fluoroacetate is naturally synthesized in some pasture plants and may be responsible for some cases of cattle and sheep poisoning. Fluoroacetate is an example of a suicide substrate (Chapter 4). Fluoroacetate is converted by **acetate-CoA ligase** to **fluoroacetyl-CoA** which is an alternative substrate for citrate synthase. The resultant product, **fluorocitrate**, inhibits aconitate hydratase.

The **operation of the pathway as a cycle** was deduced by **Hans Krebs** in 1937 from observations on the rate of oxygen consumption by suspensions of minced pigeon breast muscle. This muscle, active in flight, exhibits very high rates of oxidative metabolism and therefore was an appropriate choice for such metabolic investigations. Oxygen consumption was monitored with a **manometer**, an instrument which permits the measurement of changes in the volume of a closed system at constant pressure and temperature.

Earlier studies, mainly by **Szent-Gyorgyi** (1935), had shown that succinate, fumarate, malate and oxaloacetate stimulate the oxygen consumption by this muscle. Krebs showed that pyruvate similarly increased oxygen O_2 consumption. In addition, he observed that the oxidation of pyruvate could be markedly stimulated by oxaloacetate, *cis*-aconitate, isocitrate and 2-oxoglutarate. The effects of these substances could be abolished by the addition of **malonate**, a competitive inhibitor of succinate dehydrogenase. The addition of malonate also resulted in the accumulation of citrate, 2-oxoglutarate and succinate. The concentrations of these key intermediates were determined by the chemical methods then available. Because the addition of pyruvate and oxaloacetate to the suspension resulted in the accumulation of citrate, Krebs concluded that the pathway operated as a cycle.

the GTP formed may be readily converted into ATP by the action of nucleoside-diphosphate kinase. This reaction is not an integral part of the cycle. In some bacterial systems (and in higher plants), ADP is directly phosphorylated by a different succinate–CoA ligase.

The remainder of the cycle, termed **the dicarboxylic acid reactions,** is concerned with the regeneration of oxaloacetate (with which acetyl groups condense in the initial reaction) from **succinate** (Figure 10.4). Three reactions, **an oxidation, a hydration** and **another oxidation**, are required to convert a methylene group of succinate into a carbonyl group, a fundamental biochemical principle which is also seen during the pathway for the β-oxidation of fatty acids (Chapter 12).

Succinate is oxidized during a reaction catalysed by **succinate dehydrogenase**. Succinate dehydrogenase differs from other TCA cycle enzymes in that it is an integral component of the inner mitochondrial membrane (**Complex II**, Chapter 11) and contains both an FAD prosthetic group and iron–sulphur centres. It is imperative that FAD is the hydrogen acceptor in this reaction since the free-energy change is too small to accomplish the reduction of NAD^+. **Succinate dehydrogenase provides a direct link between the cycle and the electron-transport system. The enzyme is stereospecific and removes the hydrogen atoms from succinate to produce only the *trans* isomer, fumarate.**

Fumarate is hydrated by another stereospecific enzyme, **fumarate hydratase**, to form L-**malate** which is oxidized to **oxaloacetate** by an NAD^+-linked **malate dehydrogenase** (EC 1.1.1.37). Although the $\Delta G^{o\prime}$ value implies that the reverse reaction is thermodynamically more favourable, oxaloacetate formation is promoted by its role in the highly exergonic initial reaction of the cycle.

The energetics of the cycle

Degradation of glucose to pyruvate is accompanied by a standard free-energy change of $-171.5\,\text{kJ}\,\text{mol}^{-1}$ of which $61\,\text{kJ}\,\text{mol}^{-1}$ is conserved as ATP. Under standard conditions, complete oxidation of glucose to CO_2 and H_2O through aerobic glycolysis, the TCA cycle and oxidative phosphorylation releases $2870\,\text{kJ}\,\text{mol}^{-1}$. Approximately 94% of the energy contained within the chemical bonds of glucose is retained within the pyruvate molecule as it gains access to the mitochondrion for oxidation. The potential for energy conservation is indeed high! However, within the TCA cycle, only one substrate-level phosphorylation (succinate–CoA ligase) occurs.

A large amount of the energy resides within the reduced coenzymes generated during the oxidation reactions involving isocitrate dehydrogenase, the 2-oxoglutarate dehydrogenase complex, succinate dehydrogenase and malate dehydrogenase. Electrons are transferred to the electron-transport assemblies of the inner mitochondrial membrane and a proportion of the energy released during their transfer across the redox carriers is conserved during oxidative phosphorylation (Chapter 11).

Anaplerosis

The tricarboxylic acid cycle is concerned not only with catabolism but may also provide precursors for biosynthetic processes. These functions infer that certain intermediates are withdrawn from the pool of cycle intermediates. To maintain the operation of the cycle, lost intermediates must be replaced. In addition, fluctuations in intracellular conditions may demand enhanced TCA cycle activity which requires the augmentation of the concentrations of intermediates. The process of 'filling up' the pool of cycle intermediates is called, from appropriate Greek roots, **anaplerosis**. Since the entry of acetyl groups into the cycle requires oxaloacetate, the major anaplerotic pathways (Figure 10.6) will ultimately yield oxaloacetate:

- **In mammalian tissues,** excluding muscle, the most important anaplerotic reaction employs **pyruvate carboxylase** which contains a **biotin prosthetic group** (Figure 4.5c) responsible for the transfer of a carboxyl group. ATP provides the energy to bond covalently the carboxyl group from HCO_3^- to the biotin which subsequently transfers it when pyruvate binds to the enzyme.

- **In muscle cells,** the major pathway utilizes phospho*enol*pyruvate and **phospho*enol*pyruvate carboxykinase** which occurs both in the cytosol and mitochondrial matrix. Two routes are therefore possible in oxaloacetate synthesis, either as shown in Figure 10.6 or the phospho*enol*pyruvate may traverse the inner membrane and form oxaloacetate by the action of the mitochondrial enzyme.

- **Through the concerted action of two malate dehydrogenase enzymes,** EC 1.1.1.40 (also called the 'malic' enzyme) and EC 1.1.1.37, oxaloacetate may be produced indirectly from pyruvate.

The degradation of some **glucogenic amino acids** (Chapter 13) may also contribute to anaplerosis.

Oxaloacetate may also be generated by transaminase reactions involving the amino acid aspartate. However, this amino transfer reaction is not anaplerotic since it does not accomplish net synthesis of a TCA cycle intermediate as aspartate transaminase employs 2-oxoglutarate as a cosubstrate (Chapter 13).

Anaplerotic reactions may also be employed in anabolic functions. Through the reversal of these reactions, TCA cycle intermediates may serve as precursors of glucose (Chapter 9). This function is demonstrated in certain species of micro-organisms (and plants) which utilize the **glyoxylate cycle** in the synthesis of carbohydrate from acetyl-CoA.

In species of **aerobic and facultative bacteria** which can elaborate carbohydrates from **two-carbon substrates** such as acetate or ethanol, there is an additional pathway called the **glyoxylate cycle.** This cycle, not found in mammals and man, is in essence a bypass of some TCA cycle reactions. Some of the isocitrate produced by the first two reactions of the TCA cycle continues through the TCA cycle whilst the remainder is diverted into the bypass sequence of two reactions. Isocitrate is cleaved by **isocitrate lyase** into glyoxylate and succinate. Glyoxylate condenses with acetyl-CoA under the influence of **malate synthase** (in a reaction analogous to that catalysed by citrate synthase) to synthesize L-malate. The succinate is employed in TCA cycle reactions to produce L-malate which proceeds through the microbial gluconeogenic pathway to produce carbohydrate.

In plants, the glyoxylate cycle is located in an additional cytoplasmic organelle called the **glyoxysome.** The glyoxylate cycle also functions in some algae, fungi and protozoa.

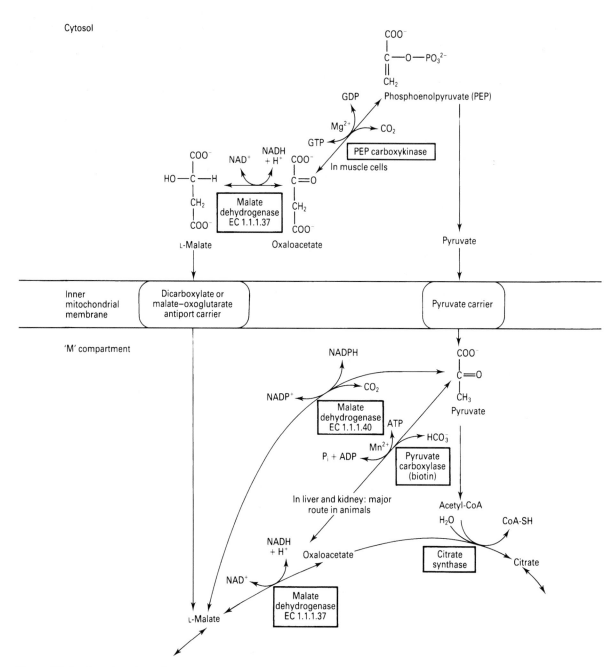

Figure 10.6 *Anaplerotic pathways*

The regulation of the TCA cycle

The activity of the **pyruvate dehydrogenase complex** controls the availability of acetyl-CoA. The pyruvate dehydrogenase of the complex is regulated through an enzyme interconversion cycle (Chapter 8) involving pyruvate dehydrogenase kinase and pyruvate dehydrogenase phosphatase which are associated with the enzyme complex. When the adenylate energy charge (Chapter 8) is high, kinase-mediated phosphorylation of pyruvate dehydrogenase diminishes acetyl-CoA production and consequently ATP production. When the adenylate energy charge is low and pyruvate is available, pyruvate dehydrogenase phosphate is dephosphorylated by the specific phosphatase to render the pyruvate dehydrogenase active. High levels of acetyl-CoA or NADH inhibit the reaction by activating the kinase but when they are present at low concentrations, the phosphatase maintains pyruvate dehydrogenase in an activated state. Since acetyl-CoA requires oxaloacetate for the condensation reaction, acetyl-CoA promotes anaplerosis by acting as a positive effector of pyruvate carboxylase.

The major factor in the regulation of the cycle flux is the [NAD$^+$]/[NADH] ratio: the ATP and ADP levels are apparently less important because mitochondrial ratios exhibit little fluctuation due to the export of ATP. High NADH concentrations allosterically inhibit three TCA cycle enzymes: citrate synthase, isocitrate dehydrogenase and the 2-oxoglutarate dehydrogenase complex. Isocitrate dehydrogenase may, in addition, be significantly regulated by the adenylate energy charge, ATP being inhibitory.

Cycle intermediates may also effect control on the activity of cycle enzymes. Succinyl-CoA demonstrates product inhibition on the 2-oxoglutarate dehydrogenase complex and inhibits citrate synthase. Oxaloacetate inhibits succinate dehydrogenase. **Intramitochondrial Ca^{2+} levels** are also considered to be important in the regulation of TCA cycle. Pyruvate dehydrogenase is activated by increasing Ca^{2+} concentrations through the effect of the cation on the regulatory phosphatase. Isocitrate dehydrogenase (NAD$^+$) and oxoglutarate dehydrogenase are stimulated more directly by Ca^{2+} ions.

Tricarboxylic acid cycle intermediates may influence the flux of other pathways, e.g. the glycolytic enzymes 6-phosphofructokinase and pyruvate kinase are inhibited by citrate and succinyl-CoA respectively.

> In **bacteria and plants**, another **anaplerotic pathway** occurs. This route employs an enzyme not found in animal tissues, **phospho*enol*pyruvate carboxylase**. This enzyme may convert phospho*enol*pyruvate into oxaloacetate without the requirement of a nucleoside triphosphate or biotin. This enzyme also has an important role in photosynthesis.

Suggested further reading

Bentley, R. (1994). A history of the reaction between oxaloacetate and acetate for citrate biosynthesis: An unsung contribution to the tricarboxylic acid cycle. *Perspectives in Biology and Medicine* **37**, 362–383.

Gruer, M.J., Artymuik, P.J. and Guest, J.R. (1997). The aconitase family: three structural variations as a common theme. *Trends in Biochemical Sciences* **22**, 3–6.

Mattevi, A., Obmolova, G., Schulze, E., Kalk, K.H., Westphal, A.H., de Kok, A. and Hol, W.G.J. (1992). Atomic structure of the cubic core of the pyruvate dehydrogenase multienzyme complex. *Science* **255**, 1544–1550.

Sahlin, K., Jorfeldt, L., Hendriksson, K.G., Lewis, S.F. and Haller, R.G. (1995). Tricarboxylic acid cycle intermediates during incremental exercise in healthy subjects and in patients with McArdle's disease. *Clinical Science* **88**, 687–693.

Holmes, F.L. (1993). *Hans Krebs: Architect of Intermediary Metabolism*, Vol. II. Oxford: Oxford University Press.

Kay, J. and Weitzman, P.D. J. (eds) (1987). *Krebs' Citric Acid Cycle – Half a Century and Still Turning*. Colchester: Biochemical Society.

Self-assessment questions

1. Dihydrolipoamide dehydrogenase features in two reactions involved in the aerobic degradation of pyruvate. Which are they?
2. Which enzyme catalyses the only substrate-level phosphorylation in the TCA cycle?
3. Compare the anaplerotic routes in muscle cells with the first bypass reaction of gluconeogenesis.
4. What advantage is conferred by employing the pyruvate–hydroxyl antiport system for the translocation of pyruvate?
5. In the TCA cycle, two oxidative decarboxylation reactions occur by different mechanisms. Identify the enzymes responsible for these reactions and show the stages of each mechanism.
6. The activity of which two enzymes of the TCA cycle produces CO_2?
7. What two variations of the TCA cycle may occur in microorganisms?
8. Which TCA cycle enzyme is inhibited by malonate?
9. Which oxidation reaction of the TCA cycle does not generate NADH?
10. Write out the reactions of the glyoxylate cycle as it occurs in *E. coli*.

Key Concepts and Facts

- The TCA cycle has catabolic and anabolic functions.

- The TCA cycle is located in the mitochondrial matrix.

- Pyruvate must be translocated from the cytosol into the matrix.

- The major substrate of the cycle is acetyl-CoA.

- Pyruvate and 2-oxoglutarate are oxidatively decarboxylated by different enzyme complexes employing the same mechanism of reaction.

- Only the equivalent of one molecule of ATP is produced per turn of the TCA cycle.

- The major source of energy from the TCA cycle is electrons harvested by the reduction of coenzymes, principally NAD^+ but also FAD.

- The continued operation of the cycle depends upon the maintenance of oxaloacetate levels.

- The operation of the TCA cycle is regulated by the levels of nucleotides, Ca^{2+} ions and substrates in the matrix.

Answers to questions (Chapter 10)

1. The pyruvate dehydrogenase complex and 2-oxoglutarate dehydrogenase complex.
2. Succinate-CoA ligase.
3. When phospho*enol*pyruvate is converted to oxaloacetate by the cytosolic PEP carboxykinase, the route by which it gains entry to the TCA cycle is a reversal of the reactions which occur in the first bypass of gluconeogenesis.
4. The maintenance of the matrix pH by balancing the charges of inward- and outward-moving substances.
5. Isocitrate dehydrogenase and the 2-oxoglutarate dehydrogenase complex. The mechanism of action for isocitrate dehydrogenase is given in Figure 10.5c. The mechanism of the 2-oxoglutarate dehydrogenase complex is as for Figure 10.2b with the following modifications: 2-oxoglutarate (structure given in Figure 10.4) is the substrate for E_1 = oxoglutarate dehydrogenase and forms α-hydroxysuccinyl thiamin diphosphate*. E_2 = dihydrolipoamide succinyltransferase then produces succinyl lipoate [replace acetyl group $(-C=O)-CH_3$ in Figure 10.2b with $-(C=O)-CH_2-CH_2-COO^-$]. Succinyl-CoA (Figure 10.4) is produced in the second stage of E_2 activity.

$$\overset{*}{E}-TDP-\underset{\underset{H}{|}}{\overset{\overset{OH}{|}}{C}}-CH_2-CH_2-COO^-$$

6. Isocitrate dehydrogenase and the 2-oxoglutarate dehydrogenase complex.
7. The glyoxylate cycle for acetate-utilizing cells and direct ADP phosphorylation.
8. Succinate dehydrogenase.
9. Succinate dehydrogenase utilizes FAD.
10. Follow the TCA cycle (Figure 10.4) as far as isocitrate.

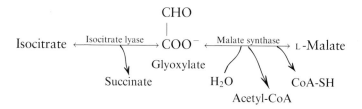

All structures not given above are available in Figure 10.4.

Chapter 11
Oxidative phosphorylation

Learning objectives

After studying this chapter you should confidently be able to:

Interrelate the two coupled components of oxidative phosphorylation, namely electron transport and ATP synthesis.

Discuss the principles of oxidation–reduction (redox) reactions.

Describe the sequence of the carriers of the respiratory chain.

Calculate the free energy released during electron transport.

Discuss the principle of, and evidence for, the chemiosmotic hypothesis.

Discuss the action of various inhibitors of oxidative phosphorylation.

Describe a model for the catalytic cooperativity by the active sites of ATP synthase.

Calculate the energy yield from the complete oxidation of fuel molecules in terms of numbers of ATP molecules.

In the **complete oxidation** of fuel molecules relatively little ATP is produced directly by substrate-level phosphorylation (Chapter 10). Irrespective of whether carbohydrates, fatty acids or amino acids serve as the metabolic fuel, most of the ATP is generated indirectly from the energy of electrons released during the reoxidation of the reduced coenzymes NADH and $FADH_2$.

During dehydrogenase-catalysed reactions, electrons are removed from substrates and transferred to **coenzymic acceptors** which, in turn, deliver the electrons to an organization of numerous proteins, called **an electron-transport assembly**. These assemblies are located, in eukaryotic cells, in the inner membrane of mitochondria (Chapter 7) or, in the case of bacteria, in the plasma membrane. Electrons are passed along an assembly by **coupled oxidation–reduction (redox) reactions** to the final acceptor, **molecular oxygen**, which is reduced in the presence of protons to water. During their transfer from component to component, a portion of the energy of the electrons is released and may be conserved by

Electron micrographs show that mitochondria in the resting state have a high matrix to intermembrane space ratio. However, when the cell demands ATP production by the mitochondria, they undergo morphological change. In active mitochondria, increased inner membrane folding markedly decreases the matrix volume with concomitant expansion of the 'O' compartment.

utilization in the phosphorylation of ADP. The reoxidation of the coenzymes by energy-yielding redox reactions is thus coupled to ATP synthesis and the overall process is called **oxidative phosphorylation.**

This chapter considers the process of oxidative phosphorylation as it occurs in eukaryotic cells. The nature of the electron transport assemblies of the inner mitochondrial membrane, the redox potentials of components, the coupling of electron-transport to ATP synthesis, the influence of various reagents which act at different sites and the energy yield during the complete oxidation of glucose are also discussed.

The role of oxidative phosphorylation

ATP must be resynthesized following its utilization in energy-dependent activities. The daily energy requirements of a 70 kg man in a sedentary occupation are considered to be approximately 10 000 kJ. The standard free energy of hydrolysis, $\Delta G^{O\prime}$, of MgATP^{2-} is estimated as -30.5 kJ mol^{-1}. This individual will therefore hydrolyse the equivalent of about 328 mol or 165 kg of ATP per day whilst his body contains only approximately 50 g of ATP. This calculation suggests that each molecule of ATP is synthesized and dephosphorylated over 3000 times each day to provide energy for this individual's activities. Oxidative phosphorylation takes place in the inner mitochondrial membrane which contains two coupled systems:

- an electron-transport chain;
- a system for ADP phosphorylation.

Electron transport

The **electron-transport chain** is a series of coupled oxidation–reduction (redox) reactions which transfer electrons to molecular oxygen.

Oxidation–reduction reactions

In redox reactions, carrier 1 in its oxidized state may accept electrons which reduce it. In the reduced state, it may donate the electrons to the oxidized form of carrier 2. In the process of the transfer, carrier 1 becomes reoxidized as carrier 2 becomes reduced. Similarly, reduced carrier 2 may donate electrons to carrier 3 and so on. In each reaction, the electron donor can only release the electrons if there is a suitable acceptor. The **electron donor** is termed the **reductant** since it reduces the acceptor and the **electron**

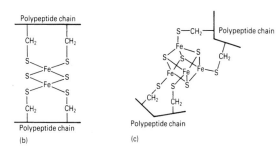

acceptor is termed the **oxidant** since it oxidizes the donor. In the electron-transport system, each electron carrier oscillates between oxidized and reduced forms which constitute **a redox couple**.

Electrons may be transferred in various ways:

- **Single-electron transfer.** Single electrons may directly reduce transition metals such as Fe^{3+} (ferric ion) to Fe^{2+} (ferrous ion) or Cu^{2+} (cupric ion) to Cu^+ (cuprous ion). Also, since hydrogen atoms contain a single electron, the transfer of a hydrogen atom effects electron transfer.

- **Two-electron transfer.** Hydride ions are composed of a hydrogen atom plus an additional electron, therefore their transfer translocates two electrons. The reduction of NAD^+ (Figure 4.5a) involves a hydride ion.

Electron donors and acceptors differ in the efficiency with which they donate or accept electrons. Their ability to transfer electrons is expressed as the **standard oxidation–reduction potential** (or **standard redox potential**), denoted by E_0, which is a constant for the redox couple dependent upon temperature, pH and the concentration of the oxidized and reduced species. The measurement of the standard redox potential of redox couples has been by three methods: a spectrophotometric method, a potentiometric method and electron spin resonance.

By convention, **standard redox potentials** refer to reactions recorded as: oxidant + electron(s) → reductant. Electrons flow from couples of higher potential to those of lower potential in an attempt to equalize the two potentials, a phenomenon termed the **electromotive force** (e.m.f.) which is measured in volts (or millivolts). Table 11.1 presents estimated standard redox potentials of some carriers. These data are not absolute values since measurements of free carriers differ from bound carriers, the values of some carriers measured in complexes differ from measurements in intact mitochondria and different solvents have been employed to solubilize different carriers. Thus, the recorded data should strictly be employed as a guide.

The **actual redox potential** (E') of any couple may be estimated from the standard redox potential and the concentrations of the oxidized and reduced species. This relationship is given by:

The **potentiometric method** for the measurement of standard oxidation–reduction potentials, E_0, utilizes **an electrochemical cell**. Such cells consist of **two half-cells**, each containing both components of a redox couple, e.g. NAD^+ and NADH, at a concentration of 1 M. Each half-cell contains an **electrode**. A test half-cell is connected to a reference half-cell by a salt-containing agar gel which serves as a **conductive bridge**. The electrodes are connected by a **voltmeter** (potentiometer) to permit the measurement of the **electromotive force** (voltage) between them.

The **reference half-cell** normally contains 1 M of a strong acid (e.g. HCl) in equilibrium with hydrogen gas (H_2) at a pressure of 1 atmosphere. The H^+/H_2 reference half-cell is assigned the value of $E_0 = 0$ V. The E_0 of all the other redox couples are compared with this reference half-cell value on the basis of the direction and magnitude of the reading on the voltmeter. Depending on whether H_2 or the test electron donor has the greater tendency to release electrons, the electrons may flow either from or to the reference half-cell. H_2 has a greater tendency to lose electrons than NADH, therefore electron flow will be towards the test half-cell.

Table 11.1 *Estimated standard redox potentials of selected respiratory chain carriers*

Carrier	E_0' (mV)	No. of electrons transferred
Reference: $2H^+ + 2e^- \rightarrow H_2$	−420	2
NAD^+	−320	2
FMN	−220	2
FAD	−220	2
Ubiquinone	+60	2*
Cytochrome b_{566}	−30	1
Cytochrome b_{562}	+70	1
Cytochrome c_1	+230	1
Cytochrome c	+240	1
Cytochrome a	+290	1
Cytochrome a_3	+385	1
$\frac{1}{2}O_2 + 2H^+ + 2e^-$	+820	2

* The complete reduction of ubiquinone to ubiquinol requires two electrons. However, this reduction occurs in two stages, each of which involves the transference of a single electron

$$E' = E_0' + \frac{RT}{nF} \ln \frac{[\text{oxidized species}]}{[\text{reduced species}]}$$

where E'= actual redox potential at pH 7.0, E_0'= *standard redox potential*, R = the gas constant = 8.3 J $K^{-1}mol^{-1}$, T = temperature in K, n = number of electrons transferred, F = the Faraday constant = 96 500 J V^{-1} and ln = natural logarithm. At 25°C, the equation reduces to:

$$E' = E_0' + \frac{59}{n} \log \frac{[\text{oxidized species}]}{[\text{reduced species}]}$$

when E' and E_0' are expressed in mV.

Isolation of the protein complexes

Electron transport involves protein complexes located in the inner mitochondrial membrane. By treatment of the inner membrane with **detergents**, the hydrophobic protein–protein and protein–lipid interactions may be disrupted and the assembly proteins released from the membrane. The most useful agent proved to be **deoxycholate** which decreases the hydrophobic interactions responsible for the integrity of the membrane. The carboxylate groups of the bile acid (Chapter 6) bestow negative charges on the proteins which create charge repulsions causing the membrane proteins to be released and solubilized in the aqueous environment. The proce-

Table 11.2 *The composition of the protein complexes of the electron-transport assemblies of bovine heart mitochondria*

Complex	Enzyme function	Electron-transfer components	No. of different polypeptide chains
I	NADH dehydrogenase (ubiquinone)	FMN, 8FeS*	>26
II	Succinate dehydrogenase (uniquinone)	FAD, cytochrome b_{560} 3 FeS, 1 Qp†	4
III	Ubiquinol-cytochrome-c reductase	Cytochrome b_{562} Cytochrome b_{566} Cytochrome c_1 1 FeS$_R$‡	10
IV	Cytochrome-c oxidase	Cytochrome a	13
V	H$^+$-transporting ATP synthase	—	>18

* FeS = iron–sulphur centre.
† Qp = a specific ubiquinone apoprotein which is required for the binding of ubiquinone.
‡ FeS$_R$ = Rieske iron–sulphur binuclear centre, named after its discoverer.

dural conditions are selected to isolate the proteins without affecting the internal structure of the protein complexes:

- **low concentrations of deoxycholate** can solubilize four protein complexes (Complexes I–IV) which may then be separated by additional techniques;
- **at a higher deoxycholate concentration** (in conjunction with salt fractionation), a fifth complex (Complex V) is released.

Each complex exhibits a **specific enzyme activity** (Table 11.2). In addition to four of these complexes, the mitochondrial electron-transport assembly contains **ubiquinone** [also called coenzyme Q or Q_{10} since it has 10 isoprenoid units (Figure 6.7b)] and **cytochrome c**. Complex V contains the active site for ADP phosphorylation; the others transport electrons and constitute the **respiratory chain**. FMN and FAD (Figure 4.5b) are prosthetic groups of NADH dehydrogenase and succinate dehydrogenase respectively. Complexes I–IV contain iron atoms. In proteins, iron may complex with sulphur atoms to form iron–sulphur centres or be present as haem (Chapter 3).

Iron-sulphur centres

Three types of iron–sulphur centres (FeS, Figure 11.1) are found in Complexes I–IV:

- **a mononuclear centre** may be formed by a single iron atom coordinating with the sulphur atoms of four cysteinyl residues of an FeS protein;
- **a binuclear centre**, denoted by 2Fe–2S, contains two iron atoms coordinated with two inorganic and four cysteinyl sulphur atoms of an FeS protein;

The pH of 1 M strong acid is pH 0. However, **standard conditions for biological systems** must relate to pH 7 and so the biological reference half-cell contains 10^{-7} M acid. The hydrogen electrode (H$^+$/H$_2$) at pH 7 gives a E_0' of -420 mV in comparison with an E_0 of 0 V for the true reference half-cell. The prime ($'$) denotes measurement at pH 7.

- **a tetranuclear centre** contains four iron atoms, four inorganic and four cysteinyl sulphur atoms.

The iron atom may exist in the ferrous or ferric state. Irrespective of the numbers of iron atoms present in an FeS centre, each centre accepts or donates only one electron at a time. Complex I contains five binuclear and three tetranuclear centres, Complex II contains two binuclear and one tetranuclear centre and Complex III has one binuclear centre.

Cytochromes

Cytochromes are proteins found in Complexes II, III and IV which effect electron transport via the prosthetic group **haem**. The structure of the haem of cytochromes b, c and c_1 is identical to that of myoglobin and haemoglobin (Figure 3.10a) but different from cytochrome a in which the substituents at positions 2 and 8 are an isoprenoid chain and a formyl group respectively. The various forms of cytochrome b are denoted by the wavelength of their spectrophotometric absorption maxima when in the reduced state. **Complex IV**, however, contains two identical haems, called a and a_3, to signify differences in their bonding to the protein. In Complex IV, there are also two copper atoms, designated Cu_A or Cu_B. Cu_A is located in subunit II whilst subunit I houses $haem_a$, Cu_B and $haem_{a_3}$. The mammalian complex has 13 subunits but the bacterial enzyme is simpler with four subunits. Cu_B and $haem_{a_3}$ are closely associated physically to function as a binuclear haem iron–copper centre at which the reduction of oxygen occurs.

The sequence of electron transport carriers

Electron transport operates by sequential redox reactions involving FMN, FAD, ubiquinone, FeS centres, haems and protein-bound copper atoms. The sequence of the carriers has been deduced from:

- **The redox potentials of the carriers.** Since electrons normally flow from more electronegative to more electropositive values, the standard redox potentials of the carriers should become progressively more positive towards the final acceptor, oxygen.
- **The use of specific inhibitors** of electron transport, e.g. rotenone, antimycin A and cyanide.
- **The use of artificial electron acceptors**, e.g. the dye 2,6-dichloro-phenol-indophenol (DCPIP; $E_0' = +220\,mV$) which can spontaneously oxidize cytochrome b_{562} ($E_0' = +70\,mV$) but not cytochrome c_1 ($E_0' = +230\,mV$).
- **The use of artificial electron donors**, e.g. ascorbate in the presence of tetramethyl-p-phenylene diamine (TMPD) delivers electrons non-enzymatically to the respiratory chain at cytochrome c.
- **Enzyme specificities.** Each complex enzyme may only catalyse the

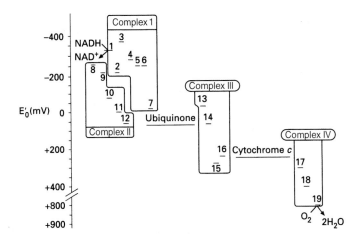

Figure 11.2 *Standard redox potentials of complex components; 1 NAD$^+$, 2 FMN, 3 FeS$_{N-1}$, 4 FeS$_{N-5}$, 5 FeS$_{N-4}$, 6 FeS$_{N-3}$, 7 FeS$_{N-2}$, 8 FeS$_{S-2}$, 9 FAD, 10 Cytochrome b$_{560}$, 11 FeS$_{S-1}$, 12 FeS$_{S-3}$, 13 Cytochrome b$_{566}$, 14 Cytochrome b$_{562}$, 15 FeS$_{R\,(Rieske)}$, 16 Cytochrome c$_1$, 17 Cytochrome a, 18 Cytochrome a$_3$, 19 O$_2$*

transfer of electrons between specific carriers so that electron transport is an ordered event.

Figure 11.2 shows the established order of the complexes and the experimental E'_0 values for their prosthetic groups. The pathways followed by electrons within the protein complexes remain the subject of intensive research. In **Complex I, NADH dehydrogenase** is orientated in the membrane so that its binding site for NADH is readily accessible from the matrix. NADH, derived from numerous dehydrogenase-catalysed reactions, reduces the FeS centres within 10 ms. It is considered that electrons pass from NADH to FMN before they are transferred across the various FeS centres. It is believed that reduced FeS$_{N-2}$ effects the reduction of **ubiquinone**. The reduction of ubiquinone is accompanied by the translocation of four protons, a process which appears to involve the FeS$_{N-2}$ centre.

Complex II transports electrons from the tricarboxylic acid cycle intermediate, succinate, to ubiquinone. As in Complex I, the substrate is oxidized on the matrix side of the enzyme. **Succinate dehydrogenase** binds its prosthetic group, FAD, covalently through a histidinyl residue. The production of fumarate in the TCA cycle involves the reduction of this protein-bound FAD to FADH$_2$ which immediately transfers the electrons to the FeS centres which, in turn, pass them to ubiquinone. The exact role of cytochrome b$_{560}$ remains uncertain. When Complex II is purified and inserted into an artificial phospholipid membrane, it fails to pump protons out of the matrix when supplied with succinate and an appropriate electron acceptor.

Ubiquinone (Figure 6.7), in addition to its role as an electron acceptor for Complexes I and II, may also receive electrons from **glycerol-3-phosphate dehydrogenase** of the glycerol phosphate shuttle (Chapter 9) and the **acyl-CoA dehydrogenases** involved in the β-oxidation of fatty acids (Chapter 12). Ubiquinone is a mobile

Reconstitution experiments were used to determine how electrons transfer from Complex I or II to Complex III and from Complex III to Complex IV. It had been shown that the complexes do not physically bind to each other.

Artificial membranes were constructed by mixing pairs of purified complexes in the presence of phospholipids and detergents. During dilution of the detergent, the phospholipids assemble into vesicles, into the membranes of which the protein complexes become incorporated. By employing different combinations of complexes and other substances, it was shown that the transfer of electrons from Complex I to Complex III and from Complex II to Complex III required the presence of ubiquinone in the membrane. Similarly, the movement of electrons from Complex III to Complex IV required cytochrome c. Additional experimental evidence indicates that both ubiquinone and cytochrome c effect their transport roles by diffusion along the membrane.

intramembranal electron carrier which is reduced in two stages to ubiquinol.

Complex III effects the transformation from two-electron to one-electron transport. **Ubiquinol-cytochrome-c reductase** catalyses electron transfer from ubiquinol to cytochrome c. Electron movement from ubiquinol to cytochrome c is rather complex and involves a **branching** of electron transport (Figure 11.3). Ubiquinol diffuses to a site, called **the Qp site**, on the intermembrane space ('O') side of Complex III and donates one electron to the FeS_R centre which transfers it to **cytochrome c_1** with which it is aggregated. This route is confirmed by the extraction of the FeS_R protein (called the Rieske protein) from the complex. This procedure prevents electron transfer from ubiquinol to cytochrome c_1 even though the FeS_R centre has a more positive E_0' than cytochrome c_1. Cytochrome c_1 transfers the electron to cytochrome c.

The second electron follows a pathway referred to as **the Q cycle**. This electron cycles through **cytochrome b_{566}** located on the 'O' side of the complex **to cytochrome b_{562}** on the 'M' side and to a molecule of ubiquinone positioned in a second binding site, called **the Qn site**. Here the ubiquinone is reduced by one electron to a **semiquinone anion**.

A second molecule of ubiquinol is oxidized at the Qp site. One electron proceeds through the FeS_R centre to cytochrome c_1 and the second electron proceeds via cytochromes b_{566} and b_{562} to reduce the semiquinone anion at the Qn site to ubiquinol. This molecule of ubiquinol is released from the Qn site and becomes part of the **ubiquinol pool** in the membrane.

These events in Complex III are coupled to the net translocation of two protons: four protons are released into the 'O' compartment during the oxidation of two ubiquinol molecules but two protons

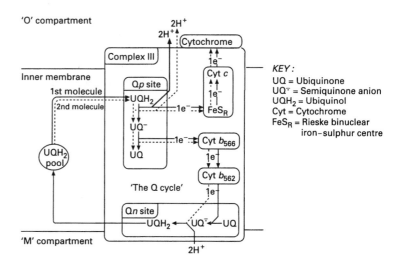

Figure 11.3 *The flow of electrons through Complex III*

are captured from the matrix in the reduction of the semiquinone anion.

Cytochrome c acquires electrons from cytochrome c_1. Cytochrome c is the only water-soluble cytochrome. Like ubiquinone, it is a mobile electron carrier. However, due to its hydrophilic nature it is not an integral part of the inner membrane but loosely associates with it to receive electrons from the FeS_R–cytochrome c_1 aggregate of Complex III. In its reduced state, it migrates along the surface of the 'O' compartment side of the membrane to Complex IV.

Within **Complex IV, cytochrome-c oxidase** accepts electrons from cytochrome c and catalyses the reduction of molecular oxygen by four electrons in the presence of four protons. Although cytochrome c is on the 'O' side of the membrane, reduction of oxygen takes place on the 'M' side and therefore the electrons delivered by cytochrome c must traverse the membrane. The carriers within Complex IV participate in one-electron transfer with a copper atom lying close to a haem group.

The primary acceptor of an electron is Cu_A which transfers it to $haem_a$ in subunit I. From $haem_a$, the electron reduces Cu_B (to Cu^+). Another electron then reduces $haem_{a_3}$ (to Fe^{2+}). When both $haem_{a_3}$ and Cu_B have been reduced, oxygen binds to reduced $haem_{a_3}$ and creates a **peroxy** (-O–O-) **bridge** between the reduced forms of $haem_{a_3}$ and Cu_B. Two electrons, one from $haem_{a_3}$ and the other from Cu_B, are transferred to the oxygen molecule as $haem_{a_3}$ and Cu_B are reoxidized. The participation of a third electron and two protons produces a molecule of water bound to Cu_B (Cu^{2+}) and generate in $haem_{a_3}$ an $Fe^{4+}O^{2-}$ species which is converted by a fourth electron into bound ferric hydroxide whilst copper hydroxide is produced from the Cu_B–H_2O complex. In the final step, two protons from the 'M' compartment interact with these hydroxides to form two molecules of water which are released from $haem_{a_3}$ and Cu_B into the matrix.

Electron transfer by cytochrome-c oxidase is associated with additional proton-translocation activity.

In the final stages of the process, i.e. post-reoxidization of $haem_{a_3}$ and Cu_B, approximately four protons are ejected from the matrix into the intermembrane space by Complex IV.

ATP synthesis

The flow of electrons along the respiratory chain is driven by the reduction in the potential energy which occurs within the electron cloud of each carrier and results in the release of small amounts of free energy.

The **complete reduction of one molecule of oxygen to water** involves four electrons. The events occurring in Complex IV continually generate incompletely reduced **species of oxygen** which are highly reactive and potentially toxic to the cell. A three-electron reduction of oxygen will produce a **hydroxyl radical** (OH·) and **a hydroxyl ion** (OH⁻). It is considered that hydroxyl radicals may damage membranes by lipid peroxidation. Hydroxyl radicals may cause breakage of DNA strands. Single-strand breaks may be repaired but double-strand breaks are irreparable, resulting in cell death during mitosis. Several reactive oxygen species have been implicated in numerous serious conditions including cancer, atherosclerosis, cerebrovascular accident (stroke) and emphysema.

Redox reactions and free energy

The magnitude of the free-energy release during electron transport is dependent upon the difference in the standard redox potentials, $\Delta E_0'$, between the two redox couples. The change in standard redox potential can be calculated from the equation:

$$\Delta E_0' = E_0' \text{ (electron acceptor)} - E_0' \text{ (electron donor)}$$

If the entire respiratory chain is considered, the acceptor is O_2 and the donor is NADH, and then

$$\Delta E_0' = +820 - (-320) \text{ mV (from Table 11.1)} = +1140 \text{ mV}$$

The **change in standard free energy** in a redox reaction is given by the equation:

$$\Delta G^{O'} = -nF\Delta E_0'$$

where $\Delta G^{O'}$ = the standard free-energy change in $J\,mol^{-1}$, n = number of electrons transferred, F = the Faraday constant = $96\,500\ J\ V^{-1}$ and $\Delta E_0'$ = change in redox potential in $mV\,mol^{-1}$.

$$\Delta G^{O'} = -2 \times 96.5 \times 1140\ J\,mV^{-1}mV\,mol^{-1}$$

$$= -220\,020\ J\,mol^{-1} = -220\ kJ\,mol^{-1}$$

The accompanying changes in free energy between members of the respiratory chain may be similarly calculated. Since, under standard conditions, the hydrolysis of ATP yields $-30.5\ kJ\,mol^{-1}$, its synthesis from ADP may be considered as requiring $30.5\ kJ\,mol^{-1}$. Therefore, the free-energy changes associated with electron transfer in Complexes I, III and IV are sufficient to enable ATP synthesis. Free-energy changes between other carriers, e.g. cytochrome c and cytochrome a, are, however, too small to support ADP phosphorylation and this energy is dissipated as heat.

Complex V

The fifth complex isolated from the inner mitochondrial membrane is the location of the **H^+-transporting ATP synthase**, the enzyme responsible for the synthesis of ATP. The mitochondrial enzyme is a large multiprotein complex, also called the **F_oF_1 complex** (Figure 11.4). Electron microscope studies of intact mitochondria have revealed knob-like structures projecting from the inner membrane into the matrix. The F_oF_1 complex comprises two moieties:

- **The F_o moiety** is so-called because in prokaryotes the analogous region binds the antibiotic oligomycin. F_o is composed of three types of polypeptide chain called a, b and c plus seven other proteins. It is believed that aggregates of between nine and 12 chains of polypeptide c span the membrane and form a channel

'M' compartment

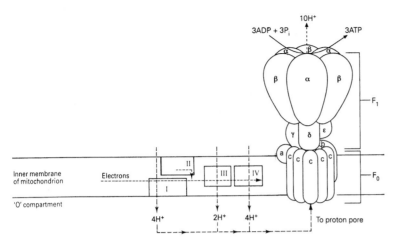

The linkage between the **consumption of O_2 by aerobic cells** and the synthesis of ATP from ADP and orthophosphate has been recognized since 1941. The relationship between phosphate and oxygen consumption, measured using the oxygen electrode, has been expressed as the **P/O ratio** which is defined as the number of molecules of phosphate incorporated into ATP per atom of oxygen utilized. Although numerous estimations of P/O ratios resulted in **non-integral values**, because of the stoichiometries of chemical reactions, the P/O ratio for the oxidation of NADH was interpreted as 3. From this figure, it was deduced that there were three sites of ATP synthesis. The first site was determined to lie between NADH and ubiquinone on the basis of experiments employing inhibitors of electron transport. There was also the consensus that the P/O ratio for the oxidation of succinate was 2. Electrons from succinate are passed to ubiquinone and thus bypass the first site of ATP synthesis. The oxidation of substrates by FAD-linked dehydrogenases permits the synthesis of only two ATP. These early judgements were utilized in the proposed **chemical coupling hypothesis** (1953) of ATP synthesis which was modelled on the glycolytic oxidation of glyceraldehyde 3-phosphate to 3-phosphoglycerate (Chapter 9).

Figure 11.4 *Principle of chemiosmotic hypothesis*

through which protons may migrate, called the **proton pore**. The proton pore is stabilized by polypeptides a and b.

- The **F_1 moiety** consists of a **head** (~9–10 nm) and **stalk** (~4.5 nm). The head consists of three α, three β and one each of γ, δ and ε polypeptide chains. Each of the β chains forms a catalytic site for the synthesis of ATP. The γ, δ and ε chains interact with the F_o moiety through the stalk which has three additional proteins. One of these proteins, the **oligomycin-sensitivity-conferring protein** (OSCP) is responsible for binding oligomycin which interferes with the function of the complex.

The synthesis of ATP from F_1-bound ADP and orthophosphate is considered not to require energy. Rather, the energy-requiring step is the release of the product, ATP. The delivery of the necessary energy is considered below.

The chemiosmotic hypothesis

The chemiosmotic hypothesis (1961) is currently favoured (Figure 11.4) although elements of another proposal, the **conformational coupling hypothesis** (1974), have been incorporated. The hypothesis proposes that electron transport ejects protons from the mitochondrial matrix into the 'O' compartment where an increasing proton concentration causes a decrease in pH. Since the inner membrane is impermeable to protons, a gradient of protons is established across the membrane. The protons attempt to flow back across the membrane to equilibrate their concentrations on both sides, a phenomenon termed **proton motive force** (p.m.f.) by analogy to electromotive force. It is believed that a specific proton pore exists in the F_o part of the ATP synthase (hence the name, H^+-transporting ATP synthase) which provides access from the 'O' compartment to the 'M' compartment. The p.m.f. drives protons through the enzyme structure with a concomitant release of free energy which is utilized in the production of free ATP.

The strength of any hypothesis depends on its accurate description through experimental evidence. Supportive evidence for the chemiosmotic hypothesis is now considered.

- **The membrane can establish a proton gradient.** This has been accomplished by measurement of the changes in pH and electrical potential across the inner mitochondrial membrane. The pH and membrane potential (E_m) both contribute to the p.m.f. which may be calculated from the following equation:

$$\Delta p = E_m - 2.3 \frac{RT}{F}{}^i\Delta^o \text{pH}$$

where Δp = proton motive force in V, E_m = membrane potential in V, R = the gas constant, T = temperature in K, F = the Faraday constant and, ${}^i\Delta^o$pH = the difference in pH from the inside of the membrane to its outside. The equation reduces to: $\Delta p = E_m - 59$ ${}^i\Delta^o$pH when expressed in mV. Note that Δp and E_m are negative values. Experimental investigations have revealed that electron transport may generate an ${}^i\Delta^o$pH of approximately 1.4 units and an E_m of -140 mV. The p.m.f. generated (-223 mV) is sufficient to account for the synthesis of three molecules of ATP.

- **The sites for proton translocation** in the respiratory chain have been located to Complex I, III and IV.

- **Oxidative phosphorylation relies upon a functionally intact inner membrane.** Although electron transport may proceed in damaged or modified membranes, the capacity for ATP generation may be destroyed. Membranes perforated by detergents permit leakage of protons into the matrix which abolishes both the gradient and ATP production.

- **Oxidative phosphorylation relies upon a complete proton circuit.** **Uncouplers** are agents which separate electron transport from ATP synthesis. Uncouplers such as *NN'*-dicyclohexylcarbodiimide (DCCD) and **oligomycin** are believed to block the proton pore and thereby destroy the continuity of the circuit with the result that ATP generation is prevented. The antibiotic **valinomycin** is an ionophore. It binds K^+ ions and acts as a mobile carrier which diffuses through membranes. By binding K^+ ions from the 'O' compartment and translocating them to the 'M' compartment, valinomycin effects the abolition of the H^+ gradient without direct interaction with the protons.

- **Generation of a proton gradient facilitates the production of ATP in the absence of electron transport.** This evidence has come from the chloroplast and a photosynthetic bacterium.

The **uncoupling of electron transport** and ATP generation is also a natural occurrence. Newborn animals and humans generate **heat** rather than ATP in specialized adipose tissue. This tissue, located in man at the back of the neck, is called **brown fat** due to the colouration bestowed by large numbers of mitochondria. In these mitochondria, electron transfer is accompanied by the usual ejection of protons out of the matrix. However, the inner membranes of brown fat mitochondria possess a protein, called **thermogenin**, which creates a proton pore additional to that of ATP synthase. This proton pore permits protons to return to the matrix without the involvement of Complex V and thereby without ADP phosphorylation. The energy released during the transport of the electrons is dissipated as heat.

The **chloroplast** is an organelle exclusive to **green tissue** in the plant kingdom. The roles of chloroplasts are the capture of electromagnetic (light) energy and its conversion into chemical energy, a process referred to as photosynthesis. Like the mitochondrion, the chloroplast is surrounded by two distinct membranes, the inner of which contains a H^+-transporting ATP synthase. By incubating chloroplasts in an acid medium (pH 4) for several hours, and rapidly transferring them to a solution of ADP and orthophosphate at pH 8, the chloroplasts produced ATP as the gradient was abolished. Similar experiments have been successfully conducted with mitochondria.

Also, the **photosynthetic bacterium** *Halobacterium halobium* contains a plasma membrane protein called **bacteriorhodopsin** which translocates protons when the bacteria are illuminated. Illumination of artificial phospholipid vesicles incorporating purified bacteriorhodopsin and the mitochondrial ATP synthase demonstrated the production of ATP in the absence of electron transport. The ATP synthesis could only be the result of the combined activity of the bacterial proton pump and the mitochondrial enzyme in the enclosed membrane.

- **Rotenone** and **amytal** abolish ATP synthesis driven by NADH-derived electrons but that initiated by $FADH_2$ continues. The sites of action of electron-transport inhibitors were identified by the 'crossover technique' in which the carriers before the blockage become more reduced and those beyond more oxidized.
- **Certain agents can abolish ATP generation by dissipation of the transmembrane proton gradient** rather than the impairment of electron transport. Such agents, e.g. **2,4-dinitrophenol** and **carbonyl cyanide-*p*-trifluoromethoxyphenylhydrazone**, are called **uncouplers** because they separate the two functional aspects of oxidative phosphorylation.
- **Ionophores**, e.g. **valinomycin** and **nigericin**, are also lipid-soluble substances which promote the transfer of cations across the membrane. Ionophores may function by insertion into the membrane to create a pore or as mobile carriers which diffuse through the membrane.
- **Certain agents can block the proton pore** of the ATP synthase, e.g. **oligomycin B** and **DCCD**.

The generation of ATP

The **MgADP$^-$ complex** is the actual substrate in ADP phosphorylation (Chapter 8). When ADP and orthophosphate were employed with purified ATP synthase in the presence of radioactively labelled water, ($H_2^{18}O$) but in the absence of a proton gradient, the ^{18}O appeared in the phosphate (Figure 11.5). The ^{18}O had become incorporated into the phosphate through the synthesis and sub-

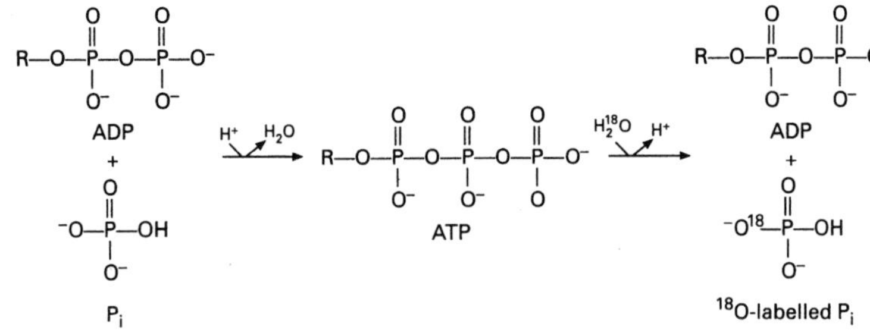

Figure 11.5 *Isotope exchange experiment showing the incorporation of labelled oxygen into phosphate by ATP synthase*

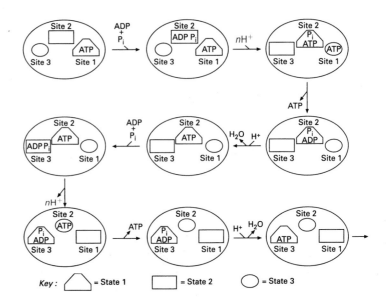

sequent hydrolysis of ATP. On synthesis, ATP had not departed from the active site but remained to be hydrolysed. Through this experiment it was realized that the proton flow does not provide the energy to form ATP but to displace it from the enzyme.

The **ATP synthase** has three catalytic sites (located on β-chains) but they are not in the same conformation at any given moment. They simultaneously cycle through three different conformational states. One state has a high affinity for ATP, a second state binds ADP and orthophosphate with low affinity and a third state has a very low affinity for ATP (Figure 11.6). Suppose ATP is bound at catalytic site 1, ADP and P_i will bind to site 2 and site 3 is currently unoccupied. The proton flow through F_O generates a conformational change in F_1. Site 1 changes into the third state. Concomitantly, site 2 is converted into the first state and site 3 adopts the conformation of the second state. ATP is released from site 1. In site 2, ADP and P_i are reversibly condensed into ATP with the release of water. There is no phosphorylated enzyme intermediate. ADP and P_i now bind to site 3. The proton flow permits

Figure 11.6 *The conformational states of the catalytic sites of ATP synthase*

the change of site 3 into the first state, site 2 assumes the third state, ATP is released and in site 3 another ATP molecule is formed by condensation, and so the process progresses. The mechanism is an example of **catalytic cooperativity**.

Transport of ATP from the matrix

Most ATP-requiring reactions occur in the cytosol and produce ADP and orthophosphate. Since most ATP is formed by mitochondrial oxidative phosphorylation (in appropriate cells) from ADP and orthophosphate, these molecules traverse the inner membrane. ATP and ADP are translocated by the specific **adenine-nucleotide-transport system**. This **antiport system** (Chapter 7) is widely distributed in the membrane and exchanges one mitochondrial ATP for one cytoplasmic ADP. The carrier selectively binds and transports ADP inwards and ATP outwards. The phosphate enters the mitochondrion via a phosphate carrier, either an antiport system which exchanges phosphate for a hydroxyl ion or the **symport system** of P_i and H^+. The effect of these transport mechanisms is that extramitochondrial ADP^{3-} and HPO_4^{2-} are exchanged for ATP^{4-} with a net gain of one proton in the 'M' compartment.

Inhibitors of oxidative phosphorylation

The experimental investigation of the entire process of oxidative phosphorylation has been assisted by the use of a variety of agents which inhibit at different stages (Table 11.3).

The numbers of ATP molecules generated via the respiratory chain

The precise relationship between the numbers of protons passing through the proton pore of the H^+-transporting ATP synthase and the numbers of ATP generated remains uncertain. The consensus opinion is that three protons pass through into the matrix for each ATP generated. Also it is widely believed that electron transport of a pair of electrons from:

- **NADH** through Complexes I, III and IV pumps out about 10 protons (estimates vary between 9 and 12 protons);
- **FAD**-linked dehydrogenases ejects about six protons since the electron pathway omits Complex I.

The transport of phosphate into the matrix results in a net gain of one proton. Therefore, assuming 10 protons are ejected from the 'M' compartment and 4 protons return for each ATP synthesized, then 10/4 molecules of ATP are produced for each pair of electrons released from NADH to reduce oxygen at the end of the respiratory

Table 11.3 *Some inhibitors of oxidative phosphorylation*

Site of inhibition	Agent	Comment
Electron transport	Rotenone } Amytal }	Prevent reduction of ubiquinone and simultaneous oxidation of Complex I FeS centres
	Antimycin A	Inhibits transfer of electron from cytochrome b_{562} to ubiquinone
	Hydrogen cyanide } Hydrogen sulphide } Azide }	Bind to Fe^{3+} of cytochrome a and a_3
	Carbon monoxide	Binds to Fe^{2+} of cytochrome a and a_3

Inner membrane	2,4-Dinitrophenol }
	Carbonyl cyanide-
	  p-trifluoromethoxy-
	  phenylhydrazone }
		Are anionic at pH 7.0, may protonate to become lipophilic and soluble in membrane. Protons are transported through membrane and H^+ gradient is abolished

	Valinomycin	Renders membrane permeable to K^+ which may abolish E_m
	Nigericin	Abolishes H^+ gradient by K^+–H^+ exchange
ATP synthase	Oligomycin	Binds to OSCP in stalk and blocks H^+ pore
	DCCD	Reacts with DCCD-binding proteolipid of F_o component and blocks H^+ pore
Adenine-nucleotide carrier	Atractyloside	Binds to external conformation to preclude ADP interaction
	Bongkrekic acid	Binds to internal conformation to preclude ATP interaction
Phosphate carrier	Mercurial reagents	Bind to sulphydryl groups

The **oxygen** consumption of a mammalian cell mainly reflects the requirement for ATP production. Under normal conditions, approximately 90% of total oxygen consumption is destined for use by the mitochondrion as an electron acceptor. The remaining 10% is employed in other oxygen-dependent activities, e.g. monooxygenase reactions. Of the oxygen consumed by the mitochondrion, $\sim$ 80% is used in ATP synthesis and $\sim$ 20% is uncoupled by the leakage of protons across the inner membrane. It has been estimated that the ATP produced is employed as follows: protein synthesis $\sim$ 30–38%; **Na^+–K^+ exchanging ATPase** $\sim$ 24–35%; gluconeogenesis $\sim$ 8.8–12.5%; **Ca^{2+}-transporting ATPase** $\sim$ 5–10%; urea synthesis $\sim$ 3.8%, and myosin ATPase (microfilament contraction) $\sim$ 2.5–10% (bold indicates a major activity in all cells). Other significant usages include mRNA synthesis and substrate cycling.

chain. A similar calculation shows that 6/4 molecules of ATP are produced by electrons emanating from $FADH_2$. Thus:

- one NADH produces about 2.5 ATP;
- one $FADH_2$ produces about 1.5 ATP.

ATP yield from the complete oxidation of glucose

Near the beginning of this chapter, the role of oxidative phosphorylation was identified as the continual resynthesis of ATP to satisfy man's energy needs. Now that oxidative phosphorylation has been discussed, it is possible to calculate energy yields from aerobic metabolic processes. The net ATP production during the aerobic degradation of pyruvate and glucose, a major fuel molecule, is shown in Table 11.4.

Each **pyruvate** molecule will ultimately produce about 12.5 molecules of ATP. Since every glucose molecule is degraded to two molecules of pyruvate, the mitochondrial processes listed account for 25 ATP per glucose molecule. Glycolysis contributes two ATP but, under aerobic conditions, reduced coenzymes participate in oxidative phosphorylation to produce another three or five ATP per glucose molecule depending upon their mode of entry into the mitochondrion. Therefore, the complete oxidation of glucose will yield $\sim$ 30 or 32 ATP depending upon the tissue in which it is

Table 11.4   *The net yield of ATP during complete oxidation of pyruvate and glucose*

Location	Reaction sequence	Product	ATP yield per pyruvate	ATP yield per glucose	
				In liver, kidney, cardiac muscle	In skeletal muscle, brain
Mitochondrion	Tricarboxylic acid cycle	1 GTP	1	2	2
		3 NADH*	7.5	15	15
		1 FADH₂†	1.5	3	3
	Pyruvate dehydrogenase complex	1 NADH	2.5	5	5
Cytosol	Glycolysis	2 ATP	—	2	2
		2 NADH‡	—	5‡	3‡
Total	—	—	12.5	32	30

*Each NADH on delivery of its electrons to the beginning of the electron-transport chain produces 2.5 ATP through oxidative phosphorylation.
†Each $FADH_2$ of Complex II of the electron-transport chain produces 1.5 ATP through oxidative phosphorylation.
‡Each NADH produced in the cytosol must circumvent the permeability barrier of the inner mitochondrial membrane by the use of shuttle mechanism (Chapter 8). The malate–aspartate shuttle yields mitochondrial NADH capable of producing 2.5 ATP whereas each $FADH_2$ produced by the glycerol–phosphate shuttle provides only 1.5 ATP.

oxidized. The complete oxidation of glucose 6-phosphate produced during glycogenolysis (Chapter 9) by skeletal muscle will yield ~ 31 ATP since only one priming phosphorylation reaction is necessary. A simple calculation [energy conserved/energy available $= 32 \times 30.5 \, \text{kJ} \, \text{mol}^{-1}/2870 \, \text{kJ} \, \text{mol}^{-1} = 976/2870 = 0.34$] reveals that approximately 34% of the available energy contained within the glucose molecule is conserved as ATP.

Suggested further reading

Boyer, P.D. (1997). The ATP synthase: a splendid molecular machine. *Annual Review of Biochemistry* **66**, 717–749.

Brand, M.D., Chien, L.-F. and Diolez, P. (1994). Experimental discrimination between proton leak and redox slip during mitochondrial electron transport. *Biochemical Journal* **297**, 27–29.

Gray, H.B. and Winkler, J.R. (1996). Electron transfer in proteins. *Annual Review of Biochemistry* **65**, 537–561.

Lanyl, J.K. (1995). Bacteriorhodopsin as a model for proton pumps. *Nature* **375**, 461–463.

Verkhovsky, M.I., Morgan, J. E., Puustinen, A. and Wikström, M. (1996). Kinetic trapping of oxygen in cell respiration. *Nature* **380**, 268–270.

Nicholls, D.G. and Ferguson, S.J. (1992). *Bioenergetics 2*. London: Academic Press.

Self-assessment questions

1. Calculate the standard free-energy change when a pair of electrons are transferred from NADH ($E_0' = -320\,\text{mV}$) to ubiquinol ($E_0' = +60\,\text{mV}$).

2. The inhibitor of oxidative phosphorylation, 2,4-dinitrophenol, permits pyruvate to be oxidized by mitochondria. Explain.

3. Calculate the net yield of ATP when one molecule of glycerol is completely oxidized by hepatocytes (liver cells).

4. Calculate the proton motive force generated by a pH gradient of 1.4 and a membrane potential of $-140\,\text{mV}$ across a membrane.

5. Produce a scheme for the production of water by the reduction of molecular oxygen in the presence of protons by cytochrome-*c* oxidase.

6. Explain why the oxidation of succinate to fumarate yields about 1.5 molecules of ATP via oxidative phosphorylation whilst oxidative decarboxylation of 2-oxoglutarate to succinyl-CoA produces about 2.5 ATP.

7. When vitamin C is employed as a respiratory chain substrate, how many ATP may be produced per molecule of vitamin C?

8. List the numbers of mononuclear, binuclear and tetranuclear iron–sulphur centres found in each protein complex of the inner mitochondrial membrane.

9. Which stages of oxidative phosphorylation are inhibited by the following: atractyloside, antimycin A, carbon monoxide, hydrogen cyanide, nigericin and oligomycin.

10. Suggest an explanation for the following observation. NAD(P)H transhydrogenase transfers electrons from NADPH to NAD^+ with subsequent transfer of the electrons to NADH dehydrogenase. This reaction requires energy although the experimental standard redox potential values suggest otherwise ($NAD^+ \rightleftharpoons NADH$: $E_0' = -320\,\text{mV}$; $NADP^+ \rightleftharpoons NADPH$: $E_0' = -324\,\text{mV}$).

Key Concepts and Facts

Electron Transfer
- Electron transport assemblies are located, in man, in the inner mitochondrial membrane.

- The respiratory chain is a series of coupled redox reactions.

- The electron-transport assemblies consist of four protein complexes.

- Ubiquinone and cytochrome c are the only mobile electron-transport carriers.

- Electrons are initially transferred as pairs but latterly as single electrons.

- During electron transport, protons are pumped out of the matrix into the intermembrane space.

- The ultimate electron acceptor in the respiratory chain is oxygen which, in the presence of protons, is reduced to form water.

ATP Synthesis
- ATP is produced within Complex V of the inner mitochondrial membrane.

- ATP is synthesized by an enzyme called H^+-transporting ATP synthase.

- The accepted hypothesis for the supply of energy to ATP synthase is called the chemiosmotic hypothesis.

- ATP may be produced in the absence of electron transport provided that a proton gradient exists.

- Energy is required by ATP synthase to effect the release of synthesized ATP.

Complete Oxidation of Glucose
- The energy from a pair of electrons from one molecule of NADH results in ~ 2.5 molecules of ATP.

- The energy from a pair of electrons from one molecule of $FADH_2$ results in ~ 1.5 molecules of ATP.

- Complete oxidation of one molecule of glucose may yield about 30 or 32 molecules of ATP depending on the tissue-specific shuttle employed.

Answers to questions (Chapter 11)

1. $\Delta E_0' = E_0'$ (electron acceptor) $- E_0'$ (electron donor) $= 60 - (-320)\,mV = +380$ mV. $\Delta G'^\circ = -nF\Delta E_0' = -2 \times 96.5 \times 380$ $J\,mV^{-1}mV\,mol^{-1} = -73.34\,kJ\,mol^{-1}$.

2. 2,4-DNP is an uncoupler of oxidative phosphorylation. In its presence, electron transport is permitted O_2 but ATP synthesis does not occur.

3. 16 ATP. Glycerol enters glycolysis at glycerone phosphate (Figure 9.8) at the expense of one ATP but generates one NADH. Thus, glycerol kinase $= -1$ ATP; glycerol-3-phosphate dehydrogenase $= 1$ NADH $= +2.5$ ATP; phosphoglycerate kinase + pyruvate kinase = + 2 ATP; pyruvate dehydrogenase $=1$ NADH $= + 2.5$ ATP; TCA cycle $= 3$ NADH $+ 1$ FADH$_2$ + 1 GTP $= +7.5 + 1.5 + 1$ ATP. Total yield = 16 ATP.

4. $\Delta p = E_m - 59\ ^i\Delta^\circ pH = -140 - 59\ (1.4) = -140 - 82.6 = -222.6\,mV$.

5.

6. Succinate dehydrogenase is a component of Complex II and its prosthetic group, FAD, transfers electrons to ubiquinone. The oxidative decarboxylation utilizes NAD$^+$. NADH passes electrons across Complex I where four protons are translocated to the 'O' compartment. Thus, NADH produces one more ATP than FADH$_2$.

7. Ascorbic acid passes electrons indirectly to cytochrome c. Four protons are pumped by cytochrome-c oxidase, enough to generate more than one ATP.

8. Complex I/II/III/IV/V have five binuclear + three tetranuclear/ two binuclear + one tetranuclear/one binuclear/none/none.

9. See Table 11.3

10. The electron transfer takes place up a concentration gradient.

Chapter 12
Lipid metabolism

Learning objectives

After studying this chapter you should confidently be able to:

Identify the tissue and intracellular locations of the major pathways of fatty acid metabolism.

Describe the key reactions of each pathway.

Discuss the important features of the activity of key enzymes of each pathway.

Compare and contrast the major features of fatty acid anabolism and catabolism.

Calculate the energy yield, in terms of numbers of ATP molecules produced, from the complete oxidation of any linear fatty acid.

Discuss alternative fates for the metabolites generated through the functioning of different pathways.

Describe the synthesis of cholesterol and its role as the precursor of steroid hormones.

Discuss the metabolism of steroid hormones.

Lipids have important functions in membrane structure and cellular metabolism. Lipids, excluding terpenes and steroids, contain fatty acid moeties (Chapter 6). **Fatty acids** are therefore important as constituents of more complex molecules, e.g. phosphoacylglycerols, and are major sources of energy for most cells. In humans and mammals, small amounts of fatty acids are stored within most cells and larger amounts are generally found in specialized storage tissues, e.g. adipose tissue. The major storage form of fatty acids is **triacylglycerols**, delivered from the diet or synthesized intracellularly. Triacylglycerols are anhydrous and can release more energy per unit weight than hydrated storage carbohydrates. For this reason, during periods of excess food consumption, energy is stored as fat. Fatty acids supply about 40% of the calorific requirements of man on a normal diet. This figure may increase to almost 100% during periods of fasting and starvation. Fatty

In 1905, a key study on the **oxidation of fatty acids** was reported. **Knoop** conducted experiments in which dogs were fed ω-**phenyl derivatives** (a hydrogen atom of the terminal methyl group was substituted by a phenyl ring) of long-chain fatty acids with either an even or odd number of carbon atoms. The excretion products were the glycine conjugates of phenylacetate or benzoate called **phenylacetylglycine** (from even numbers) **and benzoylglycine** (from odd numbers). Knoop therefore concluded that the degradation of fatty acids must involve the successive removal of two-carbon units which he considered to be **acetate**.

The elucidation of the details of the process was delayed for 46 years until the discovery of coenzyme A (CoA). This discovery stimulated research and within the following 2 years, acetyl-CoA was identified as the major product of the β-oxidation pathway, the fundamental sequence of the reactions and the intracellular location of the pathway were established.

acids constitute the major energy supply during the migration of birds and the hibernation of animals.

This chapter considers the β-oxidation pathway, the potential production of ketone bodies and their utilization, and the synthesis of fatty acids. Steroid biosynthesis is discussed through the synthesis of cholesterol and its subsequent utilization as a precursor of steroid hormones. The intravascular transport and excretion of steroid hormones are briefly described.

Lipid degradation

In man, several pathways for fatty acid catabolism exist:

- **The β-oxidation pathway,** in which the carbon atom C-3 (β-carbon) is oxidized.
- **The α-oxidation pathway** which involves the oxidation of the C-2 atom. This pathway is important in the brain and in the degradation of ingested branched fatty acids to prepare such fatty acids for entry into the β-oxidation pathway.
- **The ω-oxidation (omega) pathway** which involves the oxidation of the terminal methyl group primarily of C_6 to C_{10} fatty acids. The dicarboxylate product enters the β-oxidation pathway.

Three important aspects of fatty acid degradation are considered here:

- **the release of fatty acids from storage** and subsequent delivery to tissues;
- **the β-oxidation pathway,** the major degradative pathway for fatty acids in man;
- **ketone body metabolism** which functions when carbohydrate metabolism is depressed.

The release and delivery of fatty acids from storage

The **fatty acids for β-oxidation** may be derived from the diet, storage triacylglycerols or the turnover of membrane lipids. The mobilization of fatty acids from adipocytes occurs when the diet or glycogen reserves are insufficient to satisfy the calorific requirements of tissues. Hormonally controlled **lipases** systematically hydrolyse the ester bonds of triacylglycerols to release fatty acids and glycerol. This **lipolysis** is mediated by cAMP following the interaction of, adrenaline or glucagon, for example, with their specific receptors in the adipocyte plasma membrane (Chapter 8).

The **glycerol** by conversion to glycerone phosphate can enter the glycolytic pathway or be released into the blood circulation from which it is sequestered by the liver and kidneys for gluconeogenesis

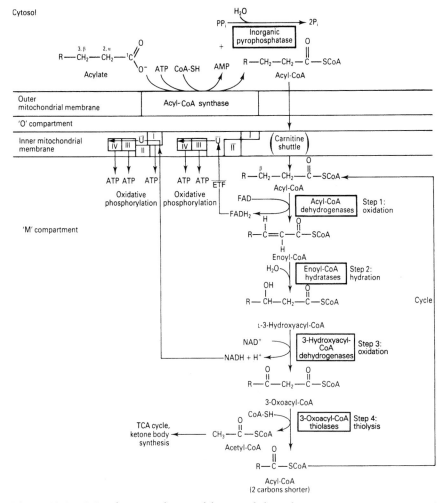

Figure 12.1 *β-Oxidation pathway of fatty acid degradation*

(Chapter 9). The fatty acids diffuse through the plasma membranes and are transported in the blood circulation as a **serum albumin–acylate complex** to the tissues requiring fatty acids for oxidation. At these tissues, the fatty acids dissociate from the complex and enter the tissue cells by diffusion. This aspect of fatty acid transport is governed by the ratio of the concentration of albumin-bound fatty acid to the intracellular concentration of fatty acid. The long-chain fatty acids delivered to the tissue cells undergo cytosolic activation by an **acyl-CoA synthase** (also called **fatty acid-CoA ligase**) before entry into the mitochondrion for oxidation.

The β-oxidation pathway

The **β-oxidation pathway** from **saturated fatty acid** to **acetyl-CoA** is shown in Figure 12.1. A long-chain fatty acid in the ionized form is activated in the cytosol by a transmembranous **acyl-CoA synthase**,

The synthesis of the **PG₂ series of prostaglandins** occurs in most mammalian tissues and commences with arachidonate, released from membranous phosphoacylglycerols by the action of **phospholipase A₂** (Chapter 6). Arachidonate undergoes conversion by the enzyme **prostaglandin H₂ synthase** which contains two catalytic activities. A **cyclooxygenase activity** performs a double dioxygenation, i.e. the addition of two molecules of oxygen to arachidonate, and cyclization to produce the intermediate **prostaglandin G₂** (PGG₂). A **hydroperoxidase activity** converts the hydroperoxy group at position C-15 of PGG₂ to a hydroxyl group to yield **prostaglandin H₂** (PGH₂). PGH₂ is the substrate for various synthases (e.g. prostaglandin F synthase) which yield PGD₂, PGF₂ₐ, PGE₂, PGI₂ and thromboxanes A₂ and B₂. Different cells and tissues produce different quantities of the prostaglandins. For example, cardiac muscle produces equivalent amounts of PGE₂, PGF₂ₐ and PGI₂ whereas PGI₂ is the principal product in the endothelial cells of blood vessels where it functions as an inhibitor of platelet aggregation to prevent blood coagulation.

the coenzyme A-binding site of which is located on the cytosolic surface of the outer mitochondrial membrane. Several acyl-CoA synthases are known:

- **long-chain-acyl-CoA synthase** which acts on C_6 to C_{20} substrates in the liver, and up to C_{24} in the brain;
- **medium-chain-acyl-CoA synthases** which act on C_4 to C_{12} substrates;
- **short-chain-acyl-CoA synthases** which are located in the mitochondrial matrix and activate C_2 and C_3 substrates.

The reaction catalysed by long-chain-acyl-CoA synthase is freely reversible and so, to drive the reaction in the desired direction, the pyrophosphate is hydrolysed by **inorganic pyrophosphatase** (Chapter 8).

Long-chain saturated acyl-CoA molecules, e.g. palmitoyl-CoA, gain entry to the mitochondrial matrix where the enzymes of the β-oxidation cycle are located by utilizing the **carnitine antiport carrier** (Figure 12.2). There are three known **carnitine O-acyltransferases**. Carnitine O-palmitoyltransferase (for C_8 to C_{18} acyl-CoA molecules), bound to the outside of the inner membrane, bonds the acyl group of palmitoyl-CoA to carnitine. The **palmitoylcarnitine** thus formed crosses the inner membrane via the carnitine antiport carrier in exchange for a free carnitine from the matrix. Another isoenzyme of carnitine palmitoyltransferase, located on the inside of

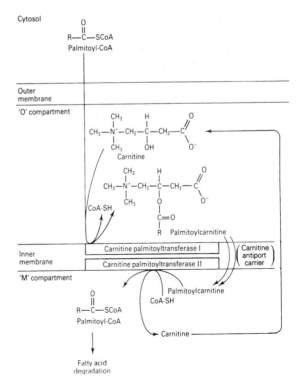

Figure 12.2 *Transportation of palmitoyl-CoA into the mitochondrion for fatty acid oxidation*

the membrane, transfers the palmitoyl group to matrix CoA. The released carnitine will subsequently be exchanged for another palmitoylcarnitine.

In the mitochondrial matrix, saturated acyl-CoA molecules are processed through a cycle of reactions in which they are successively **oxidized, hydrated, oxidized** (cf. TCA cycle, Chapter 10) **and thiolysed** (Figure 12.1). At each step of the cycle, there are multiple enzymes with differing chain-length specificities.

At step 1, there are four possible acyl-CoA dehydrogenases:

- **very-long-chain-acyl-CoA dehydrogenase (VLCAD)** which acts on C_{12} to C_{24} substrates;
- **long-chain-acyl-CoA dehydrogenase (LCAD)** for C_8 to C_{20} substrates;
- **medium-chain-acyl-CoA dehydrogenase (MCAD)** for C_4 to C_{12} substrates;
- **short-chain-acyl-CoA dehydrogenase (SCAD)** which is active on branched and unbranched C_4 and C_6 substrates.

Each of the above enzymes has an FAD prosthetic group which is reduced in the production of a **2-enoyl-CoA**. A matrix FAD-linked protein called the **electron transfer flavoprotein (ETF)** accepts the reducing equivalents from the FAD and transfers the electrons to an iron–sulphur flavoprotein located in the inner membrane. This specific oxidoreductase then delivers the electrons to ubiquinone of the respiratory chain (Chapter 11). Therefore, this step is ultimately responsible for the production of 1.5 ATP by oxidative phosphorylation.

At step 2, three **enoyl-CoA hydratases** add the elements of water to C-2 (H) and C-3 (OH) atoms of a 2-enoyl-CoA to form L-3-hydroxyacyl-CoA. **At Step 3**, two **3-hydroxyacyl-CoA dehydrogenases** with overlapping chain-length specificities catalyse the NAD-linked oxidation to form a **3-oxoacyl-CoA**. The NADH passes its electrons to Complex I and produces 2.5 ATP by oxidative phosphorylation. **At the final step (step 4)**, three enzymes catalyse the thiolytic cleavage of 3-oxoacyl-CoAs to generate acetyl-CoA and an acyl-CoA intermediate which is two carbons shorter than the acyl-CoA entering step 1. The shortened acyl-CoA re-enters the cycle at step 1.

The **long-chain specificities** of the enzymes active in steps 2, 3 and 4 are not due to discrete enzymes but are the result of constituents of a **trifunctional enzyme complex** closely associated with the inner mitochondrial membrane. The complex consists of four α-subunits and four β-subunits. Enoyl-CoA hydratase and 3-hydroxyacyl-CoA dehydrogenase activities are associated with the α-subunits which also serve in binding the complex to the inner membrane. The β-subunits contain the long-chain-3-oxoacyl-CoA thiolase activity.

If the initial saturated fatty acid contained **an even number of carbon atoms**, e.g. palmitate, the cycling would continue until C_4

Aspirin (acetylsalicylate) is a **non-steroidal anti-inflammatory drug (NSAID)**. It has been long prescribed for its **analgesic** (pain-killer) and **antipyretic** (fever-reducing) properties. Its mode of action was established in 1971. Aspirin and other NSAIDs, e.g. ibuprofen, inhibit the **cyclooxygenase** activity of **prostaglandin H_2 synthase** but have no effect on the hydroperoxidase activity. Aspirin acetylates a seryl residue, [530]serine, which is not involved in the catalytic action. O-Acetylation of this seryl residue blocks an internal channel in the enzyme through which arachidonate must pass to gain access to the catalytic site of the enzyme. It is believed that other NSAIDs also achieve their effects by interference with this channel, e.g. the carboxyl group of flurbiprofen interacts with [120]arginine.

There is evidence that low dose levels of aspirin, e.g. one tablet (75 mg) on alternate days reduces significantly the risk of cardiac arrest and thrombosis in later life. At this dosage, aspirin inhibits platelet aggregation by its action on prostaglandin H_2 synthase which reduces PGH_2 availability for the synthesis of the potent platelet aggregator, thromboxane A_2.

Aspirin inhibits the production of PGH_2 by both isoforms of the enzyme. The inducible enzyme is elevated in approximately 90% of cases of colonic carcinoma but is not expressed in non-tumour tissue. The regular use of four to six aspirin tablets per week over the long term, e.g. over 20 years, appears to reduce substantially (approximately 50%) the risk of colorectal cancer.

Figure 12.3 *Fate of propionyl-CoA produced by the β-oxidation of fatty acids with an odd number of carbons*

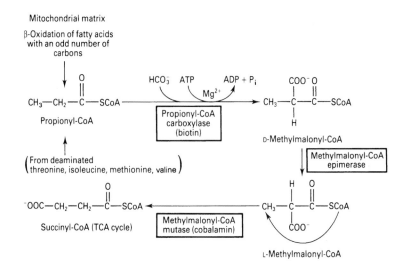

acyl-CoA (butyryl-CoA) enters step 1 and then would produce one FADH$_2$, one NADH and two acetyl-CoA molecules. Palmitoyl-CoA would be processed by steps 1 to 4 of the cycle seven times (Table 12.1). The net yield of energy as ATP from the β-oxidation of a fatty acid can be calculated as shown in Table 12.2. One molecule of palmitate may yield 106 molecules of ATP. Compare this yield with that from the complete oxidation of glucose (Table 11.4). For the energy yield from other even-numbered saturated fatty acids, adjust the number of cycles and recalculate.

If the initial saturated fatty acid contained **an odd number of carbon atoms** (mainly originating from the individual's diet), the last cycle starts from C$_5$ acyl-CoA and produces one FADH$_2$, one NADH, one acetyl-CoA and one terminal propionyl-CoA molecule.

Table 12.1 *The sequential degradation of a fatty acid* by the β-oxidation pathway*

Palmitate as substrate								*Number of cycles*
CH$_3$—CH$_2$—CH$_2$—CH$_2$—CH$_2$—CH$_2$—CH$_2$—CH$_2$—CH$_2$—CH$_2$—CH$_2$—CH$_2$—CH$_2$—CH$_2$—CH$_2$—COSCoA								
							Acetyl-CoA	First cycle
						Acetyl-CoA		Second cycle
					Acetyl-CoA			Third cycle
				Acetyl-CoA				Fourth cycle
			Acetyl-CoA					Fifth cycle
		Acetyl-CoA						Sixth cycle
Acetyl-CoA	Acetyl-CoA							Seventh cycle

* For any fatty acid, the number of cycles can be calculated by the formula:

$$\text{Number of cycles} = \frac{\text{number of carbon atoms in the fatty acid} - 2}{2}$$

Table 12.2 *The net yield of ATP during complete oxidation of a fatty acid by the β-oxidation pathway*

Fatty acid	Step no.	Number of cycles	Number of molecules of ATP gained per cycle via oxidative phosphorylation	Number of molecules of ATP gained per molecule of fatty acid
Palmitate	1	7	$FADH_2 \equiv 1.5$	10.5
	3	7	$NADH \equiv 2.5$	17.5
	4	7	Acetyl-CoA $\equiv 10$	70
	4	Terminal	Acetyl-CoA $\equiv 10$	10
	Total of ATP molecules gained			108
	Number of ATP equivalents used during activation			2*
	Net yield of ATP molecules			106

* Although only one ATP is actually used in the cytosolic activation, the product is AMP. The regeneration of ATP from this AMP would require two phosphorylation reactions and so the number of ATPs used is quoted as two equivalents.

The fate of the propionyl-CoA is entry into the TCA cycle as succinyl-CoA (Figure 12.3). Propionyl-CoA is carboxylated to form the D-stereoisomer of **methylmalonyl-CoA**. However, succinyl-CoA can only be produced by **methylmalonyl-CoA mutase** if the substrate is in the L-form. Therefore, the D-configuration is converted into L-methylmalonyl-CoA by the appropriate **epimerase**. L-Methylmalonyl-CoA is rearranged internally by the specific mutase to yield succinyl-CoA. **Methylmalonyl-CoA mutase** requires as coenzyme a form of the vitamin **cobalamin** (B_{12}). Study of the formulae of methylmalonyl-CoA and succinyl-CoA may suggest a repositioning of the carboxylate group. However, the rearrangement proceeds by the transfer of the bulky coenzyme A group. The

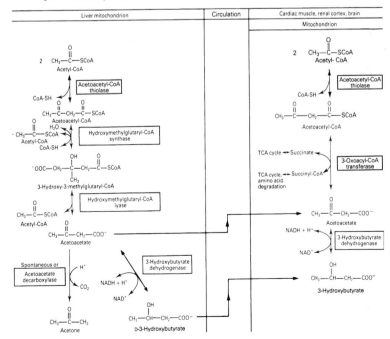

Figure 12.4 *Synthesis and utilization of ketone bodies*

catabolism of some amino acids also produces propionyl-CoA which enters the TCA cycle via this pathway.

Ketone body metabolism

The **utilization of acetyl-CoA** by the tricarboxylic acid cycle is dependent upon the availability of an appropriate intramitochondrial concentration of oxaloacetate which is maintained by anaplerotic reactions (Chapter 10). The intracellular concentration of oxaloacetate therefore depends upon the levels of certain glycolytic intermediates. If carbohydrate metabolism is depressed and fatty acid degradation predominant such as during starvation, fasting or diabetes mellitus, acetyl-CoA cannot enter the TCA cycle because oxaloacetate is employed in gluconeogenesis. Acetyl-CoA is therefore utilized by a pathway leading to **ketone body formation**. There are three so-called ketone bodies:

- acetoacetate;
- D-**3-hydroxybutyrate** which is not a ketone but derived from acetoacetate;
- acetone.

The major site of ketone body production (Figure 12.4) is the liver. Two acetyl-CoA molecules condense to form **acetoacetyl-CoA**. The enzyme catalysing this reaction is a specific 3-oxoacyl-CoA thiolase called **acetoacetyl-CoA thiolase**. Mechanistically, the step is a reversal of step 4 of the β-oxidation pathway (Figure 12.1). Although the equilibrium is unfavourable for the formation of acetoacetyl-CoA, the reaction proceeds by coupling (Chapter 8) to the next step which involves the hydrolysis of the thioester linkage of another acetyl-CoA. When fatty acid oxidation proceeds under conditions of insufficient oxaloacetate, step 4 of the final cycle and thus reversal would be bypassed, leading directly to the formation of L-**3-hydroxy-3-methylglutaryl-CoA** (HMG-CoA). (Glutarate has the formula: $^-OOC\text{-}CH_2\text{-}CH_2\text{-}CH_2\text{-}COO^-$.) The formation of HMG-CoA involves the addition of an acetate group from acetyl-CoA (and water) to one end of the acetoacetyl-CoA. The following step, the cleavage of HMG-CoA by a specific lyase, involves the removal of an acetyl-CoA from the other end to yield **acetoacetate**. 3-Hydroxybutyrate is formed by the reduction of acetoacetate. The final concentrations of 3-hydroxybutyrate and acetoacetate are dependent on the [NADH]/[NAD$^+$] ratio in the mitochondrion. **Acetone** is produced either by slow **spontaneous decarboxylation** of acetoacetate or by the action of **acetoacetate decarboxylase**. 3-Hydroxybutyrate and acetoacetate do not undergo further metabolism by the liver.

3-Hydroxybutyrate and acetoacetate diffuse from the hepatocytes into the extracellular fluid and into the blood circulation which transports them to **3-oxoacyl-CoA transferase**-containing

The degradation of **monounsaturated fatty acids** is primarily by the β-oxidation pathway. However, the presence of the double bond necessitates an additional reaction. β-Oxidation proceeds until a *cis* double bond occurs in the Δ^3-position (between C-3 and C-4). The double bond is in both the wrong conformation and the wrong position for hydration. **Enoyl-CoA isomerase** converts the double bond into a *trans*-Δ^2 bond which can be utilized by an enoyl-CoA hydratase. The normal pathway for β-oxidation continues.

The degradation of **polyunsaturated fatty acids** requires enoyl-CoA isomerase and another enzyme called Δ^2, Δ^4-**dienoyl-CoA reductase**. The latter enzyme functions when the action of an acyl-CoA **dehydrogenase** produces a Δ^2, Δ^4-dienoyl-CoA. The NADPH-dependent reductase produces a *cis*-Δ^3-enoyl CoA, the conversion of which to a *trans*-Δ^2 bond is catalysed by enoyl-CoA isomerase. The *trans*-Δ^2-enoyl-CoA proceeds through the remaining cycles of the β-oxidation pathway.

tissues which can utilize them as sources of energy. In these tissues, 3-hydroxybutyrate is converted back into acetoacetate. Acetoacetate is converted into acetoacetyl-CoA by 3-oxoacyl-CoA transferase which requires succinyl-CoA as the source of coenzyme A. Acetoacetyl-CoA yields two acetyl-CoAs by the action of acetoacetyl-CoA thiolase. Cardiac muscle and the renal cortex preferentially use these ketone bodies rather than glucose. The brain prefers glucose to satisfy its high energy demands but during starvation etc. may adapt to use acetoacetate as an energy source.

Acetone may diffuse into the blood circulation and, being volatile, may be lost during respiratory gaseous exchange in the lungs. A few studies suggest that, under certain conditions, a minor pathway may operate to convert fat to carbohydrate in the mammalian liver. However, it is generally considered that, while the glyoxylate pathway enables such transformation in plants and certain micro-organisms on a significant scale, such a facility is absent from animal tissues.

Lipid biosynthesis

In man, there are important biosynthetic pathways involved in lipid metabolism, e.g. for the provision of:

- **metabolic fuels for energy release**, e.g. fatty acid biosynthesis;
- **cholesterol**, the precursor for further biosyntheses resulting in a variety of **steroid hormones, bile salts and vitamin D**.

The synthesis of fatty acids

The **biosynthesis of saturated fatty acids** in most respects is, in essence, a reversal of the β-oxidation degradative pathway, except that:

- the **cytosol** is the location for the biosynthetic pathway;
- **citrate** is employed in the transference of acetyl-CoA across the inner mitochondrial membrane;
- **acyl-carrier protein (ACP)** functions in the biosynthetic pathway and **malonyl-ACP** donates a two-carbon unit to the growing chain;
- **condensation, reduction, dehydration and reduction** constitute the four-step cycle in biosynthesis;
- the **reductant** is NADPH;
- **chain elongation** is driven by the release of CO_2;
- the D-**isomer** of 3-hydroxyacyl derivatives participate in biosynthesis.

Precursor acetyl-CoA, produced in the mitochondrial matrix,

Diabetes is a disease characterized by excessive urination together with an insatiable thirst. The urine from patients suffering from **diabetes mellitus** tastes sweet whereas that from patients with **diabetes insipidus** tastes normal! Diabetes insipidus is a disorder due to a deficiency of **antidiuretic hormone** (ADH).

Diabetes mellitus affects approximately 30 million humans world-wide. Primary diabetes mellitus has two major forms: **insulin-dependent** (IDDM or Type I) and **non-insulin-dependent** (NIDDM or Type II). **In IDDM**, which afflicts youngsters, the **β-cells of the islets of Langerhans** in the pancreas produce insufficient insulin. In the UK, about 0.3% of the population is treated by routine intravenous injections of genetically engineered human insulin. **In NIDDM**, which befalls the older, more affluent members of society, an insensitivity to insulin develops due to a reduction in the numbers of insulin receptors. In both **IDDM and NIDDM**, there is failure to maintain an adequate uptake of glucose into the muscle, liver and adipose cells. These cells respond by increased gluconeogenesis and degradation of lipid and protein. Elevated gluconeogenesis exhausts available oxaloacetate and results in enhanced production of ketone bodies. Acetone may be detectable from the breath of IDDM patients due to the high blood levels of ketone bodies.

Figure 12.5 *Transportation of acetyl-CoA from the mitochondrion for fatty acid synthesis*

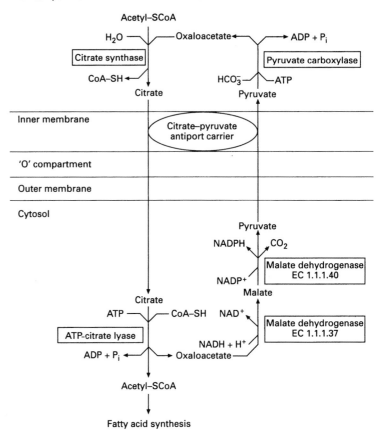

cannot pass through the inner membrane but the acetyl group is transferred across the membrane as citrate by the **citrate–pyruvate antiport carrier** (Figure 12.5). Acetyl-CoA, subsequently released from this citrate in the cytosol by the action of **ATP citrate lyase**, is utilized in the biosynthesis of fatty acids. The oxaloacetate can be reused indirectly to transfer an acetyl group of another matrix acetyl-CoA following conversion into malate then pyruvate to permit re-entry into the matrix in exchange for citrate.

Acetyl-CoA is carboxylated in the cytosol into **malonyl-CoA** by **acetyl-CoA carboxylase** (Figure 12.6) which contains the biotin (Figure 4.5c) prosthetic group essential for most carboxylation reactions. This reaction is important since it commits the acetyl-CoA to the route of fatty acid synthesis. Although HCO_3^- is required for fatty acid synthesis, its carbon atom is not a constituent of the product.

The activity of acetyl-CoA carboxylase is modulated allosterically (Chapter 4) by citrate as the positive modulator and palmitoyl-CoA as a negative modulator. The level of citrate is high when both acetyl-CoA and ATP are plentiful and available for use in fatty acid

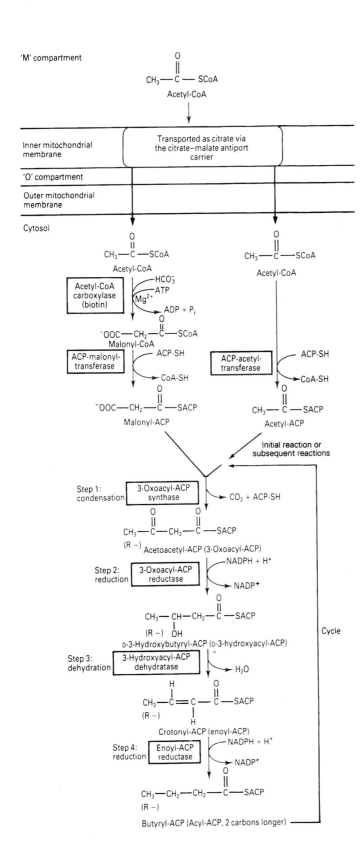

Figure 12.6 *Pathway of fatty acid synthesis*

The parameter of **body mass index** (BMI) is employed to assess the degree of obesity in humans. This index is easily calculated from the weight of the subject (in kilograms) divided by the square of the height (in metres), i.e. $kg\,m^{-2}$. A BMI for a male of 20–25 (or for a female of 19–24) is considered to be in the normal range, between 26 and 29 (25–29) is deemed overweight and > 30 (> 29) is indicative of obesity. Although it is recognized that excessive eating combined with limited exercise may result in obesity, the biochemical factors involved are now being identified.

Animal experimentation into obesity has focused on an **inbred strain of mice** which weigh about twice that of normal mice. These mice are homozygous for a mutation in a gene, called *ob*, expressed only in adipocytes which codes for the production of a 16 kDa protein called **leptin**. The *ob/ob* mice cannot synthesize leptin. Administration of leptin by injection to *ob/ob* mice corrects their obesity; after withdrawal of leptin the mice returned to their former size. It is believed that leptin is an adipose tissue hormone which signals to a region of the brain called the **hypothalamus** which controls appetite and metabolic rate. Recently, a leptin receptor which is expressed, although not exclusively, in the hypothalamus has been described. Also, a mutation in the gene encoding leptin in man has been reported in two severely obese children.

synthesis. High palmitoyl-CoA levels indicate an excess of fatty acids and that fatty acid synthesis is not desirable in the cell at that time. Palmitoyl-CoA reinforces its action on acetyl-CoA carboxylase by inhibiting citrate transport from the mitochondrion and NADPH generation by the pentose phosphate pathway.

Reactants participate in the synthetic pathway only when linked to **ACP**. Malonyl-CoA is converted into **malonyl-ACP** by a highly specific enzyme, **ACP-malonyltransferase**. Malonyl-ACP donates a two-carbon unit to elongate the acyl group attached to ACP.

In the initial step 1, malonyl-ACP condenses with acetyl-ACP formed from acetyl-CoA by the action of **ACP-acetyltransferase**. ACP-acetyltransferase is less specific than ACP-malonyltransferase and can also bond propionyl groups from propionyl-CoA to ACP to form **propionyl-ACP** in the synthesis of fatty acids with an odd number of carbons. During step 1, CO_2 is released to drive the formation of **acetoacetyl-ACP**, a reaction which otherwise would be thermodynamically unfavourable. The free energy provided by ATP in the acetyl-CoA carboxylase reaction is therefore employed in the synthesis of acetoacetyl-ACP.

In step 2, acetoacetyl-ACP is reduced by a specific **3-oxoacyl-ACP reductase**. The reducing agent is NADPH which is provided in two ways:

- by the action of an $NADP^+$-linked malate dehydrogenase (EC 1.1.1.40) which converts malate into pyruvate (Figure 12.5);
- the pentose phosphate pathway.

The product of this reaction is D-**3-hydroxybutyryl-ACP** (D-3-hydroxyacyl-ACP). After the first cycle, it is more convenient to use general names (in brackets) for the intermediates.

In step 3, D-3-hydroxybutyryl-ACP is dehydrated by a chain-length specific **3-hydroxyacyl-ACP dehydratase** to yield **crotonyl-ACP** (enoyl-ACP). **In step 4**, crotonyl-ACP is reduced by an **enoyl-ACP reductase** employing NADPH as reductant to produce **butyryl-ACP**, a compound which is two carbons longer than the acetyl-ACP which participated in step 1. The addition of a two-carbon unit requires two NADPH molecules. The butyryl-ACP re-enters the cycle at step 1 and condenses with a further malonyl-ACP. This cycling continues until **palmitoyl-ACP** is produced. Palmitoyl-ACP is hydrolysed to yield palmitate and ACP. Elongation beyond C_{16} requires requires additional enzymes present on the surface of the endoplasmic reticulum or in the mitochondria.

The enzymes of the mammalian synthetic cycle are a structurally organized multifunctional complex comprising **fatty acid synthase**, the major product of which is palmitate. Fatty acid synthase of animal systems is a dimer of two identical (molecular mass 250 kDa) polypeptide chains linked head-to-tail and each comprising three domains. The reactions at each domain are as follows:

- **the condensation reaction** of step 1 occurs at domain 1;
- **the reduction, dehydration and reduction reactions** of steps 2, 3 and 4 happen in catalytic pockets within domain 2;
- **the thioesterase activity** which liberates palmitate at the limit of chain length resides within domain 3.

The role of the **4′-phosphopantotheinyl group of ACP** is similar to that of lipoate in the pyruvate dehydrogenase complex (Chapter 10), that is to swing the product of one reaction to another catalytic site.

The **energetics** of fatty acid synthesis is not straightforward since, although ATP is apparently used only in the production of malonyl-CoA from acetyl-CoA (Figure 12.6), ATP is also required:

- **to recover acetyl-CoA from citrate** after transport across the inner mitochondrial membrane (Figure 12.5);
- **in the production of NADPH by the pentose phosphate pathway** if glucose is the source of glucose 6-phosphate. There is a reduced ATP requirement if glycogen (Chapter 9) provides the glucose 6-phosphate.

The synthesis of cholesterol

Cholesterol (Chapter 6) is synthesized from acetyl-CoA primarily in the liver, but also in the small intestine, skin and adrenals, by a metabolic pathway which is located in the cell cytosol but involves the endoplasmic reticulum. Acetyl-CoA generated in the mitochondrial matrix is transported as citrate into the cytosol (Figure 12.5) to serve as a precursor of fatty acid or cholesterol biosynthesis. Figure 12.7 shows the biosynthetic sequence of reactions as 18 acetyl-CoA molecules are converted into one molecule of cholesterol.

The initial reactions in cholesterol biosynthesis are identical to those of the synthesis of ketone bodies in the mitochondria (Figure 12.4). Two acetyl-CoA molecules are thiolated to form **acetoacetyl-CoA** which reacts with a third acetyl-CoA molecule to form L-3-hydroxy-3-methylglutaryl-CoA (HMG-CoA). HMG-CoA is reduced by four electrons donated by two NADPH to yield **mevalonate** under the influence of **HMG-CoA reductase**, a major regulatory influence in cholesterol biosynthesis.

Mevalonate is converted into two key five-carbon building blocks:

- **isopentenyl diphosphate**, the synthesis of which requires four ATP, **mevalonate kinase, phosphomevalonate kinase, diphosphomevalonate kinase** and **diphosphomevalonate decarboxylase**;
- **dimethylallyl diphosphate** which is produced by an isomerization from isopentenyl diphosphate catalysed by **isopentenyl diphosphate Δ-isomerase**.

Unsaturated fatty acids are synthesized from saturated fatty acids by the action of **desaturases** located in the endoplasmic reticulum. **Stearoyl-CoA desaturase**, utilizing mainly NADH (NADPH is less commonly employed) and O_2, catalyses the most common desaturation and functions to create a double bond between C-9 and C-10 (Δ^9). Other important desaturases operate at Δ^6 and Δ^5. When the substrate is a saturated fatty acid, the first double bond is inserted at Δ^9. When the substrate is already unsaturated, subsequent double bonds are inserted between the double bond nearest the carboxyl group and the carboxyl group itself. This means that animal tissues cannot synthesize **linoleate** with an additional double bond at Δ^{12} and **linolenate** with additional double bonds at Δ^{12} and Δ^{15} (Table 6.1). Linoleate and linolenate must be supplied in the mammalian diet, usually from plants, and are therefore called **essential fatty acids**.

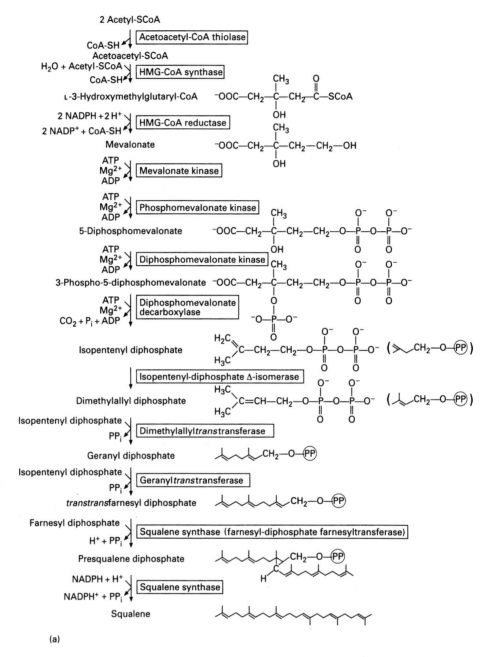

Figure 12.7 *The biosynthesis of cholesterol: (a) acetyl-CoA to squalene.*

Dimethylallyl*trans*transferase condenses one dimethylallyl diphosphate with one isopentenyl diphosphate to generate a 10-carbon intermediate, **geranyl diphosphate**. The head-to-tail addition of another isopentenyl diphosphate yields the 15-carbon compound **farnesyl diphosphate**. Both of these reactions proceed with the release of pyrophosphate, enzymic hydrolysis of which drives the reactions in the direction of farnesyl diphosphate.

(b)

Figure 12.7 *cont.*   *(b) squalene to cholesterol*

Squalene synthase is responsible for the next two reactions. Squalene synthase contains at least two catalytic activities:

- A **farnesyl-diphosphate farnesyltransferase** activity which causes two farnesyl diphosphate molecules to interact in a tail-to-tail fashion to produce the 30-carbon intermediate, **presqualene diphosphate.**

- **NADPH-linked pyrophosphate generation and rearrangement activities** which convert presqualene diphosphate into the 30-carbon compound, squalene.

Squalene is converted to **squalene 2,3-epoxide** by **squalene monooxygenase,** an enzyme bound to the endoplasmic reticulum. Squalene monooxygenase requires FAD, NADPH, molecular oxygen and a cytosolic protein called the **soluble protein activator.** Squalene 2,3-epoxide undergoes numerous bond rearrangements involving hydride ions and methyl groups, catalysed by **lanosterol synthase** to generate **lanosterol.** Another 19 reactions are required to convert lanosterol to 27-carbon cholesterol. Cholesterol may be

There are two pathways for the synthesis of phosphatidate in mammalian cells: acylation reactions from *sn*-glycerol 3-phosphate and an acylation reaction from **glycerone phosphate** which provides an alternative route to phosphatidate in adipocytes, hepatocytes and yeast, employing **glycerone-phosphate acyltransferase** located in the endoplasmic reticulum. The acylation is followed by an NADPH-linked reduction.

The **phosphatidate** is dephosphorylated by the phosphatase activity of the membrane-bound **triacylglycerol synthase complex** to yield **1,2-diacyl-*sn*-glycerol**. 1,2-Diacylglycerol may be converted to triacylglycerols by subsequent esterification at the *sn*-3 position by the **diacylglycerol acyltransferase** activity of the complex. Although the entire reaction sequence for triacylglycerol synthesis occurs in the cell cytosol, most of the enzymes are associated with the cytosolic surface of the membranes of the endoplasmic reticulum. In the intestine, however, dietary triacylglycerols are degraded by lipases to *sn*-2-monoacylglycerols which are then used to synthesize new triacylglycerols by acylation reactions catalysed by **monoacylglycerol acyltransferase** and **diacylglycerol acyltransferase**.

Phosphoacylglycerols may be produced by the addition of phosphorylcholine or phosphorylethanolamine moieties from CDP derivatives to 1,2-diacylglycerol through the action of the appropriate transferase, e.g. **diacylglycerol cholinephosphotransferase**.

Figure 12.8 *Synthesis of steroid hormones in the adrenals (plus ovaries)*

esterified by **cholesterol acyltransferase** on the cytoplasmic surface of the endoplasmic reticulum.

The metabolism of steroid hormones

Steroid hormones (Chapter 6) are synthesized from cholesterol by a set of pathways, the major reactions of which are presented in Figure 12.8. The principal site of steroid hormone syntheses is the **adrenal glands** where **aldosterone, cortisol, progesterone and testosterone** may be produced. The major site of **testosterone production** from 17α-hydroxyprogesterone is the **testes**. **Oestradiol** is not synthesized from testosterone in the adrenals but is produced primarily by the **ovaries** and, in pregnant females, the **placenta**. The testes produce some of the oestrogen

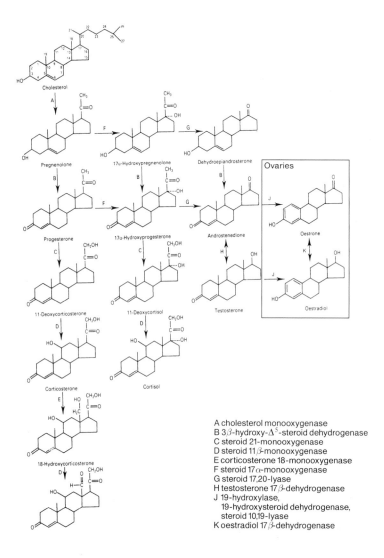

A cholesterol monooxygenase
B 3β-hydroxy-Δ⁵-steroid dehydrogenase
C steroid 21-monooxygenase
D steroid 11β-monooxygenase
E corticosterone 18-monooxygenase
F steroid 17α-monooxygenase
G steroid 17,20-lyase
H testosterone 17β-dehydrogenase
J 19-hydroxylase,
  19-hydroxysteroid dehydrogenase,
  steroid 10,19-lyase
K oestradiol 17β-dehydrogenase

found at low levels in men. Other pathways do exist. For example, testosterone may be produced by an alternative route from steroid sulphates, conjugates primarily important in the removal of steroids from the body.

In the **mitochondria of adrenal cells**, cholesterol loses its aliphatic tail by the actions of **cholesterol monooxygenase** which produces **pregnenolone** in three stages:

- hydroxylation at C-20;
- hydroxylation at C-22;
- cleavage of the tail at C-20.

Pregnenolone is converted into progesterone in the endoplasmic reticulum of adrenal cells by the oxidation of the 3β-hydroxyl group into a ketone group and isomerization of the Δ^5 double bond to the Δ^4 position. The conversion of progesterone into aldosterone occurs in the mitochondria of cells in the adrenal cortex. Hydroxylations of the C-21 methyl group and C-11 methylene group are followed by the two-stage oxidation of the C-18 methyl group into an aldehydic group to yield aldosterone.

Cholesterol monooxygenase, steroid 11β-monooxygenase and **corticosterone 18-monooxygenase** are **cytochrome P$_{450}$ enzymes** (Figure 9.9) which employ reduced ferredoxin and molecular oxygen to effect their catalyses during steroid biosynthesis. **Steroid 11β-monooxygenase** also hydroxylates steroids at the C-18 position and is responsible for the conversion of **11-deoxycorticosterone** into corticosterone and **18-hydroxycorticosterone** into aldosterone.

The mitochondria of cells in the adrenal cortex are also the location of cortisol synthesis. Cortisol is synthesized from **17α-hydroxyprogesterone** which may be synthesized from pregnenolone by two routes dependent upon the order of activity of two enzymes, **3β-hydroxy-Δ^5-steroid dehydrogenase** and **steroid 17α-monooxygenase**. The steps from 17α-hydroxyprogesterone to cortisol are identical to those from progesterone to corticosterone in the biosynthesis of aldosterone. In the adrenals and testes, 17α-hydroxyprogesterone is converted by **a steroid 17,20-lyase** into **androstenedione** from which **testosterone** is produced by a reduction catalysed by **testosterone 17β-dehydrogenase** employing NADPH as coenzyme.

In the **endoplasmic reticulum of ovarian and placental cells**, testosterone is converted into oestradiol by a series of reactions. Initially, testosterone is hydroxylated by **a 19-hydroxylase activity** and the newly formed C-19 alcohol group is oxidized by **a dehydrogenase activity** to an aldehydic group. Cleavage at C-10 by **a 10,19-lyase activity** releases the C-19 atom as **formaldehyde**. The steroid product is unstable and ring A rearranges spontaneously without enzymic involvement to become an aromatic ring

---

Leukotrienes (Chapter 6) are synthesized from **arachidonate** in polymorphonuclear leukocytes and mast cells. A single oxygen molecule is added to the C-5 position of arachidonate. An accompanying double bond shift to the Δ^6 position yields a **5-hydroperoxy derivative** (5-HPETE). This initial reaction is catalysed by the enzyme known as **5-lipoxygenase** (12- and 15- lipoxygenases yield hepoxins and lipoxins respectively). Subsequent dehydration produces the epoxide-containing **leukotriene A$_4$** (LTA$_4$). **Hydrolysis** of the allylic epoxide yields **LTB$_4$**. The addition of the tripeptide glutathione to the C-6 position of LTA$_4$ together with the formation of a hydroxyl group at the C-5 position produces **LTC$_4$**. The enzymic removal of firstly the glutamyl residue and secondly the glycyl residue yields **LTD$_4$** and **LTE$_4$** respectively.

Atherosclerosis, a degenerative disease of large and medium-sized arteries, is characterized by lipid deposition and fibrosis. A high serum cholesterol level is considered to be one of the main risk factors. The reduction of serum cholesterol levels may be achieved by the inhibition of intracellular cholesterol biosynthesis. Two important families of compounds under development as 'anticholesterol agents' are the **squalestatins** and the **zaragozic acids** which are potent inhibitors of squalene synthase.

with a C-3 β-hydroxyl group. The catalysts for these reactions are sometimes termed 'the aromatase complex'.

Aldosterone, cortisol, oestradiol and testosterone are major secretory products. They are synthesized in response to the interaction of cell-surface receptors with circulatory protein hormones of pituitary (a gland in the brain) origin called **tropic hormones** or **tropins**. There is no appreciable storage of steroid hormones in the endocrine glands. The hormones are synthesized as required and secreted into the blood circulation where transport proteins may be involved in their distribution to target tissues:

- **cortisol-binding globulin** (**transcortin**) carries cortisol, corticosterone and progesterone;

- **sex hormone-binding globulin** transports **testosterone** and **oestrogen**.

Steroid hormones permeate the plasma membranes of target cells to bind to specific cytoplasmic or nuclear receptors (Chapter 8). Many target cells, however, reduce the Δ^4 double bond of testosterone to yield **5α-dihydrotestosterone** which has a higher affinity for the androgen receptor.

The liver is the major site for the inactivation of steroid hormones mainly by stereospecific reduction and/or methylation. These metabolites are conjugated through their hydroxyl groups to sulphate or glucuronate to promote urinary excretion.

Suggested further reading

Eaton, S., Bartlett, K. and Pourfarzam, M. (1996). Mammalian mitochondrial β-oxidation. *Biochemical Journal* **320**, 345–357.

Faergeman, N.J. and Knudsen, J. (1997). Role of long-chain fatty acyl-CoA esters in the regulation of metabolism and in cell signalling. *Biochemical Journal* **323**, 1–12.

Flier, J.S. (1995). The adipocyte: storage depot or node on the energy information superhighway? *Cell* **80**, 15–18.

Hampton, R., Dimster-Denk, D. and Rine, J. (1996). The biology of HMG-CoA reductase: the pros of contra-regulation. *Trends in Biochemical Sciences* **21**, 140–145.

Zammit, V.A. (1996). Role of insulin in hepatic fatty acid partitioning: emerging concepts. *Biochemical Journal* **314**, 1–14.

Self-assessment questions

1. Calculate the energy yield, in numbers of molecules of ATP, when one molecule of : (a) a C_{12} saturated fatty acid; (b) a C_{17} saturated fatty acid; (c) a C_{12} unsaturated fatty acid are completely oxidized.

2. Distinguish between the biological roles of serum albumin and chylomicrons.

3. Cholesterol contains 27 carbon atoms but its biosynthesis uses 36 carbon atoms in the form of acetyl groups. Account for the 18 acetyl-CoA molecules required for the biosynthesis of cholesterol.

4. Assuming that malate molecules enter the mitochondria via the citrate–pyruvate antiport carrier, calculate the number of NADPH molecules which must be provided from the pentose phosphate pathway during the synthesis of palmitate.

5. In cholesterol biosynthesis, two acetyl-CoA molecules are condensed by acetoacetyl-CoA thiolase into acetoacetyl-CoA in the cytosol. Why is this reaction not employed in fatty acid biosynthesis?

6. Construct a list of differences between the pathways for β-oxidation and the biosynthesis of fatty acids.

7. In fatty acid synthesis, explain the statement that 'there is a reduced ATP requirement if glycogen provides the glucose-6-phosphate' rather than glucose for NADPH generation by the pentose phosphate pathway.

8. Using structural formulae, draw the reaction by which a C_{18} saturated fatty acid is converted into a C_{18} monounsaturated fatty acid.

9. Identify some of the enzymes involved in steroid biosynthesis from the following descriptions: (a) it catalyses the reduction of the C-17 ketone group of androstenedione to produce the male sex hormone; (b) it catalyses the hydroxylation of the C-11 methylene group of 11-deoxycortisol; (c) it catalyses the oxidation of a C-18 primary alcohol group into a C-18 aldehydic group in aldosterone biosynthesis; (d) it converts the 3β-hydroxyl group of 17α-hydroxypregnenolone into 17α-hydroxyprogesterone.

10. What are the functions of the $4'$-phosphopantotheinyl group of ACP and lipoate in the pyruvate dehydrogenase complex?

Key Concepts and Facts

Lipid Degradation

- The β-oxidation pathway occurs in the mitochondrial matrix and involves coenzyme A derivatives of fatty acids.

- Carnitine serves as a vehicle for the translocation of acyl groups into the mitochondrial matrix.

- The β-oxidation pathway involves cycles of oxidation, hydration, oxidation and thiolysis, each step being catalysed by multiple enzymes with different chain-length specificities.

- Each cycle of the β-oxidation pathway generates one NADH, one $FADH_2$ and one acetyl-CoA which are employed to generate ATP via oxidative phosphorylation.

- Acetyl-CoA may be converted into ketone bodies by the liver when oxaloacetate is not available.

Lipid Biosynthesis

- The biosynthesis of fatty acids occurs in the cytosol and involves acyl-carrier-protein derivatives.

- Citrate is the vehicle for translocation of acetyl groups into the cytosol.

- Malonyl-ACP donates two-carbon units to each biosynthetic cycle.

- Biosynthesis of fatty acids involves cycles of condensation, reduction dehydration and reduction, the enzyme specification being located on a single polypeptide chain.

- In the liver, acetyl-CoA molecules provide the carbon atoms for the five-carbon building blocks called isopentenyl diphosphate and dimethylallyl diphosphate, used in the synthesis of lanosterol.

The Metabolism of Steroid Hormones

- The major site of steroid hormone biosynthesis is the adrenal glands.

- Steroid hormone biosynthesis involves numerous monooxygenase, dehydrogenase and lyase activities.

- Steroid hormones are inactivated by the liver and excreted as conjugates in the urine.

Answers to questions (Chapter 12)

1. (a) 78 ATP. Use Table 12.1 to calculate the number of cycles, then use the layout of Table 12.2 to complete the calculation; (b) 100 ATP. Remember the cycle terminates in propionyl-CoA; (c) 78 ATP. The additional steps do not utilize or produce ATP.

2. Serum albumin transports fatty acids released from triacylglycerols in adipose tissue to tissues which cannot satisfy their energy requirements from dietary sources or glycogen reserves. Chylomicrons (Chapter 6) transport triacylglycerols of dietary origin from the small intestine to adipose tissue.

3. See Figure 12.7. An intermediate presqualene diphosphate is synthesized from two farnesyl diphosphates. Each farnesyl diphosphate is produced from one dimethylallyl diphosphate plus two isopentenyl diphosphates which in turn are produced from the intermediate mevalonate, the synthesis of which utilizes three acetyl-CoA molecules, i.e. $2 \times 3 \times 3 = 18$ acetyl-CoA. Note that the six carbon atoms are lost as CO_2 at the decarboxylase step and also three carbons are lost as methyl groups in the lanosterol to cholesterol stage.

4. 6 NADPH. Synthesis of palmitate requires eight two-carbon units. Eight NADPH are generated when eight acetyl-CoA are translocated from the mitochondrion to the cytosol. The pentose phosphate pathway provides the remainder, i.e. $14 - 8 = 6$, provided that malate molecules are not returned to the mitochondria via the citrate–malate antiport carrier. For each malate returned in this way, an additional NADPH must be provided by the pentose phosphate pathway.

5. The thiolase reaction, although reversible, favours the cleavage reaction. In cholesterol biosynthesis, subsequent reactions, i.e. those catalysed by HMG-CoA reductase and the kinases, drive the thiolase-catalysed condensation. In fatty acid biosynthesis, however, the thiolase condensations should occur at the entry into each consecutive cycle. Eight such reactions are clearly energetically unfavourable and therefore, in energetic terms, it is better that a favourable reaction is repeatedly employed.

6. β-Oxidation vs. synthesis: activation in cytosol vs. chain elongation driven by release of CO_2; occurs in mitochondria vs. cytosol; transport across inner membrane involves carnitine vs. citrate; use of CoA derivatives vs. ACP derivatives; four-step cycle of oxidation, hydration, oxidation and thiolysis vs. four-step cycle of condensation, reduction, dehydration and reduction; stereochemistry regarding L-hydroxybutyryl-CoA vs. D-hydroxybutyryl-ACP; generates reduced coenzymes (NADH and FADH$_2$) vs. uses reduced coenzyme (NADPH); provides energy vs. uses energy; releases two-carbon units in the form of acetyl-CoA vs. adds two-carbon units from malonyl-ACP; presence of a multisubunit trifunctional enzyme complex vs. multidomain polypeptide chain.

7. Glycogenolysis produces mainly glucose 6-phosphate by the action of phosphorylase and phosphoglucomutase. There is no ATP requirement in these reactions. However, some glucose is produced by debranching and requires ATP and hexokinase for phosphorylation.

8.

$$CH_3-(CH_2)_{16}-\overset{\overset{\displaystyle O}{||}}{C}-SCoA \xrightarrow[\substack{O_2 \qquad \text{Stearoyl-CoA} \\ \text{desaturase}}]{\substack{NADH+H^+ \qquad\qquad NAD^+ \\ \\ 2H_2O}} CH_3-(CH_2)_7-CH=CH-(CH_2)_7-\overset{\overset{\displaystyle O}{||}}{C}-SCoA$$

9. (a) Testosterone 17β-dehydrogenase; (b) steroid 11β-monooxygenase; (c) steroid 11β-monooxygenase; (d) 3β-hydroxy-Δ^5-steroid dehydrogenase.

10. To provide a flexible 'arm' to move intermediates from one catalytic site to another in the enzymic complex.

Chapter 13

Amino acid metabolism and protein synthesis

Learning objectives

After studying this chapter you should confidently be able to:

Discuss mechanisms for the deamination of amino acids during their catabolism.

Identify the fates of the carbon skeletons of amino acids.

Discuss the transport of ammonia from peripheral tissues to the liver in man.

Detail the reactions of the urea cycle and their intracellular compartmentalization.

State the significance of the classification of amino acids as essential and non-essential.

Compare and contrast the mechanisms by which mRNA is translated into polypeptide chains in prokaryotic and eukaryotic cells.

Describe the roles of amino acid-tRNA ligases.

Discuss the roles of the various protein factors involved in the initiation, elongation and termination phases of translation.

Review co- and post- translational modifications to polypeptide chains.

α-Amino acids are the monomeric building blocks of proteins. **Glutamate and glutamine** are also the only source of nitrogen atoms available to mammals for the biosynthesis of other α-amino acids and all other biologically important non-protein nitrogen-containing compounds, e.g. amines, haem, purine and pyrimidine bases.

Excess dietary amino acids, unlike glucose or fatty acids, are not stored. Amino acids which are surfeit to the demands of synthetic pathways are not excreted but are utilized as sources of energy, either directly or indirectly. About 10–15% of human energy

Amino acids are the sources of all nitrogen and some carbon atoms of **heterocyclic compounds** (Figure 2.2). The atoms of the **pyrimidine ring** are derived from two amino acids, aspartate and glutamine, and CO_2. Atoms N-1, C-4, C-5 and C-6 come from aspartate, C-2 from CO_2 and N-3 from glutamine.

The atoms of the **purine ring** are derived from three amino acids, aspartate, glutamine and glycine, CO_2 and formyl groups. Atom N-1 comes from aspartate, N-3 and N-9 from glutamine, C-4, C-5 and N-7 are the framework atoms of glycine and C-6 from CO_2. Atoms C-2 and C-8 are donated by two **formylation reactions** in which different **folate derivatives**, N^{10}-formyltetrahydrofolate and N^5, N^{10}-methenyltetrahydrofolate respectively, are formyl group donors.

Biosynthesis does not produce free heterocyclic compounds but nucleotides. Although purines contain a pyrimidine ring, the synthetic pathways are distinct with the imidazole ring being initially constructed. Since synthesis of pyrimidine and purine nucleotides *de novo* (anew) is energetically expensive, heterocyclic bases from dietary sources or recycled from the turnover of nucleic acids by the **salvage pathways,** involving **hypoxanthine-guanine phosphoribosyltransferase,** facilitate considerable savings in ATP.

requirements are derived from the oxidation of amino acids. It is, however, only the chains of carbon atoms, called **carbon skeletons,** which are useful as metabolic fuels and not the α-amino groups. **Deamination** of some amino acids results in the production of toxic ammonia. Ammonia is converted to **urea**, a non-toxic product at physiological levels, which provides a convenient soluble vehicle for the disposal of amino nitrogen atoms.

In man, $\sim 50\%$ of body protein is replaced every 5–6 months. This turnover involves a controlled balance between degradation and synthesis. The liver is the major site for both the biosynthesis and breakdown of amino acids in man. Since there are 20 amino acids found in mammalian proteins, there are about 20 pathway branches concerned with their catabolism and a similar number involved in their anabolism. For this reason, only the underpinning principles of amino acid metabolism are considered here.

A cell in general will utilize thousands of different proteins which constitute over half of the total dry mass of the cell. Proteins are central to the cell's well-being, growth and development. Proteins are the final recipients of the information contained within the exons of the genome. RNA is transcribed from the gene and in mammalian cells is processed into mRNA which directs the assembly of amino acids into the primary structure of specific proteins. mRNA is translated by the ribosomes from which a polypeptide chain emerges.

This chapter considers the degradation of amino acids, disposal of amino nitrogen as urea and the *de novo* synthesis of amino acids for protein synthesis. The chapter also discusses the employment of amino acids in the translation of mRNA into a polypeptide chain.

Amino acid metabolism

There are significant differences in the metabolism of amino acids in micro-organisms, plants and animals. Only their metabolism in mammals will be discussed here.

Degradation of amino acids

The **initial reaction** in the liver may involve **deamination** by:

- **transamination** reactions which collect the α-amino groups in a single substance, namely glutamate (Figure 13.1a);

- **oxidative deamination** by glutamate dehydrogenase (Figure 13.1b) and relatively minor processes involving L- and D-amino acid oxidases;

- **direct deamination** by serine dehydratase and threonine dehydratase.

Transamination is the predominant mechanism of the removal of α-amino groups from most L-amino acids (Figure 13.1a). The

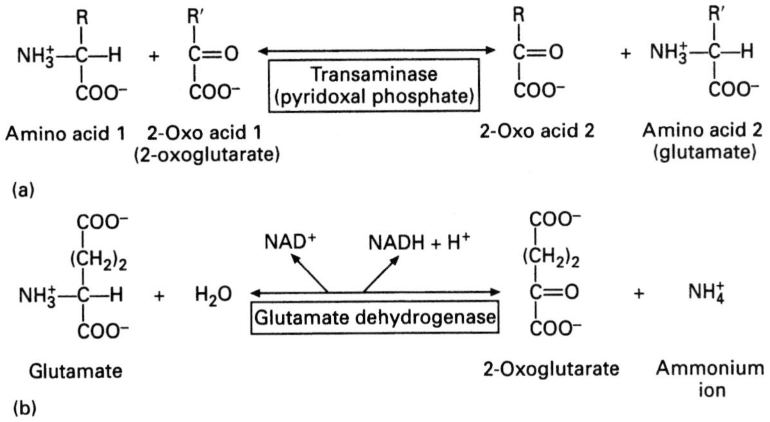

Figure 13.1 *Deamination reactions in amino acid metabolism: (a) transamination; (b) glutamate dehydrogenase reaction*

transaminases contain **pyridoxal phosphate**, a derivative of the vitamin pyridoxine (B_6), as a prosthetic group. This prosthetic group plays a crucial role in the mechanism of action of these enzymes. In man, the reactant 2-oxo acid is usually 2-oxoglutarate which is converted to glutamate as the amino acid product. Since the reaction is readily reversible, its product must be continuously removed to permit complete deamination of the reactant amino acid. Glutamate is therefore deaminated by a mechanism which is not dependent upon transamination, i.e. by **glutamate dehydrogenase**. Glutamate dehydrogenase is extremely important in the formation of urea. Although readily reversible, its primary role in man is the NAD^+-dependent deamination of glutamate.

L-**Amino acid oxidase** activity is low in tissues, including the liver and kidney. D-**Amino acid oxidase** is, however, present at high concentrations especially in the kidney and functions in the deamination of D-amino acids of bacterial origin (Chapter 5).

Not all L-α-amino acids undergo transamination. Small amounts of serine and threonine may be directly deaminated by specific dehydratases. These pyridoxal phosphate-dependent enzymes are so called because, in their mode of action, the substrate is initially dehydrated before subsequent deamination. The bulk of the serine and threonine is, however, processed by more complex degradative pathways.

Deamination yields the carbon skeletons of the amino acids which are independently catabolized into major metabolic intermediates (Table 13.1). The intermediates may participate in the tricarboxylic acid cycle (Chapter 10) to produce energy mainly through oxidative phosphorylation (Chapter 11). When the demand for energy is low, those carbon skeletons which are potential sources of malate may be employed in gluconeogenesis. Malate, an intermediate in the first bypass reaction of gluconeogenesis (Chapter 9), may be translocated into the cytosol and give rise

Alkaptonuria is a relatively rare disease with an incidence of 1 in 100,000. Originally called **black urine disease** on account of the urine of patients turning dark upon standing, alkaptonuria was the first disease identified as **an inherited disease**. In 1898, Archibald Garrod identified **homogentisic acid**, an intermediate in phenylalanine degradation, as the substance responsible for the above colour change. Homogentisic acid polymerizes to produce the blackish pigment which is deposited in cartilage and other connective tissues. Garrod hypothesized that the increased excretion of homogentisic acid resulted from a deficiency of the enzyme which was responsible for its degradation and coined the term 'inborn error of metabolism'. The deficient enzyme was identified in the 1950s as **homogentisate 1,2-dioxygenase** which cleaves the aromatic ring of homogentisate. In 1996, the gene which encodes this enzyme was cloned. Sequencing provided final proof that mutations in this gene were responsible for the loss of enzymic activity in alkaptonuric patients.

Table 13.1 *The fate of the carbon skeletons of deaminated amino acids*

Carbon skeleton	Major metabolite(s) produced
Alanine Glycine Serine Cysteine	Pyruvate*
Threonine	Pyruvate + succinyl-CoA†
Tryptophan	Pyruvate + acetoacetyl-CoA‡
Arginine Proline Histidine Glutamine Glutamate	2-Oxoglutarate†
Valine Methionine	Succinyl-CoA
Isoleucine	Succinyl-CoA + acetyl-CoA‡
Phenylalanine Tryosine	Fumarate† + acetoacetyl-CoA
Asparagine Aspartate	Oxaloacetate†
Lysine	Acetoacetyl-CoA
Leucine	Acetyle-CoA + acetoacetyl-CoA

* End product of glycolysis.
† Tricarboxylic acid cycle intermediate.
‡ Fatty acid oxidation intermediate.

to phospho*enol*pyruvate. Other amino acids may produce acetyl-CoA and/or acetoacetyl-CoA which may be further metabolized to ketone bodies (Chapter 12). Amino acids may therefore be classified in terms of their catabolism into:

- **Glucogenic**, i.e. those yielding pyruvate or tricarboxylic acid cycle intermediates.

- **Ketogenic**, i.e. those serving as precursors of ketone bodies. Leucine is the only truly ketogenic amino acid. (Lysine may appear to qualify for inclusion into this class but experimental evidence shows that it is not strongly ketogenic.)

- **Both glucogenic and ketogenic**, namely isoleucine, tyrosine, phenylalanine and tryptophan.

In man, the ammonium ions are converted into urea in the liver. However, peripheral tissues may degrade amino acids. Any release of ammonia into the blood circulation is potentially dangerous because the brain is very sensitive to ammonia which may cause mental retardation, coma or death. Ammonia is therefore transported to the liver from other tissues as:

- **Glutamine.** In most tissues, glutamate is aminated to **glutamine** by the action of **glutamate-ammonia ligase** in an ATP-utilizing reaction. Glutamine is electrically neutral and can pass through the plasma membrane. Glutamine acts as a non-toxic vehicle for delivery of ammonia to the liver where cytosolic **glutaminase** deaminates glutamine, the released NH_4^+ ions being available for urea synthesis.

- **Alanine.** In muscle cells, alanine is produced by the **glucose–alanine cycle**. Muscle derives most of its energy from glucose by glycolysis (Chapter 9). The generated pyruvate is transaminated with glutamate to yield alanine which is transported via the bloodstream to the liver where a transamination in the reverse direction occurs. The resultant glutamate molecules are acted upon by glutamate dehydrogenase to yield NH_4^+ ions for urea synthesis.

The urea cycle

Urea is synthesized by the first metabolic pathway to be elucidated. The cyclic pathway was discovered, in outline, by **Krebs and Henseleit** in 1932. A major function of the liver is urea biosynthesis but enzymes of the pathway also occur in kidney, skin and brain plus some other cells where their primary purpose is to produce arginine. The **urea cycle** (Figure 13.2) operates across two intracellular compartments:

- **the mitochondrial matrix** in which the initial reaction occurs;
- **the cytosol**, the site of the other three reactions and urea production.

The substrate of the urea cycle is **carbamoyl phosphate** produced in the mitochondrial matrix by the action of **carbamoyl-phosphate synthase (ammonia)**. Note that a different enzyme called carbamoyl-phosphate synthase (glutamine-hydrolysing) participates in pyrimidine biosynthesis which occurs in the cytosol. The mitochondrial reaction utilizes an ammonium ion (NH_4^+), delivered into the mitochondrion as glutamate by the action of the glutamate–aspartate and glutamate–hydroxyl ion antiport carriers. **Oxidative deamination** of glutamate by **glutamate dehydrogenase** releases an NH_4^+ ion. The NH_4^+ ion and a bicarbonate ion constitute the carbamoyl group in an energy-demanding (two ATP) reaction. The **flux of the urea cycle** is regulated by carbamoyl-phosphate synthase (ammonia) in two ways:

- **allosteric regulation** dependent upon the positive modulator N-acetylglutamate which is synthesized from glutamate and acetyl-CoA by amino-acid acetyltransferase;
- **fluctuations in enzyme levels** resultant from modulations in the expression of its gene induced by the protein content of the diet.

In the first reaction of the cycle, the carbamoyl group is transferred from carbamoyl phosphate to **ornithine** by **ornithine carbamoyl-**

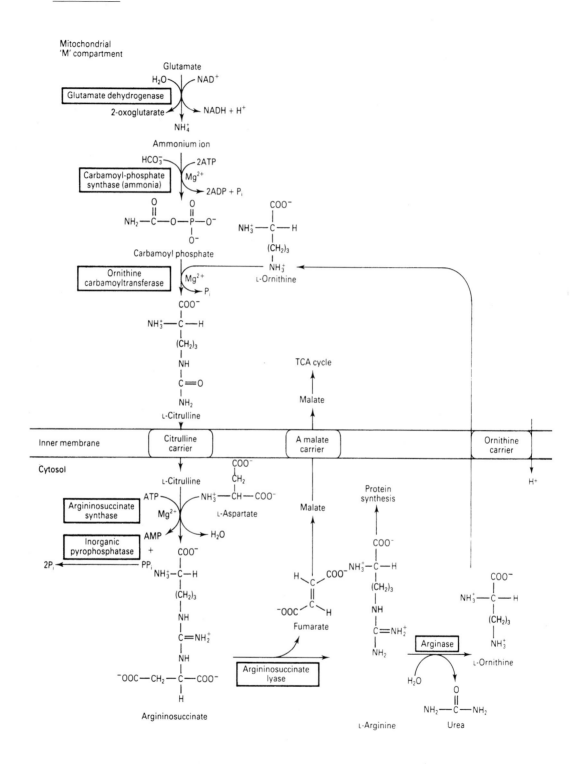

Figure 13.2   *The urea cycle*

transferase to yield **citrulline**. Neither of these amino acids are known to occur in natural proteins.

The remainder of the cycle reactions occur in the cytosol. Citrulline is therefore transported by a specific uniport carrier across the inner mitochondrial membrane. The carbonyl carbon atom of citrulline and the amino group of **aspartate** form a covalent linkage in a condensation reaction to form **argininosuccinate**. This reaction, catalysed by **argininosuccinate synthase**, is readily reversible but is driven forward by the irreversible hydrolysis of the pyrophosphate by-product. The aspartate is mainly derived from glutamate by the action of aspartate transaminase.

Argininosuccinate is cleaved by **argininosuccinate lyase** into **arginine** and **fumarate**. Arginine feeds back as a positive modulator of amino-acid acetyltransferase and, through the effects on this enzyme, arginine indirectly regulates the activity of carbamoyl-phosphate synthase (ammonia). The arginine concentration therefore regulates the synthesis of arginine and determines the rate at which amino nitrogen is excreted from the body. Fumarate, which conserves the carbon atoms of the aspartate, may be converted by cytosolic molecules of fumarate hydratase (Chapter 10) into malate which is primarily translocated into the mitochondrial pool of tricarboxylic acid cycle intermediates. Although in theory some cytosolic malate may be converted into aspartate via oxaloacetate and a transaminase reaction, experimental evidence indicates that the fumarate yields glucose. The aspartate is clearly derived from alanine by transamination.

The final reaction of the cycle involves the hydrolysis of arginine by **arginase** to yield **urea** and ornithine. The cycle is completed by the translocation of ornithine to the mitochondrion where carbamoylation produces another citrulline. The sources of the atoms of the urea molecule are as follows:

- **Both nitrogen atoms** are donated by glutamate. One atom enters the cycle via aspartate whilst the other enters in carbamoyl phosphate.

- **The carbon atom** is derived from the bicarbonate ion resulting from oxidative decarboxylation reactions (e.g. in the tricarboxylic acid cycle).

- **The oxygen atom** comes from the water molecule participating in the arginase reaction.

Urea is therefore a vehicle for the disposal of both NH_4^+ and HCO_3^- ions. The cost of urea synthesis is four ATP; two in the synthesis of carbamoyl phosphate and two equivalents in the synthesis of argininosuccinate. In the latter case, although only one ATP is used, it is hydrolysed to AMP from which two phosphorylation reactions are required to resynthesize ATP.

Urea diffuses readily across the plasma membrane of liver cells into the blood circulation. Small amounts of urea are secreted in

Arginine is the substrate from which **nitric oxide (NO)** is synthesized. NO is a very toxic gas which, being a free radical, has a short life. After about 6–10 s NO is converted into nitrates and nitrites by O_2 and H_2O. NO has a wide range of important biological activities including the regulation of arterial diameter upon its synthesis by vascular endothelium, a bacteriocidal agent in phagocytic cells especially macrophages, a neurotransmitter in the brain and an inhibitor of platelet aggregation.

NO is synthesized by the action of three isoforms of the enzyme **nitric oxide synthase (NOS)** which are the products of three distinct genes. Both NOS I and NOS III are tissue constituents, NOS I being first identified in neurones, whereas NOS III was originally found in endothelial cells. The enzymic activities of both isoenzymes are dependent upon elevated levels of calcium ions. On the other hand, NOS II is an inducible, Ca^{2+}-independent enzyme, expressed in a range of cell types, e.g. hepatocytes, macrophages and neutrophils. The three isoenzymes require, in addition to L-arginine, NADPH and O_2 as cosubstrates and five cofactors (or prosthetic groups), namely FAD, FMN, calmodulin, tetrahydrobiopterin and haem.

sweat but most is eliminated from the body in the urine following filtration by the **kidney glomeruli**, although significant quantities of urea may be passively reabsorbed with water by the proximal tubules. It is estimated that each human excretes $\sim 10\,\text{kg}$ urea per annum. Urea is the major nitrogenous constituent of urine when the diet contains normal quantities of protein. Where the diet contains low levels of or lacks protein, the decline in urinary urea concentrations reflects the control exercised on carbamoyl-phosphate synthase levels. During starvation, when muscle protein is degraded to produce substrate molecules for gluconeogenesis, the production of ammonia increases with a concomitant rise in the throughput of the urea cycle. Defects in the function of carbamoyl-phosphate synthase, ornithine carbamoyltransferase and arginase result in **hyperammonaemia** (elevated blood ammonia concentrations) with concomitant effects on the brain.

Biosynthesis of amino acids

On the basis of nutritional experiments, amino acids have been classified (Table 13.2) as:

- **non-essential amino acids** which may be synthesized *de novo* by the organism;
- **essential amino acids** which cannot be synthesized *de novo* by the organism.

The **non-essential amino acids**, in general, have short synthetic pathways: the longest pathway produces glycine from choline by five reactions. The liver contains the enzymes necessary to synthesize amino acids either by the same route as in plants or at the

Table 13.2   *Essential and non-essential amino acids for rat and man*

Essential	Non-essential
Isoleucine	Alanine
Leucine	Asparagine
Lysine	Aspartate
Methionine	Cysteine
Phenylalanine	Glutamate
Threonine	Glutamine
Tryptophan	Glycine
Valine	Proline
Arginine*	Serine
Histidine*	Tyrosine

* Arginine and histidine are essential amino acids in young animals and children because, although the metabolism of adults can satify protien-synthesis requirements, the synthetic pathways do not produce enough amino acids for normal growth.

expense of other amino acids through transamination reactions. (Plants can synthesize all 20 amino acids found in their proteins.)

Essential amino acids are not synthesized because the liver is deficient in at least one of the enzymes involved in the analogous plant pathway. Although the complete amino acid in some cases need not be supplied, the carbon skeletons of these amino acids must be provided in the diet. Proteins from animal sources, e.g. meat, milk and eggs, are very effective in the support of the maintenance and growth of man and have been referred to as 'first-class proteins'. Others, frequently from plant sources, do not contain all the essential components and have been called 'second-class proteins'. A second-class protein may lack, or contain inadequate quantities of, one or several amino acids.

Protein synthesis

The current understanding of the processes involved in protein synthesis has developed from studies in prokaryotic systems to the more complex eukaryotic systems. The knowledge of the prokaryotic mechanisms is therefore more advanced. For this reason, this section will consider the translation events within both types of cells with guidance from prokaryotic systems.

Translation

Translation of the mRNA is a relatively rapid event. In prokaryotes, about 15 amino acids per second may be polymerized into a growing polypeptide chain. In eukaryotes, the rate of incorporation is about three to five amino acids per second. Translation involves two compartments:

- **cytosol** where individual amino acids are enzymically attached to their specific tRNAs (Figure 2.13) by **amino acid-tRNA ligases** (also called aminoacyl-tRNA synthetases);
- **ribosomes** in which the amino acids are correctly positioned according to the base sequence of a mRNA template and polymerized into polypeptide chains.

The **attachment** of each of the 20 amino acids occurring in proteins to its corresponding tRNA(s) is by esterification catalysed by one of 20 different ligases which is specific for both the amino acid and the tRNA (Figure 13.3). The ligases link an amino acid to the free $2'$-OH (class I enzymes) or $3'$-OH (class II enzymes) group of the ribose of the adenosine at the $3'$-end of tRNA molecules. The first of two steps involves adenylylation of the amino acid in which the carboxyl group of the amino acid and the α-phosphate group of the ATP form an anhydride linkage with the release of pyrophosphate. The aminoacyl-adenylate remains enzyme-bound for the second step in which the aminoacyl moiety forms an ester linkage

> **Nutritional studies in rats** have indicated that mammals cannot synthesize all the amino acids required for protein synthesis. Such studies were conducted by maintenance of growing rats on diets deficient in one amino acid and monitoring for weight gain. Studies in man employing similarly constructed diets considered the short-term maintenance of a **positive nitrogen balance,** i.e. intake of nitrogen exceeds nitrogen excretion, which suggests that nitrogen is being retained for protein synthesis. A **negative nitrogen balance** during the experimental period could indicate that tissue proteins are being degraded in an attempt to supply the omitted amino acid for the synthesis of proteins required for major functions. Under normal dietary conditions, nitrogen balance is maintained.

Immunoglobulin molecules
(Figure 3.14) of a single class, e.g.
IgG, exhibit a variety of
specificities in antigen binding.
The human genome does not
contain millions of genes
dedicated to the coding of
millions of antibody molecules.
Rather the germ-line DNA
contains numerous groups of
exons from which individual
exons are rearranged in different
combinations.

For example, **the κ light-chain**
is derived from a selection of one
from 40 exons in the V region, one
from five exons in the J region and
the single exon from the C region
of the antigen-receptor gene
complex on chromosome 2. The
selection occurs at an early stage
in B-cell differentiation. If the
B-cell DNA contains the $V_{30}J_3C$
set, then following transcription,
pre-mRNA processing and the
translation of the mRNA, the
resultant κ chain will have a
different antigenic specificity from
a molecule derived from the
$V_{18}J_4C$ set but the same class-
dependent biological properties.
Similar processes apply to the λ
light-chains. However, heavy-
chain exon rearrangements
include an additional D region.

Many proteins are constructed
from exons which derive amino
acid sequences found in a variety
of different proteins, e.g. the
fibronectin type I repeat sequence
is found in tissue plasminogen
activator.

with the appropriate tRNA. Cleavage of this ester bond ($\Delta G^{\circ\prime} = -29.3$ kJ mol^{-1}) provides the energy for the ribosomal formation of a peptide bond. The cleavage of pyrophosphate renders the overall reaction irreversible (Chapter 8).

In addition to their ability to load the tRNA with an amino acid, amino acid-tRNA ligases are capable of recognizing inappropriate attachments, i.e. they have a **proof-reading function**. If an incorrect amino acid has been attached, it may be removed by the hydrolysis of the enzyme-bound aminoacyl-adenylate intermediate. Once the anhydride linkage is cleaved, the amino acid and AMP dissociate from the active site so that the tRNA may be reloaded with the correct molecule. The selectivity of these ligases is largely responsible for the maintenance of the fidelity of protein synthesis.

The **ribosomes** exist as separate subunits (Figure 2.14) unless protein synthesis is in operation. Ribosomes undergo repeated assembly and disassembly depending upon the need for new protein molecules. Translation consists of three consecutive phases:

- **the initiation phase** in which a functional mRNA-ribosome complex is assembled;

- **the elongation phase** in which the mRNA template is read and positioned amino acids are polymerized;

- **the termination phase** in which the ribosome dissociates into subunits and the nascent polypeptide chain is released.

The differences in the prokaryotic and eukaryotic mechanisms relate to:

- **the factors** involved at each phase (Table 13.3);

- **the sequence of interactions** between the small ribosomal subunit, initiation factors, initiator tRNA and mRNA;

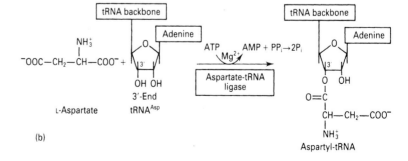

Figure 13.3 *The loading of tRNA molecules with their corresponding amino acid: (a) general equation; (b) aspartate reaction*

Table 13.3 *Factors involved in translation*

Factors	Prokaryotes	Eukaryotes
Initiation factors	IF-1, IF-2, IF-3	eIF-1, eIF-2, eIF-2B, eIF-3 eIF-4A, eIF-4B, eIF-4C, (eIF-4E), eIF-4F, (eIF-4G), eIF-5, eIF-6
Elongation factors	EF-Tu, EF-Ts, EF-G	eEF-1, eEF-2
Release factors	RF-1, RF-2, RF-3	eRF-1, (eRF-3)

- the **structures** of mRNA, ribosomal subunits (Chapter 2) and initiator tRNAs.

The initiation phase of translation in prokaryotes

Initiation in prokaryotes involves the formation of a 30S initiation complex to which the large subunit (50S) then interacts to form a **70S initiation complex** (Figure 13.4). The first event concerns one of two types of methionyl-tRNA^{Met} molecules. Both tRNAs are loaded with methionine by the same enzyme, methionine-tRNA ligase. One of these methionyl-tRNA^{Met} molecules reads internal AUG triplets (Table 2.7) to insert methionyl residues into the polypeptide chain whereas the other, called **initiator-tRNA** (methionyl-tRNA$_i^{Met}$), plays a crucial role only in the initiation of translation. The methionyl residue is N-formylated by methionyl-tRNA formyltransferase to yield **N-formylmethionyl-tRNA^{Met}**.

An **initiation factor**, **IF-2**, a member of the superfamily of G-proteins (Chapter 8), binds a molecule of GTP and selectively binds an initiator-tRNA molecule to form a ternary complex. IF-1 and IF-3 are bound to the free 30S subunit and prevent ribosomal assembly. The 30S subunit binds mRNA and the ternary complex. mRNA binding to the 30S subunit is directed by the essential IF-3. IF-2 guides the ternary complex into the correct position so that the initiator-tRNA is located at the AUG start codon. The 30S subunit aligns with the start region of the mRNA through its 16S rRNA. Near the 3′-end of 16S RNA is a pyrimidine-rich sequence, e.g. AUUCCUCC, which base-pairs with a complementary purine-rich sequence of eight bases, e.g. UAAGGAGG, on the mRNA called the **Shine–Dalgarno sequence** or the ribosome-binding site. Only six out of eight nucleotides are required to match to permit recognition. The Shine–Dalgarno sequence occurs about 10 bases upstream from the AUG sequence. The complex of 30S subunit, initiator-tRNA, IF-2–GTP, IF-1 and IF-3 is termed the **30S pre-initiation complex**.

In the **final step in initiation**, IF-3 dissociates from the 30S subunit and thus permits the GTP-dependent interaction of this assembly with a 50S ribosomal subunit. On association of the two subunits, IF-1 is liberated simultaneously from the ribosome and is followed

Figure 13.4 *The formation of the prokaryotic initiation complex*

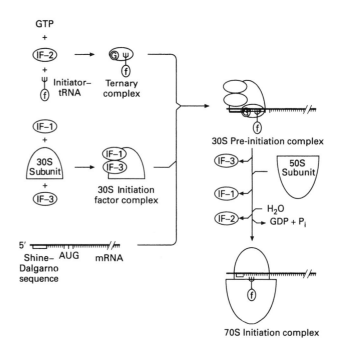

by IF-2, the release of which requires the hydrolysis of bound GTP by a ribosomal protein. On release, IF-1 and IF-3 may attach to another 30S subunit and IF-2 may form another ternary complex to initiate the formation of another 30S pre-initiation complex. The hydrolysis of GTP promotes a conformational change in the intact ribosome which, together with the dissociation of the initiation factors, allows the 70S initiation complex to accept the delivery of an aminoacyl-tRNA and thereby enter the **elongation cycle**.

The elongation phase of translation in prokaryotes

According to the current **three-site model of chain elongation** (Figure 13.5), the formation of the 70S initiation complex provides three distinguishable ribosomal sites called **P** (for peptidyl-tRNA binding site), **A** (for aminoacyl-tRNA binding site) and **E** (for exit site). During subunit association, the AUG start codon with its bound initiator-tRNA becomes positioned within the P site. The elongation cycle commences with the occupancy of the P site with the appropriate loaded tRNA, the A site contains the second codon on the mRNA and the E site lies empty.

The loaded aminoacyl-tRNA may only interact with the A site as an aminoacyl-tRNA:elongation factor, EF-Tu–GTP complex. The anticodon of the aminoacyl-tRNA forms hydrogen bonds with the complementary codon and is positioned to be incorporated into the *C*-terminus of the nascent polypeptide chain. Once the tRNA is positioned within the A site, the GTP is hydrolysed and the EF-Tu–GDP complex dissociates from the ribosome. The affinity of EF-Tu

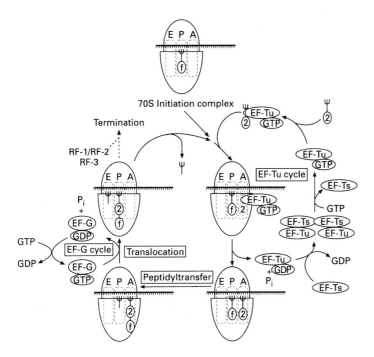

Figure 13.5 *The three-site model of the elongation phase of translation in prokaryotes*

for guanine nucleotides is too strong for regulation by the cytoplasmic [GTP]/[GDP] ratio. An additional factor, EF-Ts, is required for the exchange of GDP for GTP. A tetrameric intermediate, EF-Tu: (EF-Ts)$_2$: EF-Tu, in which EF-Ts molecules are closely associated but EF-Tu molecules make very limited contact, is formed during the exchange. The binding of GTP to EF-Tu displaces EF-Ts. The EF-Tu–GTP complex is thus regenerated.

The A site also contains a **decoding centre** (δ-centre) where the accuracy of the anticodon of the incoming aminoacyl-tRNA for the codon is examined. Only if the anticodon and codon are complementary will the aminoacyl-tRNA remain bound to site A, otherwise it is released. The mechanism of proof-reading contributes to the fidelity of protein synthesis.

The dissociation of EF-Tu–GDP from the ribosome permits the bound aminoacyl-tRNA to make contact with the **peptidyltransferase activity**. The peptidyl-tRNA housed in the P site is transferred to the aminoacyl-tRNA in the A site. The peptidyltransferase activity is **ribozymic** and is also responsible for formation of the peptide bond. The 23S rRNA appears capable of peptide bond formation in the absence of ribosomal protein. The reaction of the tRNA-linked peptidyl chain with the α-amino group of the adjacent aminoacyl-tRNA requires no additional energy since the cleavage of the ester bond between the peptide and the tRNA provides the energy for peptide bonding.

The deacylated (unloaded) tRNA in the P site is moved to the E site and the peptidyl-tRNA, which has the growing polypeptide

A number of **antibiotics** function by interference with the mechanism of **bacterial protein or peptidoglycan synthesis. Rifamycin** binds to the β-subunit of bacterial RNA polymerase to inhibit transcription. The **aminoglycosides, e.g. gentamycin and kanamycin**, act by binding to the 30S subunit of the bacterial ribosome, preventing its association with the 50S subunit and thereby inhibiting the assemblage of an active ribosome. The binding of the 30S subunit to mRNA is not affected. The therapeutically useful **tetracyclines** also bind to the 30S subunits but distort the subunit so that aminoacyl-tRNA molecules cannot align with the pertinent mRNA codon and thus protein synthesis is hindered. The **macrolides, e.g. erythromycin** bind to the 50S subunit and prevent elongation by peptidyltransferase and/or ribosomal translocation. **Chloramphenicol** also binds to the 50S subunit but prevents the attachment of the loaded end of the aminoacyl-tRNA to its binding site, an action which inhibits the peptidyltransferase and peptide bonding.

The β-**lactams, e.g. cephalosporins, monobactams and penicillins**, inhibit the last reaction in the synthesis of the peptidoglycan of the bacterial cell wall, namely the transpeptidation reaction which crosslinks the peptide R groups of the peptidoglycan backbone.

attached to it, is transferred from the A site to the P site. This is called **translocation** during which the movement of the tRNAs, under the influence of EF-G, pulls the mRNA so that the mRNA advances one nucleotide triplet so that a new codon is delivered to the A site. Translocation requires EF-G which binds to the ribosome as a EF-G–GTP complex. The hydrolysis of GTP provides the energy for translocation and for the subsequent dissociation of EF-G from the ribosome.

The release of deacylated tRNA from the E site confers a conformational change-induced high-affinity state on the A site which may now receive an aminoacyl-tRNA complementary to the recently positioned codon. One elongation cycle, in which the polypeptide chain is increased by one amino acid residue and the mRNA template moved by one codon through the protein synthesis machinery, is completed. The elongation cycle continues as described until translocation introduces a **stop codon** (UAA, UAG or UGA; Table 2.7) into site A. Since there are no natural tRNAs capable of recognizing these codons, translation enters the termination phase.

A single mRNA may be processed simultaneously by a number of ribosomes to increase the rate of protein synthesis. The structure so formed is called a **polyribosome** or polysome. Since mRNA molecules are translated in the $5' \rightarrow 3'$ direction, the ribosome bound nearest to the $5'$-end displays the shortest polypeptide chain.

The termination phase of translation in prokaryotes

In the **prokaryotic termination phase**, release factors directed specifically by the stop codons bind to the ribosomes. RF-1 responds to the triplets UAA and UAG whilst RF-2 responds to UAA and UGA when the codons occupy the A site. Recent evidence suggests that RF-1 and RF-2 do not enter the A site but bind near it. The stop codons apparently interact with a specific sequence in rRNA to form an mRNA: rRNA hybrid with which the protein factors may interact. RF-3–GTP also binds to the 50S subunit. RF-1 or RF-2 causes a change in the peptidyltransferase activity so that the *C*-terminal residue of the nascent polypeptide chain may be transferred, in an energy-requiring reaction, from the P site peptidyl-tRNA to a molecule of water. This process requires RF-3, a GTPase, which hydrolyses its bound GTP to release the necessary energy. In this way, the carboxyl end of the polypeptide chain is freed from its anchor, tRNA, and is released from the ribosome. The RF factors, GDP and tRNA are soon released. The remaining ribosome is unstable. The dissociation of the 50S subunit is promoted by the binding of IF-1 and particularly IF-3 to the 30S subunit. The free subunits may participate in the translation of another mRNA.

Translation in eukaryotes

The **mechanism of translation** in eukaryotes is analogous to that described for prokaryotes. In the initiation phase, an 80S initiation complex is constructed from a 40S ribosomal subunit, a 60S subunit and eukaryotic mRNA via the action of a larger number of initiation factors (denoted as eIFs; Table 13.3). The eukaryotic mRNA has been processed from a pre-mRNA and equipped with a $5'$-^{7}methylguanine cap (^{7}mGpppN) and a poly (A) tail (Figure 2.14b). Although recruitment of the small subunit to mRNA in prokaryotes is essentially directed by the interaction between the 16S rRNA and Shine–Dalgarno sequences on mRNA, such sequences do not exist on eukaryotic mRNAs. Therefore, the 40S subunit binds to the mRNA through protein–protein and protein–RNA reactions.

Initiation starts with a ternary complex formed by eIF-2, GTP and initiator-tRNA. Eukaryotic initiator-tRNA is a methionyl-tRNA$_i^{Met}$. The methionyl residue, however, is not formylated. A 40S subunit is prevented from association with the large subunit by eIF-3. eIF-4F consists of two subunits, eIF-4E which interacts with the cap and eIF-4G which may bind eIF-3. Prior to 40S subunit binding, eIF-4A may bind to eIF-4G. eIF-4A has an **ATP-dependent helicase activity** which unwinds any secondary structure in the mRNA. The 40S subunit is recruited to the $5'$-end of the mRNA via the association of the cap with eIF-4E, eIF-4G and eIF-3. The interaction of the ternary complex with the 40S subunit produces a **40S pre-initiation complex** (actually 43S) which contains some additional factors, e.g. eIF-1 and eIF-4B form a complex with eIF-4A to assist in mRNA binding. eIF-2-bound GTP is hydrolysed by eIF-5, and eIF-2 and eIF-3 are released from the complex. The 60S subunit has bound eIF-6 which prevents its association with the 40S subunit to form the **80S initiation complex** in which the initiator-tRNA is aligned with an AUG start codon. During assembly, the remaining IFs are freed.

The **chain elongation phase** is analogous to that in prokaryotes except that eukaryotes employ only two elongation factors. However, eEF-1 consists of two active components, eEF-1α, which functions as EF-Tu, and eEF-1$\beta\gamma\delta$ which performs the EF-Ts function. eEF-2 is the equivalent of EF-G. **Chain termination** in eukaryotes requires only one release factor, eRF-1. However, others exist, e.g. eRF-3 is essential for cell viability. eRF-1 performs the role of both RF-1 and RF-2 when a termination codon occupies the A site.

Co- and post-translational modifications and protein folding

The **products of translation** are rarely the final form in which the protein demonstrates its biological activity. Polypeptide chains undergo enzyme-catalysed **co- and post-translational modifications**

Ricin, a plant glycoprotein and one of the most toxic compounds known, is produced by the castor oil plant (*Ricinus communis*). Ricin was employed by secret agents in 1978 to murder a London-based Bulgarian defector as he waited for a bus on Waterloo Bridge. Georgi Markov was pierced by a special umbrella tip which injected a metallic microsphere coated with ricin into his leg. He died 4 days later in hospital.

Ricin is a heterodimer. It gains entry into cells by the **lectin properties** of its B-chain. Lectins are a class of proteins which bind to specific carbohydrate moieties displayed by cell surface glycoproteins and glycolipids. On binding, ricin gains entry to the cell by endocytosis (Chapter 7). Following the cleavage of an interchain disulphide bond, chain A gains access to the cytosol where it catalytically inactivates large numbers of ribosomes by removing a conserved adenine from 28S rRNA without damage to the nucleic acid framework. This adenine is necessary for the functions of the 60S subunit during the elongation phase. It is estimated that one ricin molecule is enough to kill a eukaryotic cell. The ingestion of five castor seeds by a child has proved fatal.

which, together with protein folding, produce the functional protein. The removal of certain sequences in prokaryotic and eukaryotic proteins are two examples of cotranslational processes:

- **The *N*-formylmethionyl residue.** The *N*-formylmethionyl residue is the *N*-terminal aminoacyl residue in all prokaryotic polypeptide chains undergoing synthesis but when the growing chains reach about 10 amino acids in length, the *N*-terminal oligopeptides are cleaved so that the mature proteins of prokaryotes lack the formylmethionyl residue.

- **The signal sequence** is removed in the RER (Chapter 7).

Other co- and post-translational modifications (Chapter 7) in some proteins include:

- **hydroxylation** e.g. prior to glycosylation in procollagen chains (Chapter 3);

- **glycosylation**, in the production of glycoproteins (Chapter 7);

- **phosphorylation,** a mechanism employed in the regulation of protein function including enzymes (Chapter 8) and other proteins, e.g. eIF-2, eIF-3, eIF-4B, eIF-4F and EF-2;

- **ADP-ribosylation** of nuclear proteins, e.g. DNA polymerases, histones H1, H2B, and cytoplasmic proteins, e.g. EF-2;

- **methylation** of the nitrogen atoms of basic amino acids (K, R and also H) and the carboxyl groups of acidic amino acids (D and E);

- **oxidation** which may lead to modifications in secondary and tertiary structure due to changes in hydrogen bonding arrangements.

The commonest post-translational modification is **proteolysis**. An important function of proteolytic cleavage is in the activation of digestive enzymes, e.g. **chymotrypsin**, and protein hormones, e.g. insulin, which are synthesized as longer inactive precursors called **pro-proteins**. Cleavage at specific peptide bonds produces a conformational change in the tertiary structure which places amino acid R-groups in the required positions for biological activity. Chymotrypsin is synthesized as inactive **chymotrypsinogen**, a single polypeptide chain of 245 residues containing five intrachain disulphide bonds. Its **activation by trypsin** involves removal of two dipeptides from positions 14-15 (Ser-Arg) and 147-148 (Thr-Asn) to yield polypeptide chains A, B and C conjoined by two disulphide bonds.

Protein folding is directed by the information contained within the amino acid sequence which determines bonding capabilities (Chapter 3), e.g. hydrophobic interactions, hydrogen bonding and ionic bonding. Proteins may commence folding whilst being synthesized by the ribosomes. However, the folding of proteins generally involves the participation of molecular chaperone proteins in the RER (Chapter 7).

Suggested further reading

Buckingham, R.H., Grentzmann, G. and Kisselev, L. (1997). Polypeptide chain release factors. *Molecular Microbiology* **24**, 449–456.

Green, R. and Noller, H.F. (1997). Ribosomes and translation. *Annual Review of Biochemistry* **66**, 679–716.

Lohse, P.A. and Szostak, J.W. (1996). Ribozyme-catalysed amino-acid transfer reactions. *Nature* **381**, 442–444.

Sachs, A.B., Sarnow, P. and Hentze, M.W. (1997). Starting at the beginning, middle and end: translation initiation in eukaryotes. *Cell* **89**, 831–838.

Watford, M. (1991). The Urea Cycle. A two-compartment system. *Essays in Biochemistry* **26**, 49–58.

Lewin, B. (1997). *Genes VI*. Oxford: Oxford University Press.

Self-assessment questions

1. What is the usual fate of glutamate formed by transaminase-catalysed reactions?
2. In translation, what are the roles of the following protein factors: (a) IF-2; (b) IF-3; (c) eIF-4G; (d) eIF-6; (e) eEF-1α; (f) RF-2?
3. What is the fate of fumarate produced by argininosuccinate lyase?
4. What is the significance of the Shine–Dalgarno sequence?
5. Which of the chemical groups of the aminoacyl residue of methionyl-tRNA$_i^{Met}$ is formylated at the beginning of prokaryotic translation?
6. Prior to peptidyltransfer, at which ribosomal sites are the following bound: (a) aminoacyl-tRNA; (b) peptidyl tRNA?
7. Identify two stages in which proof-reading occurs to ensure the fidelity of translation.
8. Which enzyme attaches arginine to a specific tRNA molecule?
9. By reference to Figure 13.2, trace the origins of the carbon and nitrogen atoms of urea.
10. What molecule is used as the vehicle for the transport of amino nitrogen from skeletal muscle cells to the liver?

A **mutation** is a heritable change in the nucleotide sequence of genomic DNA. Such changes may occur as an **error in replication** or are inducible by a variety of **chemical and physical agents**. Mutations may be classified according to the nature or consequence of the change. The term **point mutation** indicates a variation in only a single base-pair. A point mutation may be the result of a base substitution, a base insertion or a base deletion, although the term is frequently applied to base substitutions. **Multiple mutation** signifies a difference in two or more base-pairs from the natural sequence.

In **protein-coding genes**, alterations in the primary structure of the protein product may result from mutation. The functioning of the protein may remain unaffected by base substitutions if internal bonding arrangements remain unchanged. Insertions or deletions are harmful because they may cause **frame-shift mutations**, so called because the subsequent bases are read in different triplet combinations, resulting in alteration of amino acids from this point towards the C-terminus. Mutations may occur in regulatory genes, in which case the mutation exerts its effect by modifying the functioning of these sequences.

Key Concepts and Facts

Amino Acid Metabolism

- Transamination is the major mechanism for the deamination of amino acids.

- Amino acids are either glucogenic or ketogenic or both depending upon the metabolic fate of their carbon skeletons.

- Ammonia is transported to the liver from most peripheral tissues as glutamine.

- Urea is synthesized primarily in the liver to eliminate ammonia from the body.

- The urea cycle operates across two subcellular compartments, the cytosol and mitochondrial matrix.

- Arginine produced in the urea cycle may also be utilized in protein synthesis.

- Essential amino acids cannot be synthesized *de novo* by man.

Protein Synthesis

- mRNA is translated into polypeptide chains.

- Amino acid-tRNA ligases attach the correct amino acids to specific tRNAs in the cytosol.

- Ribosome subunits exist separately unless protein synthesis is in operation.

- Translation consists of initiation, elongation and termination phases.

- There are major mechanistic differences in protein synthesis in prokaryotic and eukaryotic cells.

- The initiation phase generates an initiation complex in which the initiator-tRNA is formylated in prokaryotes.

- The elongation phase involves three ribosomal sites called P, A and E.

- The transfer of peptidyl-tRNA from the P site to the A site is catalysed by a ribozyme.

- A single mRNA may be read simultaneously by a number of ribosomes.

- Following translation, polypeptide chains undergo further processing.

Answers to questions (Chapter 13)

1. Glutamate is deaminated by glutamate dehydrogenase to release an ammonium ion, a substrate for carbamoyl-phosphate synthase (ammonia).

2. (a) Binds a GTP and an initiator-tRNA molecule to form a ternary complex in prokaryotes; (b) keeps prokaryotic subunits apart with assistance from IF-1; (c) binds eIF-3; (d) prevents the association of large with small ribosomal subunits in eukaryotes; (e) by binding GTP and complexing with aminoacyl-tRNA, it permits the aminoacyl-tRNA to bind to site A in eukaryotes; (f) reponds to codons UAA or UGA in site A by binding to the ribosome to modify the prokaryotic peptidyl-transferase activity.

3. Experimental evidence shows that it is used in gluconeogenesis.

4. This is a purine-rich sequence of eight bases on the mRNA to which prokaryotic small ribosomal subunits bind through a pyrimidine-rich sequence in its 16S rRNA.

5. The α-amino group.

6. (a) Site A; (b) site P.

7. On attachment of the amino acid to the tRNA by the appropriate amino acid-tRNA ligase and when the aminoacyl-tRNA is in the A site of the ribosome.

8. Arginine-tRNA ligase.

9. C is from bicarbonate, one N comes from glutamate via glutamate dehydrogenase and the other from aspartate formed by a transamination involving glutamate.

10. Alanine.

Index

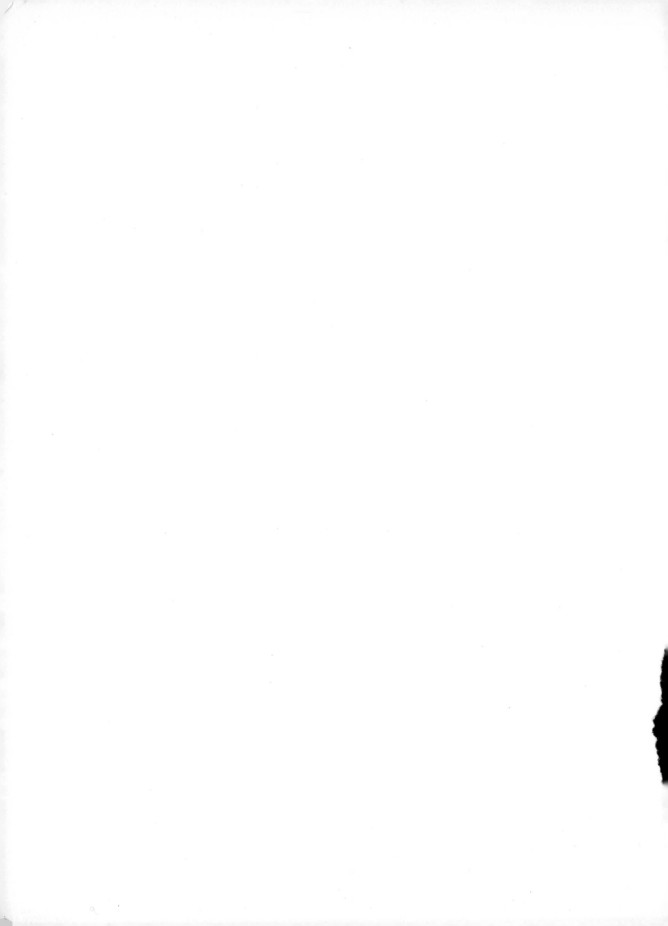